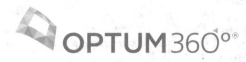

Evaluation and Management Coding Advisor

Advanced guidance on E/M code selection for traditional documentation systems

2021

optum360coding.com

Optum360 Notice

Evaluation and Management Coding Advisor is designed to provide accurate and authoritative information in regard to the subject covered. Every reasonable effort has been made to ensure the accuracy and completeness of the information within these pages. However, Optum360 makes no guarantee, warranty, or representation that this publication is accurate, complete, or without errors. It is understood that Optum360 is not rendering any legal or other professional services or advice in this publication and that Optum360 bears no liability for any results or consequences that may arise from the use of this book.

Our Commitment to Accuracy

Optum360 is committed to producing accurate and reliable materials.

To report corrections, please email accuracy@optum.com. You can also reach customer service by calling 1.800.464.3649, option 1.

American Medical Association Notice

CPT © 2020 American Medical Association. All rights reserved.

Fee schedules, relative value units, conversion factors and/or related components are not assigned by the AMA, are not part of CPT, and the AMA is not recommending their use. The AMA does not directly or indirectly practice medicine or dispense medical services. The AMA assumes no liability for data contained or not contained herein.

CPT is a registered trademark of the American Medical Association.

Copyright

Acknowledgments

Gregory A. Kemp, MA, *Product Manager*
Stacy Perry, *Manager, Desktop Publishing*
Leanne Patterson, CPC, *Subject Matter Expert*
Nichole VanHorn, CPC, CCS-P, *Subject Matter Expert*
Tracy Betzler, *Senior Desktop Publishing Specialist*
Hope M. Dunn, *Senior Desktop Publishing Specialist*
Katie Russell, *Desktop Publishing Specialist*
Kimberli Turner, *Editor*

Subject Matter Experts

Leanne Patterson, CPC

Ms. Patterson has more than 15 years of experience in the healthcare profession. She has an extensive background in professional component coding, with expertise in E/M coding and auditing and HIPAA compliance. Her experience includes general surgery coding, serving as Director of Compliance, conducting chart-to-claim audits, and physician education. She has been responsible for coding and denial management in large, multi-specialty physician practices, and most recently has been part of a team developing content for educational products related to ICD-10-CM. Ms. Patterson is credentialed by the American Academy of Professional Coders (AAPC) as a Certified Professional Coder (CPC).

Nichole VanHorn, CPC, CCS-P

Ms. VanHorn has more than 20 years of experience in the healthcare profession. Her areas of expertise include CPT and ICD-10-CM coding in multiple specialties, auditing, and education. Most recently she served as Clinical Auditor for a multi-specialty group. Ms. VanHorn was responsible for the oversight of the physician coding and education section of the Corporate Compliance Program. She has been an active member of her local American Academy of Professional Coders (AAPC) chapter for several years and has also served as an officer.

At our core, we're about coding.

Essential medical code sets are just that — essential to your revenue cycle. In our ICD-10-CM/PCS, CPT®, HCPCS and DRG coding tools, we apply our collective coding expertise to present these code sets in a way that is comprehensive, plus easy to use and apply. Print books are inexpensive and easily referenced, created with intuitive features and formats, such as visual alerts, color-coding and symbols to identify important coding notes and instructions — plus great coding tips.

Find the same content, tips and features in a variety of formats. Choose from print products, online coding tools, data files or web services, as well as from various educational opportunities.

Your coding, billing and reimbursement product team,

Ryan Nichole Greg LaJuana
Ken Julie
Regina Marianne Denise Leanne
Jacqui Anita Debbie Elizabeth Nann
Karen

Put Optum360 medical coding, billing and reimbursement content at your fingertips today. Choose what works for you.

- Print books
- Online coding tools
- Data files
- Web services

Visit us at **optum360coding.com** to browse our products, or call us at **1-800-464-3649, option 1** for more information.

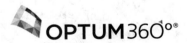

What if you could go back in time?

How much time do you think you spend researching elusive codes? Too much, probably. Time you would like to have back. We can't give time back, but we can help you save it. Our all-in-one coding solutions consolidate specialty coding processes so you can find information more easily and quickly. Each specialty-specific procedure code includes its official and lay descriptions, coding tips, cross-coding to common ICD-10-CM codes, relative value units, Medicare edit guidance, *CPT Assistant*® references, CCI edits and, when relevant, specific reimbursement and documentation tips.

With tools available for 30 specialties, we're sure you'll find the right resource to meet your organization's unique needs, even if those needs are allergy, anesthesia/pain management, behavioral health, cardiology, cardiothoracic surgery, dental, dermatology, emergency medicine, ENT, gastroenterology, general surgery, hematology, laboratory/pathology, nephrology, neurology, neurosurgery, OB/GYN, OMS, oncology, ophthalmology, orthopaedics, pediatrics, physical therapy, plastics, podiatry, primary care, pulmonology, radiology, urology or vascular surgery.

Say good-bye to time wasted digging for those elusive codes.

Your coding, billing and reimbursement product team,

Ryan Nichole Greg LaJuana
Ken Julie
Regina Marianne Denise Leanne
Jacqui Anita Debbie Elizabeth Nann
Karen

Put Optum360 medical coding, billing and reimbursement content at your fingertips today. Choose what works for you.

Print books

Online coding tools

Data files

Web services

Visit us at **optum360coding.com** to browse our products, or call us at **1-800-464-3649, option 1** for more information.

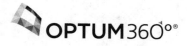

A lot goes into coding resources.
We know.

Most think that coding, billing and reimbursement includes only your essential code sets, but that leaves out reference products. An important part of the revenue cycle, reference tools provide clarity — along with coding and billing tips — to deepen medical coding knowledge, make the coding process more efficient and help reduce errors on claims. Optum360 offers reference tools for facility, physician and post-acute markets, in addition to physicians-only fee products that inform the best business decisions possible for practices.

There's a lot that goes into coding, billing and reimbursement. Make sure your organization isn't leaving anything to chance.

Your coding, billing and reimbursement product team,

Ryan   Nichole   Greg   LaJuana
Regina   Ken   Julie   Denise   Leanne
Jacqui   Marianne
Anita   Debbie   Elizabeth   Nann
Karen

Put Optum360 medical coding, billing and reimbursement content at your fingertips today. Choose what works for you.

Print books

Online coding tools

Data files

Web services

Visit us at **optum360coding.com** to browse our products, or call us at **1-800-464-3649, option 1** for more information.

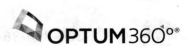

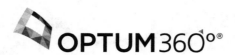 OPTUM360°®

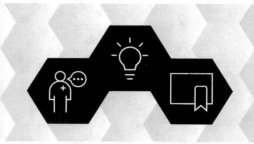

Optum360 Learning
LEARN. PRACTICE. APPLY.

Education suiting your specialty, learning style and schedule

Optum360® Learning is designed to address exactly what you and your learners need. We offer several delivery methods developed for various adult learning styles, general public education, and tailor-made programs specific to your organization — all created by our coding and clinical documentation education professionals.

Our strategy is simple — education must be concise, relevant and accurate. Choose the delivery method that works best for you:

eLearning

- **Web-based** courses offered at the most convenient times
- **Interactive**, task-focused and developed around practical scenarios
- **Self-paced** courses that include "try-it" functionality, knowledge checks and downloadable resources

Instructor-led training

On-site or remote courses built specifically for your organization and learners
- CDI specialists
- Coders
- Providers

Webinars

Online courses geared toward a broad market of learners and delivered in a live setting

No matter your learning style, Optum360 is here to help you

 Visit **optum360coding.com/learning**

 Call **1-800-464-3649, option 1**

 You've worked hard for your credentials, and now you need an easy way to maintain your certification.

Contents

Changes to E/M Coding and Documentation Under the CY 2020 Physician Fee Schedule Final Rule

The CPT editorial panel had four goals when they outlined their objective for changes to E/M office visits. One of these, easing administrative burden, was a shared goal with the Centers for Medicare and Medicaid Services (CMS), which established some administrative burden relief with documentation changes implemented in CY2019. The American Medical Association (AMA) and CMS have both taken further steps to achieve administrative burden relief, as well as other goals, such as decreasing unnecessary documentation for patient care and decreasing the need for audits through changes in guidelines.

2021 Changes to E/M Office/Other Outpatient and Prolonged Service Coding and Guidelines

Changes to the most reported E/M codes (99201–99215) first adopted by the AMA were finalized by CMS in the 2020 physician fee final rule. CMS is adopting the new coding and guidance framework issued by the AMA. CMS states that they believe it will accomplish greater administrative burden reduction than their original policies finalized for CY 2021.

Changes Coming to E/M Codes 99201–99215

Effective January 1, 2021, and aligning with changes adopted by the CPT Editorial Panel in early 2019, CMS has finalized the following changes to coding and guidelines for 99202–99215:

- Providers allowed to choose the level of visit based solely on total time or level of medical decision making (MDM).
- History and physical examination will no longer be scored and used to select the level of office/outpatient E/M visit; however, a medically appropriate history and physical examination should still be performed to demonstrate patient complexity and medical necessity.
- Deletion of 99201.
- Revised code descriptors for 99202–99215 as they will appear in the 2021 edition of CPT.
- Times included in the code descriptors have been revised and are listed as a range of time. For example, 99202 currently states, "typically, 20 minutes are spent face-to-face." Beginning in 2021, 99202 states, "15-29 minutes of total time is spent on the date of the encounter."

CPT Code	CY2021 Code Descriptions
99201	N/A. Code deleted.
99202	Office or other outpatient visit for the evaluation and management of a new patient, which requires a medically appropriate history and/or examination and straightforward medical decision making. When using time for code selection, 15-29 minutes of total time is spent on the date of the encounter.
99203	Office or other outpatient visit for the evaluation and management of a new patient, which requires a medically appropriate history and/or examination and low level of medical decision making. When using time for code selection, 30-44 minutes of total time is spent on the date of the encounter.
99204	Office or other outpatient visit for the evaluation and management of a new patient, which requires a medically appropriate history and/or examination and moderate level of medical decision making. When using time for code selection, 45-59 minutes of total time is spent on the date of the encounter.
99205	Office or other outpatient visit for the evaluation and management of a new patient, which requires a medically appropriate history and/or examination and high level of medical decision making. When using time for code selection, 60-74 minutes of total time is spent on the date of the encounter.
99211	Office or other outpatient visit for the evaluation and management of an established patient that may not require the presence of a physician or other qualified health care professional. Usually, the presenting problem(s) are minimal.
99212	Office or other outpatient visit for the evaluation and management of an established patient, which requires a medically appropriate history and/or examination and straightforward medical decision making. When using time for code selection, 10-19 minutes of total time is spent on the date of the encounter.
99213	Office or other outpatient visit for the evaluation and management of an established patient, which requires a medically appropriate history and/or examination and low level of medical decision making. When using time for code selection, 20-29 minutes of total time is spent on the date of the encounter.
99214	Office or other outpatient visit for the evaluation and management of an established patient, which requires a medically appropriate history and/or examination and moderate level of medical decision making. When using time for code selection, 30-39 minutes of total time is spent on the date of the encounter.
99215	Office or other outpatient visit for the evaluation and management of an established patient, which requires a medically appropriate history and/or examination and high level of medical decision making. When using time for code selection, 40-54 minutes of total time is spent on the date of the encounter.

- Removed required face-to-face element. Time now includes face-to-face and non-face-to-face time (e.g., reviewing test results beforehand, documenting clinical information in the medical record).

- Adoption of MDM criteria as revised by the CPT Editorial Panel, including a new table for determining the appropriate level of MDM. The new table replaces the current CMS Table of Risk. The Editorial Panel used elements from the Table of Risk when designing the new table, which includes three main topics: the number of problems addressed, amount of data reviewed, and risk of complications and/or morbidity or mortality. To review the new MDM table, go to https://www.ama-assn.org/system/files/2019-06/cpt-revised-mdm-grid.pdf.

- Concept of medical decision making and time do not apply to 99211.

- Updated E/M valuations proposed by the AMA's RVS update committee (RUC). The new valuations include some fairly significant increases in work RVUs for some of these codes, and at this time are still being reviewed. CMS has made recommendations regarding several valuations linked to the office and other outpatient services codes and seeks stakeholder comment on these in the CY2021 PFS Proposed Rule. CY2021 PFS Final Rule was not released at the time of this publication, refer to https://www.cms.gov/Medicare/Medicare-Fee-for-Service-Payment/PhysicianFeeSched/PFS-Federal-Regulation-Notices to review final comments/changes to these proposals.

- Addition of a new add-on code (99417) for prolonged office visits when time is used for code level selection, including face-to-face and non-face-to-face time of at least 15 additional minutes for level five office visits (99205, 99215).

Established Patient Office/Outpatient E/M Visit (Total Practitioner Time, When Time is Used to Select Code Level)	CPT Code
40-54 minutes	99215
55-69 minutes	99215x1 and 99417x1
70-84 minutes	99215x1 and 99417x2
85 or more minutes	99215x1and 99417x3 or more for each additional 15 minutes

New Patient Office/Outpatient E/M Visit (Total Practitioner Time, When Time is Used to Select Code Level)	CPT Code
60-74 minutes	99205
75-89 minutes	99205x1 and 99417x1
90-104 minutes	99205x1 and 99417x2
105 or more minutes	99205x1 and 99417x3 or more for each additional 15 minutes

- CMS will no longer reimburse separately for codes 99358-99359 in association with office E/M services.

- Per CMS, the revisions to these office/outpatient encounters will still not adequately reflect resources used with certain primary care and specialty care services. They are soliciting further public comments on the use of HCPCS add-on code GPC1X. Specifically, information regarding what aspects of the definition of the code are unclear, how

CMS might address those concerns, and how they might refine their original utilization assumptions for the code.

CY2021 PFS Final Rule was not released at the time of this publication, refer to https://www.cms.gov/Medicare/Medicare-Fee-for-Service-Payment/PhysicianFeeSched/PFS-Federal-Regulation-Notices to review final comments/changes to these proposals.

HCPCS Code	Proposed Code Descriptor	Total Time (mins)	Work RVU
GPC1X	Visit complexity inherent to evaluation and management associated with medical care services that serve as the continuing focal point for all needed health care services and/or with medical care services that are part of ongoing care related to a patient's single, serious, or complex chronic condition. (Add-on code, list separately in addition to office/ outpatient evaluation and management visit, new or established	11	0.33

For more information on the changes, refer to the CY 2020 Physician Fee Schedule Final Rule: https://www.federalregister.gov/documents/2019/11/15/2019-24086/medicare-program-cy-2020-revisions-to-payment-policies-under-the-physician-fee-schedule-and-other.

Chapter 1: An Introduction and Overview of E/M Coding

The evaluation and management (E/M) service codes, although some of the most commonly used codes by physicians of all specialties, are among the least understood. These codes, introduced in the 1992 CPT® book, were designed to increase accuracy and consistency of use in the reporting of levels of cognitive encounters. This was accomplished by defining the E/M codes based on the degree that certain elements common to cognitive services are addressed or performed and reflected in the medical record documentation. E/M codes have specific elements identified that must be documented to meet the level of care reported.

At the same time the E/M codes were introduced, the American Medical Association (AMA), in conjunction with other organizations, released general documentation guidelines. Over time the link between good patient care and good documentation has been realized. Documentation has gained importance not only for substantiating the services rendered for reimbursement but also for continuity of care with so many providers choosing specialty medicine, an increase in the use of electronic health record systems, the greater specificity found in ICD-10-CM coding, and even litigation support.

ORIGIN AND DEVELOPMENT OF EVALUATION AND MANAGEMENT CODES

The AMA and the Centers for Medicare and Medicaid Services (CMS) developed the evaluation and management service codes in an effort to provide a more objective framework to represent services provided to patients and more clearly define work performed by the provider. These E/M codes were developed to replace codes that described brief, intermediate, and comprehensive visits in order to classify medical visits not only on the basis of time but also by the site of service, type of patient, and patient status.

Medicare physician payment was originally based on a calculation of the customary, prevailing, and reasonable cost.

In 1985, Congress authorized the development of a Medicare physician fee schedule (MFPS) based on the physician resources expended while rendering a medical service (e.g., skill, knowledge, specialty training, and time). Medicare's resource based relative value scale (RBRVS) measures the resources (i.e., physician work, practice expense, and malpractice expense) expended when physicians perform services and procedures. The resource costs of evaluation and management services were analyzed extensively as part of Medicare's RBRVS study.

Because studies determined that the duration of the face-to-face encounter with the patient was directly linked to the total amount of work, which did not increase proportionately with encounter time, CMS set the relative value

OBJECTIVES

This chapter discusses:

- General overview of coding and documentation of evaluation and management (E/M) services
- The history and origin of E/M coding
- Telehealth and E/M coding
- The development of E/M codes
- The definitions of E/M services and the current E/M documentation guidelines pertaining to them
- Audit risks
- Types of documentation issues
- The format of this book

DEFINITIONS

customary, prevailing, and reasonable charge, Categories that were the basis for Medicare's reimbursement rates before the resource based relative value scale (RBRVS) was implemented. These rates were based on the lowest charge of the three categories rather than the relative values of each service, which caused wide variations in Medicare payments among physicians and specialties. "Customary" is the term that described a clinician's historical charges while "prevailing" represented the charges of other providers in the same specialty type residing in the same general locality and "reasonable" was the lowest charge of all three categories.

FOR MORE INFO

Additional information on the *Physicians' Current Procedural Terminology* (CPT®) can be found at https://www.ama-assn.org/practice-management/cpt-current-procedural-terminology.

units (RVU) for the work involved in E/M services by using "intraservice" time as the basis for each code.

E/M codes became an integral part of the AMA's CPT book and have constituted the first section of the book since 1992. Because these codes represent the services most frequently performed by providers (e.g., office, emergency department, inpatient visits), they are placed, for convenience, at the beginning of the book. The E/M section contains the codes applicable to all services commonly referred to as "visits." The following categories comprise the Evaluation and Management section of the CPT book as shown in the table below.

 KEY POINT

The E/M code reported is based upon the following:

- Location of the service
- Patient status
- Type of service
- Level of key component documentation
  - history
  - physical exam
  - medical decision making
- Contributory components
  - time
  - counseling
  - coordination of care
  - nature of presenting problem

CPT Section	Code Range
Office or Other Outpatient Services	99202–99215
Hospital Observation Services	99217–99220, 99224–99226
Hospital Inpatient Services	99221–99223, 99231–99239
Consultations	99241–99255
Emergency Department Services	99281–99288
Critical Care Services	99291–99292
Nursing Facility Services	99304–99318
Domiciliary, Rest Home, or Custodial Care Services	99324–99337
Domiciliary, Rest Home (e.g., Assisted Living Facility), or Home Care Plan Oversight Services	99339–99340
Home Services	99341–99350
Prolonged Services	99354–99360, 99415–99417
Case Management Services	99366–99368
Care Plan Oversight Services	99374–99380
Preventive Medicine Services	99381–99429
Non-Face-to-Face Services	99421–99423, 99441–99458
Digitally Stored Data Services/Remote Physiologic Monitoring and Physiologic Monitoring Treatment Services	99453–99454, 99091, 99457–99458, 99473–99474
Special E/M Services	99450–99458
Newborn Care Services	99460–99463
Delivery/Birthing Room Attendance and Resuscitation Services	99464–99465
Inpatient Neonatal Intensive Care Services and Pediatric and Neonatal Critical Care Services	99466–99486
Cognitive Assessment and Care Plan Services	99483
Care Management Services	99439, 99487–99491
Psychiatric Collaborative Care Management Services	99492–99494
Transitional Care Management Services	99495–99496
Advance Care Planning	99497–99498

CPT Section	Code Range
General Behavioral Health Integration Care Management	99484
Other E/M Services	99499

The classification system for E/M services is divided into three factors:

- Place of service—The setting in which the services were provided to the patient (e.g., office or other outpatient facility, hospital inpatient).
- Patient status—Status of the patient (e.g., new or established patient, outpatient, inpatient)
- Type of service—The reason the service is performed (e.g., consultation, inpatient admission, office visit, etc.)

General E/M guidelines precede the Evaluation and Management section of the CPT book. Guidelines specific to a particular subsection within the E/M section are also provided for additional clarification. The information contained in the guidelines provides definitions, explanations of terms, time-based instruction as applicable, and any other information unique to that set of codes necessary for appropriate E/M code assignment.

E/M codes were designed to increase accuracy and consistency when reporting the various levels of patient encounters and were jointly developed by the AMA and CMS. The AMA and CMS have, over time, developed guidelines for the use of evaluation and management codes to supplement the information found in the CPT book. The level of visit is based on the extent of the clinical history taken, the level of physical examination performed, and the complexity of medical decision making. In 1995, CMS published guidelines on how to appropriately document and quantify the provider's evaluation and plan of care for patients. These guidelines were expanded in 1997 to recognize that certain specialists like ophthalmologists, would not need to perform a cardiovascular or gastrointestinal exam, but, instead would need to perform a focused, complex, single-system examination. Both sets of guidelines are valid, and providers may choose either set to assist them in their documentation.

Although the number of E/M codes is a relatively small percentage of the total Physicians' Current Procedural Terminology (CPT®) codes, they represent some of the most frequently reported services by physicians of all specialties and other qualified healthcare providers.

E/M services represent such a significant percentage of all billed services that every year, the Office of Inspector General (OIG) includes some evaluation and management services in the agency's annual work plan as an area of continued investigative review.

The OIG continually reviews the accuracy of E/M coding with emphasis on documentation. Documentation has always been an area of concern for the OIG. The key to making the determination of accuracy will be the medical record documentation. Although these statements link correct coding of E/M and attendant documentation, there is enough separation of these two concepts, correct coding and documentation, to illustrate an important point that this guide will repeatedly reference, that documentation should support the level of service assigned, but does not always dictate the correct code in terms of work performed. Any federal review will likely focus on documentation as the determinant of correct coding, but in fact the level of

 KEY POINT

The history and exam elements are supporting elements to the medical decision making.

 FOR MORE INFO

A copy of the complete 1995 and 1997 Evaluation and Management Coding Guidelines can be found in appendix C and appendix D, respectively.

documentation merely supports, or does not support, the correctly assigned level of work performed.

Reimbursement for E/M services, and passing an audit of these services, is ultimately dependent on supporting documentation in the patient's medical chart and upon a determination that the services rendered were medically necessary. The latter aspect of medical necessity is linked to both the diagnosis code assigned and a determination of whether the documented elements are consistent with the problems addressed.

TELEHEALTH SERVICES

As technology and healthcare changes, the way that providers render care has also changed. Telemedicine continues to grow as a way to deliver appropriate healthcare to patients who might have difficulty being able to see a doctor in the traditional manner and is helping to facilitate greater access to healthcare for patients in medically underserved communities as well as to patients who desire traditional care delivered in a more modern, timely manner.

Telehealth services are largely evaluation and management services including, but not limited to teleconsultations via telecommunication systems for patients. The teleconsultations most often involve a primary care practitioner with a patient at a remote site and a consulting medical specialist at an urban or referral facility. The primary care practitioner is usually requesting advice from the consulting physician about the patient's conditions or treatment.

Coverage Criteria

The Medicare, Medicaid, and Improvement and Protection Act (BIPA) of 2000 expanded Medicare payment and coverage for telehealth services furnished on or after October 1, 2001. Coverage and payment for telehealth includes consultation, office visits, end stage renal disease (ESRD) related services, individual psychotherapy, pharmacologic management, and neuro-behavioral status examination delivered via a telecommunications system. Eligible geographic areas will include both rural health professional shortage areas and counties not in a metropolitan statistical area (MSA). Also, those sites serving as telemedicine demonstration projects as of December 31, 2000, are included. BIPA also allows the use of asynchronous "store and forward" technology that was previously forbidden.

Billing and Coding Rules

An originating site is the location of the eligible Medicare beneficiary at the time the service is being furnished via a telecommunications system. Originating sites authorized by law include the following:

- Physician or practitioner's office
- Hospital
- Critical access hospital (CAH)
- Rural health clinic (RHC)
- Federally qualified health center (FQHC)
- Community mental health center (CMHC)
- Skilled nursing facility (SNF)
- Hospital-based or CAH-based renal dialysis center

✓ **QUICK TIP**

There has been a temporary expansion of telehealth services due to the COVID-19 Public Health Emergency (PHE). More details can be found starting on page 5.

Independent renal dialysis facilities are not eligible originating sites.

Effective January 1, 2014, geographic eligibility for an originating site is established for each calendar year based upon the status of the area as of December 31st of the prior calendar year.

To be eligible for payment, interactive real-time audio and video telecommunications must be used and the patient must be present and participating in the conference. The entirety of the interaction between the physician and patient during a real-time telehealth service must be commiserate with the amount of time and nature sufficient to meet the key components or requirements of the service if performed face to face. As a result of the public health emergency (PHE) declaration, temporary policy changes were made to allow easier implementation and access to telehealth services during the PHE. Effective March 1, 2020 CMS added additional services to their comprehensive list of covered telehealth services for the duration of the PHE. The following list are those telehealth services covered by Medicare. Services listed as temporary are only covered by Medicare for the duration of the PHE. Telehealth services guidelines, as well as the list of covered services, are continuing to evolve. For the most current changes, refer to https://www.cms.gov/Medicare/Medicare-General-Information/Telehealth.

Code	Status
77427	Temporary addition during PHE
90785	
90791	
90792	
90832	
90833	
90834	
90836	
90837	
90838	
90839	
90840	
90845	
90846	
90847	
90853	Temporary addition during PHE
90875	Temporary addition during PHE —Added 4/30/20
90951	
90952	Temporary addition during PHE
90953	Temporary addition during PHE
90954	
90955	
90956	Temporary addition during PHE —Added 4/30/20

Code	Status
90957	
90958	
90959	Temporary addition during PHE
90960	
90961	
90962	Temporary addition during PHE
90963	
90964	
90965	
90966	
90967	
90968	
90969	
90970	
92002	Temporary addition during PHE —Added 4/30/20
92004	Temporary addition during PHE —Added 4/30/20
92012	Temporary addition during PHE —Added 4/30/20
92014	Temporary addition during PHE —Added 4/30/20
92507	Temporary addition during PHE
92508	Temporary addition during PHE —Added 4/30/20
92521	Temporary addition during PHE
92522	Temporary addition during PHE
92523	Temporary addition during PHE
92524	Temporary addition during PHE
92601	Temporary addition during PHE —Added 4/30/20
92602	Temporary addition during PHE—Added 4/30/20
92603	Temporary addition during PHE —Added 4/30/20
92604	Temporary addition during PHE —Added 4/30/20
94002	Temporary addition during PHE —Added 4/30/20
94003	Temporary addition during PHE —Added 4/30/20
94004	Temporary addition during PHE —Added 4/30/20
94005	Temporary addition during PHE —Added 4/30/20
94664	Temporary addition during PHE —Added 4/30/20
96110	Temporary addition during PHE —Added 4/30/20
96112	Temporary addition during PHE —Added 4/30/20
96113	Temporary addition during PHE —Added 4/30/20
96116	
96121	Temporary addition during PHE —Added 4/30/20
96127	Temporary addition during PHE —Added 4/30/20
96130	Temporary addition during PHE

Code	Status
96131	Temporary addition during PHE
96132	Temporary addition during PHE
96133	Temporary addition during PHE
96136	Temporary addition during PHE
96137	Temporary addition during PHE
96138	Temporary addition during PHE
96139	Temporary addition during PHE
96156	
96158	Temporary addition during PHE —Added 4/30/20
96159	
96160	
96161	
96164	
96165	
96167	
96168	
96168	
96170	Temporary addition during PHE —Added 4/30/20
96171	Temporary addition during PHE —Added 4/30/20
97110	Temporary addition during PHE
97112	Temporary addition during PHE
97116	Temporary addition during PHE
97150	Temporary addition during PHE —Added 4/30/20
97151	Temporary addition during PHE —Added 4/30/20
97152	Temporary addition during PHE —Added 4/30/20
97153	Temporary addition during PHE —Added 4/30/20
97154	Temporary addition during PHE —Added 4/30/20
97155	Temporary addition during PHE —Added 4/30/20
97156	Temporary addition during PHE —Added 4/30/20
97157	Temporary addition during PHE —Added 4/30/20
97158	Temporary addition during PHE —Added 4/30/20
97161	Temporary addition during PHE
97162	Temporary addition during PHE
97163	Temporary addition during PHE
97164	Temporary addition during PHE
97165	Temporary addition during PHE
97166	Temporary addition during PHE
97167	Temporary addition during PHE
97168	Temporary addition during PHE
97530	Temporary addition during PHE —Added 4/30/20

Code	Status
97535	Temporary addition during PHE
97542	Temporary addition during PHE —Added 4/30/20
97750	Temporary addition during PHE
97755	Temporary addition during PHE
97760	Temporary addition during PHE
97761	Temporary addition during PHE
97802	
97803	
97804	
99201	
99202	
99203	
99204	
99205	
99211	
99212	
99213	
99214	
99215	
99217	Temporary addition during PHE
99218	Temporary addition during PHE
99219	Temporary addition during PHE
99220	Temporary addition during PHE
99221	Temporary addition during PHE
99222	Temporary addition during PHE
99223	Temporary addition during PHE
99224	Temporary addition during PHE
99225	Temporary addition during PHE
99226	Temporary addition during PHE
99231	
99232	
99233	
99234	Temporary addition during PHE
99235	Temporary addition during PHE
99236	Temporary addition during PHE
99238	Temporary addition during PHE
99239	Temporary addition during PHE
99281	Temporary addition during PHE
99282	Temporary addition during PHE
99283	Temporary addition during PHE

Code	Status
99284	Temporary addition during PHE
99285	Temporary addition during PHE
99291	Temporary addition during PHE
99292	Temporary addition during PHE
99304	Temporary addition during PHE
99305	Temporary addition during PHE
99306	Temporary addition during PHE
99307	
99308	
99309	
99310	
99315	Temporary addition during PHE
99316	Temporary addition during PHE
99324	Temporary addition during PHE —Added 4/30/20
99325	Temporary addition during PHE —Added 4/30/20
99326	Temporary addition during PHE —Added 4/30/20
99327	Temporary addition during PHE
99328	Temporary addition during PHE
99334	Temporary addition during PHE
99335	Temporary addition during PHE
99336	Temporary addition during PHE
99337	Temporary addition during PHE
99341	Temporary addition during PHE
99342	Temporary addition during PHE
99343	Temporary addition during PHE
99344	Temporary addition during PHE
99345	Temporary addition during PHE
99347	Temporary addition during PHE
99348	Temporary addition during PHE
99349	Temporary addition during PHE
99350	Temporary addition during PHE
99354	
99355	
99356	
99357	
99406	
99407	
99441	Temporary addition during PHE —Added 4/30/20
99442	Temporary addition during PHE —Added 4/30/20
99443	Temporary addition during PHE —Added 4/30/20

Code	Status
99468	Temporary addition during PHE
99469	Temporary addition during PHE
99471	Temporary addition during PHE
99472	Temporary addition during PHE
99473	Temporary addition during PHE
99475	Temporary addition during PHE
99476	Temporary addition during PHE
99477	Temporary addition during PHE
99478	Temporary addition during PHE
99479	Temporary addition during PHE
99480	Temporary addition during PHE
99483	Temporary addition during PHE
99495	
99496	
99497	
99498	
0373T	Temporary addition during PHE —Added 4/30/20
S9152	Temporary addition during PHE —Added 4/30/20
0362T	Temporary addition during PHE —Added 4/30/20
90785	
G0108	
G0109	
G0270	
G0296	
G0396	
G0397	
G0406	
G0407	
G0408	
G0410	Temporary addition during PHE —Added 4/30/20
G0420	
G0421	
G0425	
G0426	
G0427	
G0436	
G0437	
G0438	
G0439	
G0442	

Code	Status
G0443	
G0444	
G0445	
G0446	
G0447	
G0459	
G0506	
G0508	
G0509	
G0513	
G0514	
G2086	
G2087	
G2088	
G9685	Temporary addition during PHE —Added 4/30/20

Telehealth services are reimbursed when the technology is designated as a real-time interactive audio and video telecommunications system; to attest that the telehealth services furnished have been provided with this specific technology, CMS established two HCPCS modifiers to be used with the appropriate CPT code. These include modifier GT if the conference is via interactive audio and video telecommunications system or modifier GQ if via an asynchronous telecommunications system.

Asynchronous telecommunication and, therefore, the use of modifier GQ is restricted only to demonstration programs in Alaska and Hawaii. Providers, physicians, and practitioners who are affiliated with these demonstration programs may receive payment when using an asynchronous telecommunication system.

For payers that do not recognize these HCPCS modifiers, CPT modifier 95 was established to be used with certain CPT codes defined as synchronous telemedicine services. A list of applicable CPT codes for reporting real time telehealth services with modifier 95 can be found in Appendix P of the CPT manual.

Reimbursement Issues
The payment for the professional service from a distant site will be equal to what would have been paid without the use of telemedicine.

As a condition of Medicare payment for telehealth services, the physician or practitioner at the distant site must be licensed to provide the service. Medicare practitioners eligible to bill for covered telehealth services are:

- Physicians
- Nurse practitioners
- Physician assistants
- Nurse midwives

 KEY POINT

For more information on telehealth technology requirements during the PHE, refer to page 12. Additional information can also be found in the CMS FAQ at https://www.cms.gov/files/document/03092020-covid-19-faqs-508.pdf.

 KEY POINT

Effective January 1, 2018, providers submitting codes for telehealth services to Medicare administrative contractors (MAC) are not required to append modifier GT to the CPT or HCPCS code. The use of telehealth POS code 02 is sufficient to certify that the reported service meets the telehealth requirements.

- Clinical nurse specialists
- Certified registered nurse anesthetists
- Clinical psychologists
- Clinical social workers
- Registered dietician or nutrition professional

Effective January 1, 2017, CMS created a new place of service (POS) code 02 Telehealth: the location where health services and health related services are provided or received, through telecommunication technology, for use by clinicians to indicate that the service provided is an approved telehealth service furnished from a distant site.

Effective January 1, 2018, claims for telehealth services submitted by providers to MACs are not required to have modifier GT appended to the CPT code. Per CMS, the use of POS code 02 confirms that the encounter meets the telehealth requirements.

Coding Examples

Payer does not accept modifier GT for telehealth services:
For 60 minutes of psychotherapy delivered via telemedicine, append CPT code 90837 with modifier 95 and use the originating place of service code 02.

MAC's that have been accepting modifier GT for telehealth services:
For 60 minutes of psychotherapy delivered via telemedicine, report CPT code 90837 and use the originating place of service code 02.

Originating sites, those sites where the telehealth service is being provided to the patient, are paid an originating site facility fee for telehealth services. HCPCS Level II code Q3014 Telehealth originating site facility fee, describes this fee and should be submitted to the MAC as a separately billable Part B payment.

In November 2018, CMS announced via the 2019 Medicare Physician Fee Schedule Final Rule (MPFS) that CMS will be paying for more telehealth services. The agency established two new codes that will cover prolonged preventive services for Medicare beneficiaries. CMS is continuing efforts to ensure access, particularly for patients in rural areas, to access Medicare telehealth services by adding more codes for telehealth coverage, reimbursing for more services, and facilitating easier billing requirements for clinicians through the creation of new codes. In doing so, CMS has an ongoing focus committed to patient-centered, innovative quality, and efficient care.

TEMPORARY EXPANSION OF TELEHEALTH SERVICES DUE TO COVID-19 PUBLIC HEALTH EMERGENCY

On March 17, 2020, the Centers for Medicare and Medicaid Services (CMS) announced the emergent and temporary expansion of telehealth services. CMS is expanding the telehealth benefit on a temporary and emergency basis under the 1135 waiver authority and Coronavirus Preparedness and Response Supplemental Appropriations Act. Beginning March 6, 2020, and continuing through the duration of the Public Health

---

✍ FOR MORE INFO

Information pertaining to reporting telehealth services and POS code 02 may be found at:

https://www.cms.gov/Regulations-and-Guidance/Guidance/Transmittals/2017Downloads/R3929CP.pdf.

Emergency (PHE), Medicare can reimburse telehealth services, including office, hospital, and other visits furnished by physicians and other practitioners to patients anywhere in the United States, including the patient's place of residence. Many services have been temporarily added to the Medicare list of eligible telehealth services (refer to page 5), and some frequency limitations and other requirements have been removed. These changes have been made to encourage the substitution of in-person services, thus reducing exposure risks for patients, practitioners, and the community at large. These telehealth services are not limited to patients with COVID-19 but must be considered reasonable and necessary.

All healthcare practitioners who are authorized to bill Medicare for their services may also furnish and bill for telehealth services during the PHE, including physical therapists, occupational therapists, speech language pathologists, licensed clinical social workers, and clinical psychologists. Telehealth services should include the same level of documentation that would ordinarily be provided if the services were furnished in person.

The following areas have been revised for the duration of the PHE site of service:

- Originating site
  - telehealth services can be provided to patients wherever they are located, including their home.
- Distant site
  - physicians/practitioners should report the place-of-service (POS) code that would have applied if the service had been provided in person. The provider is permitted to furnish the telehealth service from their home.

Telehealth technology requirements:

- For the duration of the COVID-19 pandemic, "interactive telecommunications system" is defined as multimedia communications equipment that includes, at a minimum, audio and video equipment permitting two-way, real-time interactive communication between the patient and distant-site physician or practitioner, including video-enabled phones.
- CMS is allowing some telehealth services to be provided using audio-only communications technology (telephones or other audio-only devices). These include telephone E/M services, certain counseling behavioral healthcare, and educational services, to name a few. For the duration of the PHE, Medicare is also reimbursing codes 99441–99443 for practitioners who can independently bill for E/M services. These CPT codes can be used for new and established patients. Report the place of service code that would have applied if the service had occurred in person for these telephone-only telehealth service codes. Reimbursement for these codes increased for dates of service on or after March 1 to align with the payment rates for levels two to four established office E/M services (99212–99214).
- Penalties will not be enforced for noncompliance with regulatory requirements under the Health Insurance Portability and Accountability Act (HIPAA) against physicians and other practitioners providing telehealth services to patients in good faith through everyday

 KEY POINT

For more information, refer to COVID-19 Frequently Asked Questions (FAQs) on telehealth and other Medicare Fee-for-Service (FFS) Billing, see https://www.cms.gov/files/document/03092020-covid-19-faqs-508.pdf.

communication technologies, such as Facebook Messenger video chat, Google Hangouts video, FaceTime, or Skype.

During the PHE, the CPT telehealth modifier, modifier 95, should be applied to claim lines that describe services furnished via telehealth. Modifiers CR (catastrophe/disaster related) and DR (disaster related) are not necessary for Medicare telehealth services.

Many Medicare services that are typically furnished in person may be provided via telehealth during a waiver for the public health emergency (PHE), including emergency department codes (99281–99285), critical care codes (99291–99292), and observation codes (99217–99220, 99224-99226, and 99234–99236). CMS continues to evaluate and make appropriate additions of services to the Medicare telehealth list. This current and evolving list of services is available at https://www.cms.gov/Medicare/ Medicare-General-Information/Telehealth/Telehealth-Codes. The current list of audio-only services are included in this list.

ABOUT THIS BOOK

Evaluation and Management Coding Advisor is a reference guide to help providers select the correct code based on work, and to assist staff and compliance personnel in efforts to ensure that their medical record documentation substantiates the level of E/M service code selected. The guide can also be used as a training tool to help staff educate providers regarding the type and detail of documentation that is necessary.

The guide will provide:

- The American Medical Association's definition of the key components of the E/M codes, as found in the CPT book, and the documentation criteria that must be met or exceeded in order to support a particular E/M code. This text will familiarize readers with the basics.
- An analysis of the difference between correct coding and supporting documentation. This includes in-depth discussion of the medical decision making component and should result in an increase in E/M coding accuracy. This will include both AMA-proposed revisions and current CMS guidelines.
- A section prior to each range of E/M codes that will outline real-world issues with particular code types.
- Samples of proper medical documentation for both the level of service and the medical necessity for the service with documentation indicators as required by CMS. Optum360 editors will endeavor to provide realistic samples as well as "perfect" notes.
- The potential for decreased audit liability by presenting guidelines for appropriate medical record documentation, including an explanation of the Subjective Objective Assessment Plan (SOAP) format, an alternative documentation format of Subjective, Nature of presenting problem, Objective, Counseling and/or coordination of care, Assessment, Medical decision making, and Plan (SNOCAMP); and examples of supporting documentation and standard abbreviations
- A reference for each code comparing the 1995 and 1997 versions of the E/M documentation guidelines.

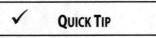

QUICK TIP

The most notable differences between 1995 and 1997 guidelines are in the exam section.

In addition to being a resource for solving day-to-day coding and documentation problems, the *Evaluation and Management Coding Advisor* can be used as a teaching tool for in-service education and as a source book for seminars, E/M coding and documentation training programs, and college and university courses.

Evaluation and Management Coding Advisor does not replace the CPT code book, nor does it contain all the E/M coding guidelines created by the AMA. Rather, it is to be used to understand proper code selection and the linkage to medical record documentation.

PHYSICIAN OR OTHER QUALIFIED HEALTHCARE PROFESSIONAL

The AMA's CPT book advises coders that the procedures and services listed throughout the book are for use by any qualified physician or other qualified healthcare professional or entity (e.g., hospitals, laboratories, or home health agencies).

The use of the phrase "physician or other qualified healthcare professional" was adopted to identify a healthcare provider other than a physician. This type of provider is further described in the CPT book as an individual "qualified by education, training, licensure/regulation (when applicable), and facility privileging (when applicable)" who performs a professional service within his/her scope of practice and independently reports that professional service." The professionals within this definition are separate from "clinical staff." The CPT book defines clinical staff as "a person who works under the supervision of a physician or other qualified healthcare professional and who is allowed, by law, regulation, and facility policy to perform or assist in the performance of a specified professional service, but who does not individually report that professional service." Keep in mind that there may be other policies, guidance, or payer policies that can affect who may report a specific service.

CONTENTS

Organization
Evaluation and Management Coding Advisor is a resource for physicians and their staff with helpful sections to assist physicians in validating medical documentation and enable staff to verify support of the selected E/M code.

The 1997 version of the E/M documentation guidelines for both general multisystem physical examinations and single-system examinations is provided, together with a comparison of the 1995 and 1997 versions of the E/M documentation guidelines. Providers may use either version of the E/M guidelines; both are currently supported by CMS for audit purposes.

The Building Blocks of Evaluation and Management Coding
This section defines the components that must be considered when selecting an E/M code. Decision making is covered in some depth as well as a description of the content of each component, as defined by the AMA and federal guidelines.

 QUICK TIP

Misuse of modifiers with E/M services has been, and continues to be, carefully reviewed by CMS and other payers as well as the OIG.

Modifiers that may be used with an E/M code are provided in this section, as well as the steps for selecting an E/M code. In addition, this section contains a list of terms commonly used in defining the E/M codes.

The Elements of Medical Documentation

Documentation principles are presented in this section, as well as information on how to evaluate medical chart documentation. This information is the result of a collaborative effort by representatives from national health information, medical societies, and insurance industry associations.

This section also explains components of the SOAP format, a method of medical chart documentation. It does not provide comprehensive instruction in using the SOAP format; it merely introduces the concept and states what is required for each component.

An alternative method of documentation—SNOCAMP—also is explained. This system offers greater support of the general approach that the nature of the presenting problem and decision making are primary in determining code levels. This format, developed by Walter L. Larimore, MD, allows for easier identification of each E/M code component with particular attention paid to those elements that drive the provider thought process, and allows for a useful way to document this in the medical record.

Adjudication of Claims by Third-Party Payers

This section outlines what third-party payers expect to find documented in the medical chart for a particular level of service. The guidelines presented are not comprehensive, nor specific to a particular third-party payer. However, some documentation requirements presently enforced under the Medicare program are included. We have also included review sheets that can be used by auditors to evaluate a provider's documentation and correct code assignment. These are available at the level of the 1997 single system specialty exams as well as the general multi-system exam level. Examples of the 1995 guidelines are also included.

EM Code Types: Coding, Common Issues, and Documentation

This section is organized by E/M code type into 13 chapters numbered 5 through 16, with chapter 17 covering HCPCS Level II G codes applicable to evaluation and management coding. Each chapter contains general guidance on code selection, a discussion of issues that may surround particular codes (when applicable), a summary of individual code requirements, and sample documentation. When possible, Optum360 will provide both a complete note—samples of medical documentation taken from real-life clinical vignettes and patient presentations, with all elements clearly specified—and the more common "economical version" that many physicians currently provide. Each may be compliant but the difference in detail will illustrate varying approaches to documentation. The shorter notes typically represent the use of the 1995 exam guidelines while the longer notes support 1997 documentation requirements.

The information in these sections may be used to compare whether the E/M code documented in similar clinical scenarios in the typical physician practice resembles the documentation samples provided, or whether another code would be more appropriate for billing based on documentation deficiencies or surpluses. In addition, ICD-10-CM guidance as it relates to

E/M coding including examples of details necessary in the E/M documentation for appropriate code selection has been provided.

Chapter 18, "Coding and Compliance," evaluates a variety of E/M compliance issues, both new and ongoing, that have been or currently are being investigated or scrutinized by different authoritative agencies including the OIG and recovery audit contractors (RAC). Issues discussed contain the investigating agency, details of the investigation, and applicable guidelines related to the E/M codes under investigation, as well as suggested strategies medical practices may employ to ensure compliance when reporting these specific E/M codes

Knowledge Assessments

Chapter 19 provides the answers to and rationales for the knowledge assessments found in chapters 1 through 18.

Appendixes

Four appendixes are included in this publication. Each appendix provides valuable information for applying the E/M documentation guidelines and offers insight into potential areas of concern, such as fraud and abuse. Appendixes included in the book are:

- Appendix A: Physician E/M Code Self Audit Forms, as well as the documentation worksheets from Medicare contractor Novitas Solutions
- Appendix B: Crosswalk for 1995 and 1997 E/M Documentation Guidelines
- Appendix C: 1995 E/M Documentation Guidelines
- Appendix D: 1997 E/M Documentation Guidelines
- Glossary

Commonly used terms are found throughout the chapters and in a glossary at the back of this book.

HOW TO USE *EVALUATION AND MANAGEMENT CODING ADVISOR*

To identify a particular E/M code, select an E/M level of service code from the CPT book. Next, locate this code in the E/M code types section of *Evaluation and Management Coding Advisor*.

The subsections within E/M code types are in numeric order according to the CPT book, and most subsections contain the following information:

- Quick comparison
  - at-a-glance chart for a quick review of all of the codes in that particular CPT code series and associated decision making, history, and exam requirements
- General guidelines
  - instructional notes for correct E/M code assignment within subset
- Common issue
  - outlines questions frequently associated with a code range or single code
- Documentation requirements
  - divides each CPT code into its key and non-key elements
    — history

 QUICK TIP

Providers should check with the hospitals with which they are affiliated or privileged for a listing of the acceptable abbreviations.

— physical examination

— medical decision making/ problem severity

— counseling and/or coordination of care is the only situation in which time spent becomes a factor in coding and documentation with the exception of time-based codes (e.g., critical care)

- total encounter time associated with each code when time is considered contributory will be listed as well. If counseling and coordination of care take up more than 50 percent of the time spent during the face-to-face visit, and the length of the visit, the amount of time spent in counseling, and the extent of counseling and/or coordination of care are documented in the chart, the correct code is based on the time indicated in the code narrative.

• Sample documentation
  - complete real-life clinical vignettes to assist in verifying the level of service and medical necessity for each CPT code in the series.
  - textbook- style notes, as well as samples, when practical, that provide a more real-life style of documentation

Review the coding and documentation requirements for the code selected. If the history, physical examination, and medical decision making documented in a chart being reviewed do not match the levels required for that particular code, locate a more appropriate code by reviewing the quick comparison chart or the code detail of the next code, higher or lower.

Pay careful attention to the level of decision making. A code that was assigned was correct relative to this area, but the components of either history or exam are insufficiently documented. This is a common failing. (Refer to the section entitled "The Building Blocks of E/M Coding" for definitions of terms.)

Note: Some sections may also contain additional information or instruction from a Medicare contractor, CMS, or other agency titled under the header "Special Instructions" or "Special Notice."

Follow these steps to validate medical documentation in a chart being reviewed

1. Identify the components in the medical record documentation (see the following example).

2. Select an E/M code from the CPT code book based on the key components of the documentation.

3. Review in the E/M code types section the documentation requirements and samples of documentation for the code selected.

If the documentation does not include all of the necessary components to support the level of E/M code that has been chosen, it may be necessary for the physician/qualified healthcare professional to complete the chart note with correct details of the patient encounter, if appropriate, or select the documented E/M code for billing purposes.

✓ QUICK TIP

Review the practices policy for correcting documentation or creating an addendum.

Correcting documentation in "real time" is generally accepted; late entries for the purpose of filling documentation gaps to support billing a particular code level is not. If it takes a few charts being billed at a lower code level based on missing or insufficient documentation to get a provider's attention, this may prove a good lesson in the long run. The goal should be to teach the provider to recognize the key elements of services as they are provided and be certain that they are documented in the normal course of documentation.

When reviewing documentation, make a point of looking for the following items that are often missing from chart notes:

- Chief complaint
- HPI elements (e.g., duration, timing)
- Review of systems
- Past, family, and/or social history
- Specific organ systems, if any, which were reviewed
- Differential diagnoses
- Diagnostic or therapeutic services that were ordered or performed
- The number, status, and management of conditions evaluated

Check for additional instructions under "General Guidelines," or situations that may be relevant in the common issues section. Such instructions include whether a modifier is necessary or what information may need to be reported separately. Consult the provider if chart documentation may not support medical necessity for services. While medical necessity is based on the judgment of the clinician, the chart documentation must clearly support the need for services provided.

The following medical documentation represents physician care consistent with a level IV ED service (99284) and is based on a general multisystem examination (1997 guidelines):

QUICK TIP

Emergency department E/M services are reported with codes 99281–99285.

QUICK TIP

The 1997 guidelines state a detailed exam requires one of the following:

- Twelve bullet points from two or more organ systems

- At least two bullet points from at least six organ systems

Sample Documentation

History: the patient is a 19-year-old female who presents to the emergency department with a chief complaint of abdominal pain **chief complaint**. The pain started approximately two days prior to her evaluation and has persisted **duration**. The pain increased in severity the morning of admission to the emergency department [severity]. The patient describes the pain as bilateral and lower in the abdominal area **location**. The patient also experienced nausea and two episodes of vomiting **associated symptoms**. She denies other GI problems **ROS**. She has recently noted abnormal menstrual periods over the last two or three months. She also noted an occasional or intermittent vaginal discharge **ROS**. She admits to being sexually active with no form of birth control being used **social history**. She has no other significant past or family medical history germane to her complaints **past and family history**.

Physical examination: the patient is a slender young female, well developed and well nourished. Her temperature is 100.5 degrees, blood pressure is 122/76, pulse is 64, respiratory rate is 26 **constitutional—2 bullet points**. Well oriented to time and place; somewhat anxious **psychiatric—2 bullet points**. Heart showed regular rate and rhythm; no murmurs **cardiovascular—1 bullet point** and lungs were clear to auscultation and percussion **respiratory—2 bullet points**. Abdominal exam revealed a soft abdomen with decreased bowel sounds, and bilateral lower abdominal pain to deep palpation. The pain was greater in the right lower quadrant and there were signs of local rebound tenderness. No masses or hepatosplenomegaly were noted. Rectal exam was benign **gastrointestinal—3 bullet points**. Pelvic exam revealed a tender but normal cervix with minimal vaginal discharge. No bleeding was noted. There was right adnexal pain but no masses were noted **genitourinary (female)—3 bullet points**. Extremities revealed no edema **cardiovascular—1 bullet point**.

Laboratory and procedures: Routine CBC, electrolytes, amylase and UA, as well as serum pregnancy tests were performed **tests ordered**. The results of these tests revealed a white blood count of 11,500 and a negative b-HCG. Other tests were unremarkable. In view of the patient's condition, she underwent a routine ultrasound study of her lower abdominal and pelvic regions. The ultrasound revealed a right side ovarian cyst and was otherwise unremarkable **minimal diagnostic procedures ordered**.

Impression: abdominal pain secondary to ovarian cyst **moderate diagnosis options**.

Treatment: The patient was treated in the emergency department with intravenous fluids and parenteral pain medications **moderate management options selected**. Her course improved in the department and her pain resolved. Her vital signs remained stable. She was discharged after a total stay in the emergency department of two and one half hours. The patient was referred to her gynecologist for immediate follow-up **moderate management options**.

- The history includes an extended history of present illness (HPI) with four elements documented. There are notes for problem-pertinent reviews of systems (ROS) of at least two systems—gastrointestinal (GI) and genitourinary (GU). In addition, a complete social and past medical history has been taken. These history elements define a detailed history.

- The examination is categorized as "detailed" since at least 12 bullet points from two or more organ systems were performed and documented.

- Medical decision making (MDM) is classified as being of moderate complexity because the physician evaluated an undiagnosed new problem with an uncertain prognosis and ordered and reviewed several laboratory tests, and because the risk associated with intravenous pain medication is considered moderate.

The exam above was supportive of a detailed exam using the 1997 "elemental" approach to the physical exam.

Under the 1995 guidelines the sample exam documented below would also have supported the detailed level with the following documentation:

Sample Documentation

WDWN, vitals stable, A & O x3, somewhat anxious, Chest CTA, CV RRR, ABD soft no HSM, tender to deep palpation RLQ, local rebound tenderness rectal benign. Pelvic no bleeding or masses, minimal discharge, some right adnexal pain. No edema.

KNOWLEDGE ASSESSMENT CHAPTER 1

See chapter 19 for answers and rationale.

1. What are the methods of documentation mentioned?
   a. Subjective, Objective, Assessment, and Plan (SOAP) format
   b. Subjective, Nature of presenting problem, Objective, Counseling and/or coordination of care, Assessment, Medical decision making, and Plan (SNOCAMP)
   c. Who, What, When, Where, Why, and How (5 W and H) format
   d. Both a and b

2. How is using a documentation method beneficial?
   a. Using a standardized documentation format expedites the revenue cycle process
   b. Using a standardized documentation format ensures a lower medical malpractice premium
   c. Using a standardized documentation format can help decrease audit liability
   d. Using a standardized documentation format has not been proven to be beneficial

3. What are the primary differences between the 1995 and the 1997 documentation guidelines?
   a. There are no differences
   b. The 1995 guidelines do not outline history requirements and the 1997 history component is well defined
   c. The 1997 guidelines use a detailed bullet point format for exam and the 1995 focuses on body areas and organ systems
   d. The decision making for 1997 is determined solely on the table of risk

4. Why are E/M services considered the dominant source of revenue for most providers?
   a. They are among the most frequently billed services
   b. They have high reimbursement values
   c. Providers can bill all high levels of care
   d. These services are not monitored

5. What can providers use to assess overall coding patterns?
   a. Reimbursement rates from payers
   b. Coder productivity
   c. Payer requests for documentation
   d. Benchmark data

6. Which modifier should be reported to indicate to a payer that service was provided via synchronous telemedicine?

a. 25

b. 57

c. 95

d. 97

Chapter 2: The Building Blocks of E/M Coding

The levels of evaluation and management (E/M) services define the wide variations in skill, effort, time, and medical knowledge required for preventing or diagnosing and treating illness or injury, and promoting optimal health. These codes are intended to represent provider work—mostly cognitive work. Because much of this work revolves around the thought process, and involves the amount of training, experience, expertise, and knowledge that a provider may bring to bear on a given patient presentation, the true indications of the level of this work may be difficult to recognize without some explanation.

At first glance, selecting an E/M code appears to be complex, but the system of coding medical visits is actually fairly simple once the requirements for code selection are learned and used.

LEVELS OF E/M SERVICES

Codes for E/M services are categorized by the place of service (e.g., office or hospital) or type of service (e.g., critical care, observation, or preventive medicine services). Many of the categories are further divided by the status of the medical visit (e.g., new vs. established patient or initial vs. subsequent care).

A **new patient** is defined by the American Medical Association (AMA) and Centers for Medicare and Medicaid Services (CMS) as one who has *not* received any professional services from a provider of the exact same specialty and subspecialty from the same group practice within the last three years. An **established patient** is defined as one who *has* received a professional service from a provider of the exact same specialty and subspecialty from the same group practice within the last three years. If the patient is seen by a physician who is covering for another physician, the patient will be considered the same as if seen by the physician who is unavailable.

DETERMINING THE LEVEL OF SERVICE FOR OFFICE OR OTHER OUTPATIENT E/M SERVICES

Effective January 1, 2021, the AMA and CMS have adopted new guidelines and code descriptions for reporting E/M codes for new and established office or other outpatient services (99202–99215). Note that 99201 has been deleted and is no longer valid for dates of service after December 31, 2020.

Per CMS CY2020 Physician Fee Schedule (PFS) Final Rule and CPT guidelines, the history and examination will no longer be used to select the code level for these services. These services will include a medically appropriate history and/or physical examination, the number of body systems/areas examined or reviewed as part of the history and examination will no longer apply. The history and examination are still required and

OBJECTIVES

This chapter discusses:
- The levels of evaluation and management (E/M) services
- Component sequence and code selection
- How to identify elements of the key components
- How to use AMA tables
- How to recognize contributory components
- The relationship between E/M coding and appropriate ICD-10-CM code selection
- Definitions of common terms
- Why documentation of the key and contributing components is important

should be documented, but the nature and extent of the history and/or physical examination will be determined by the treating clinician based on clinical judgement and what is deemed as reasonable, necessary, and clinically appropriate.

Selecting the level of office or other outpatient visit (99202–99205 and 99212–99215) should be based on the redefined levels of medical decision making (MDM) or total time spent by the clinician on the day of the encounter, including face-to-face and non-face-to-face activities. Keep in mind that medical necessity is still the overarching criterion for selecting a level of service in addition to the individual requirements of the E/M code.

Medical Decision Making: Office or Other Outpatient E/M Services

MDM is used to establish diagnoses, assess the status of a condition, and select a management option(s). MDM for these services is defined by three elements detailed in the redefined MDM table published in the CPT E/M guidelines. Two noteworthy changes in the redefined table are that new and established patient levels are scored the same and new and established codes require two out of three elements for any given code.

The three elements of the table will look familiar but do differ slightly from the existing MDM elements.

- Number and complexity of problems addressed during the encounter
- Amount and/or complexity of data to be reviewed and analyzed
- Risk of complications and/or morbidity or mortality of patient management

Number and Complexity of Problems Addressed During the Encounter

CPT now includes definitions to assist in the selection of the different levels of problems listed in the MDM table.

- Minimal problem: A problem that may not require the presence of the physician or other qualified healthcare professional, but the service is provided under the physician's or other qualified healthcare professional's supervision (see 99211).
- Self-limited or minor problem: A problem that runs a definite and prescribed course, is transient in nature, and is not likely to permanently alter health status.
- Stable, chronic illness: A problem with an expected duration of at least one year or until the death of the patient.
- Acute, uncomplicated illness or injury: Recent or new short-term problem with low risk of morbidity for which treatment is considered. There is little to no risk of mortality with treatment, and full recovery without functional impairment is expected.
- Chronic illness with exacerbation, progression, or side effects of treatment: A chronic illness that is acutely worsening, poorly controlled, or progressing with an intent to control progression and requiring additional supportive care or requiring attention to treatment for side effects but that does not require consideration of hospital level of care.
- Acute illness with systemic symptoms: An illness that causes systemic symptoms and has a high risk of morbidity without treatment.

KEY POINT

Level one established visit (99211) describes and only includes visits performed by clinical staff; the concept of MDM does not apply.

KEY POINT

The four levels of MDM are consistent with the current guidelines: Straightforward, Low, Moderate, and High.

- Acute, complicated injury: An injury that requires treatment that includes evaluation of body systems that are not directly part of the injured organ, extensive injuries, or the treatment options are multiple and/or associated with risk of morbidity.
- Chronic illness with severe exacerbation, progression, or side effects of treatment: The severe exacerbation or progression of a chronic illness or severe side effects of treatment that have significant risk of morbidity and may require hospital level of care.
- Acute or chronic illness or injury that poses a threat to life or bodily function: An acute illness with systemic symptoms, an acute complicated injury, or a chronic illness or injury with exacerbation and/or progression or side effects of treatment that poses a threat to life or bodily function in the near term without treatment.
- Undiagnosed new problem with uncertain prognosis: A problem in the differential diagnosis that represents a condition likely to result in a high risk of morbidity without treatment.

Level 3: Number and Complexity of Problems Addressed

Code	Level of MDM	Number and Complexity of Problems Addressed at the Encounter
99203 99213	Low	Low • Two or more self-limited or minor problems or • One stable, chronic illness or • One acute, uncomplicated illness or injury

Note: Each level has the same requirements for new or established patients.

Amount and/or Complexity of Data to be Reviewed and Analyzed

The second element listed for determining the level of service is no longer based on counting points for each test category or specific task. Each level has the same requirements for new or established patients. The four levels for this category are consistent with the current guidelines: minimal, limited, moderate, and extensive.

This MDM element includes medical records, tests, and other information that must be obtained, reviewed, ordered, and/or analyzed for the visit, including information obtained from multiple sources or interprofessional correspondence and interpretation of tests that aren't reported separately. Ordering and subsequently reviewing test results are considered part of the current encounter, not a subsequent encounter.

CPT now includes definitions of certain elements used within the data category of the MDM table to help with the interpretation of these elements.

- Test: Imaging, laboratory, psychometric, or physiologic data.
- External: Records, communications, and/or test results from an external physician, other qualified healthcare professional, facility, or healthcare organization.
- Independent historian(s): Individual (e.g., parent, guardian, surrogate, spouse, witness) who provides a history in addition to a history provided by the patient who is unable to provide a complete or reliable

history (e.g., due to developmental stage, dementia, or psychosis) or because a confirmatory history is judged to be necessary.

- Appropriate source: Professionals who are not healthcare professionals but may be involved in the management of the patient (e.g., lawyer, parole officer, case manager, teacher). It does not include discussion with family or informal caregivers.

Level 3: Amount and/or Complexity of Data Reviewed and Analyzed

Code	Level of MDM	Amount and/or Complexity of Data to be Reviewed and Analyzed *Each unique test, order, or document contributes to the combination of two or combination of three in Category 1 below.*

99203
99213
	Low	**Limited**
		(Must meet the requirements of at least one of the two categories.)
		Category 1: Tests and documents
		• Any combination of two from the following:
		   – review of prior external note(s) from each unique source*
		   – review of the result(s) of each unique test*
		   – ordering of each unique test*
		or
		Category 2: Assessment requiring an independent historian(s)
		(For the categories of independent interpretation of tests and discussion of management or test interpretation, see moderate or high)

Note: Each level has the same requirements for new or established patients.

Risk of Complications and/or Morbidity or Mortality of Patient Management

The third element listed for determining the level of service includes decisions made during the encounter associated with the patient's problems, diagnostic procedures, and treatments. This includes potential management options selected, and those considered but not selected, after shared MDM with the patient and/or family. Shared MDM involves eliciting patient and/or family preferences, patient and/or family education, and explaining risks and benefits of management options.

The four levels for this category are consistent with the current guidelines: minimal, low, moderate, and high. The minimal and low categories no longer include examples and the examples for moderate and high risk have been revised.

CPT now includes definitions of certain elements used within the data category of the MDM table to help with the interpretation of these elements.

- Risk: The probability and/or consequences of an event. The assessment of the level of risk is affected by the nature of the event under consideration. Definitions of risk are based upon the usual behavior and thought processes of a physician or other qualified healthcare professional in the same specialty. For the purposes of MDM, level of risk is based upon consequences of the problem(s) addressed at the encounter when appropriately treated. Risk also includes MDM related to the need to initiate or forego further testing, treatment, and/or hospitalization.

- Morbidity: A state of illness or functional impairment that is expected to be of substantial duration during which function is limited, quality of life is impaired, or there is organ damage that may not be transient despite treatment.

- Social determinants of health: Economic and social conditions that influence the health of people and communities. Examples may include food or housing insecurity.

- Drug therapy requiring intensive monitoring for toxicity: A drug that requires intensive monitoring and is a therapeutic agent that has the potential to cause serious morbidity or death. The monitoring is performed for assessment of these adverse effects and not primarily for assessment of therapeutic efficacy.

Level 3 and 4: Risk of Complications and/or Morbidity or Mortality of Patient Management

Code	Level of MDM	Risk of Complications and/or Morbidity or Mortality of Patient Management
99203 99213	Low	**Low risk of morbidity from additional diagnostic testing or treatment**
99204 99214	Moderate	**Moderate risk of morbidity from additional diagnostic testing or treatment** *Examples only:* • Prescription drug management • Decision regarding minor surgery with identified patient or procedure risk factors • Decision regarding elective major surgery without identified patient or procedure risk factors • Diagnosis or treatment significantly limited by social determinants of health

Note: Each level has the same requirements for new or established patients.

2021 Medical Decision Making Table (Codes 99202–99205 and 99212-99215)

CPT E/M Office and Other Outpatient Services Revisions to Level of Medical Decision Making (MDM) (Revisions effective January 1, 2021)

Code	Level of MDM (Based on 2 out of 3 Elements of MDM)	Elements of Medical Decision Making		
		Number and Complexity of Problems Addressed	Amount and/or Complexity of Data to be Reviewed and Analyzed	Risk of Complications and/or Morbidity or Mortality of Patient Management
99211	N/A	N/A	N/A	N/A
99202 99212	Straightforward	**Minimal** • **1** self-limited or minor problem	**Minimal or none**	**Minimal risk of morbidity from additional diagnostic testing or treatment**

99203 99213	Low	**Low**
		 • **2** or more self-limited or minor problems;
		 or
		 • stable chronic illness;
		 or
		 • **1** acute, uncomplicated illness or injury
			Limited
			 (Must meet the requirements of at least 1 of the 2 categories)
			 Category 1: Tests and documents
			 • Any combination of 2 from the following:
			   – Review of prior external note(s) from each unique source*;
			   – Review of the result(s) of each unique test*;
			   – Ordering of each unique test*
			 or
			 Category 2: Assessment requiring an independent historian(s)
			 (For the categories of independent interpretation of tests and discussion of management or test interpretation, see moderate or high)
				Low risk of morbidity from additional diagnostic testing or treatment

*Each unique test, order, or document contributes to the combination of 2 or combination of 3 in Category 1.

		Elements of Medical Decision Making		
Code	Level of MDM (Based on 2 out of 3 Elements of MDM)	Number and Complexity of Problems Addressed	Amount and/or Complexity of Data to be Reviewed and Analyzed	Risk of Complications and/or Morbidity or Mortality of Patient Management
99204 99214	Moderate	**Moderate** • **1** or more chronic illnesses with exacerbation, progression, or side effects of treatment; **or** • **2** or more stable chronic illnesses; **or** • **1** undiagnosed new problem with uncertain prognosis; **or** • **1** acute illness with systemic symptoms; **or** • **1** acute complicated injury	**Moderate** *(Must meet the requirements of at least 1 out of 3 categories)* **Category 1: Tests, documents, or independent historian(s)** • Any combination of 3 from the following: – Review of prior external note(s) from each unique source*; – Review of the result(s) of each unique test*; – Ordering of each unique test*; – Assessment requiring an independent historian(s) **or** **Category 2: Independent interpretation of tests** • Independent interpretation of a test performed by another physician/other qualified health care professional (not separately reported); **or** **Category 3: Discussion of management or test interpretation** • Discussion of management or test interpretation with external physician/other qualified health care professional\appropriate source (not separately reported)	**Moderate risk of morbidity from additional diagnostic testing or treatment** *Examples only:* • Prescription drug management • Decision regarding minor surgery with identified patient or procedure risk factors • Decision regarding elective major surgery without identified patient or procedure risk factors • Diagnosis or treatment significantly limited by social determinants of health

Each unique test, order, or document contributes to the combination of 2 or combination of 3 in Category 1.

Code	Level of MDM (Based on 2 out of 3 Elements of MDM)	Elements of Medical Decision Making		
		Number and Complexity of Problems Addressed	Amount and/or Complexity of Data to be Reviewed and Analyzed	Risk of Complications and/or Morbidity or Mortality of Patient Management

99205 99215	High	**High**
		• **1** or more chronic illnesses with severe exacerbation, progression, or side effects of treatment;
		or
		• **1** acute or chronic illness or injury that poses a threat to life or bodily function
			Extensive
			(Must meet the requirements of at least 2 out of 3 categories)
			Category 1: Tests, documents, or independent historian(s)
			• **Any combination of 3 from the following:**
			  – Review of prior external note(s) from each unique source*;
			  – Review of the result(s) of each unique test*;
			  – Ordering of each unique test*;
			  – Assessment requiring an independent historian(s)
			or
			Category 2: Independent interpretation of tests
			• Independent interpretation of a test performed by another physician/other qualified health care professional (not separately reported);
			or
			Category 3: Discussion of management or test interpretation
			• Discussion of management or test interpretation with external physician/other qualified health care professional/appropriate source (not separately reported)
				High risk of morbidity from additional diagnostic testing or treatment
				Examples only:
				• Drug therapy requiring intensive monitoring for toxicity
				• Decision regarding elective major surgery with identified patient or procedure risk factors
				• Decision regarding emergency major surgery
				• Decision regarding hospitalization
				• Decision not to resuscitate or to de-escalate care because of poor prognosis

Each unique test, order, or document contributes to the combination of 2 or combination of 3 in Category 1.

Time as the Basis for Code Selection

Effective January 1, 2021, time alone may be used to select the appropriate code level for 99202–99205 and 99212–99215. Time alone may be used to report these services regardless of whether counseling and/or coordination of care was provided or dominated greater than 50 percent of the encounter. These services do require a face-to-face encounter, but face-to-face and non-face-to-face time personally spent by the provider on the date of the encounter count toward the total reported time.

The time defined in the code descriptor is used for selecting the appropriate level of service. Applicable time spent on the date of the encounter should be documented in the medical record when it is used as the basis for code selection.

A shared or split visit occurs when a physician and other qualified healthcare professional(s) jointly provide the face-to-face and non-face-to-face work related to the encounter. When time-based reporting of shared or split visits

 KEY POINT

Per CMS, medical necessity is still the overarching criterion for selecting a level of service in addition to the individual requirements of the E/M code.

is allowed, the time personally spent by the physician and other qualified healthcare professional(s) evaluating and managing the patient on the date of the encounter is added together to determine total time. If two or more providers meet with or discuss the patient, only one provider should count this time toward the total time of the split/shared visit.

Determining the Level of E/M Service for Hospital Observation, Hospital Inpatient, Consultations, Emergency Department, Nursing Facility, Domiciliary, Rest Home or Custodial Care, Home Services

The narrative descriptions for the levels of most E/M services, excluding 99202–99205 and 99212–99215, include seven components. The key components—history, examination, and medical decision making—are most often used to select the appropriate level of service code. Information regarding at least two of the three key components for inpatient or outpatient follow-up visits—and all three for consults and inpatient or outpatient initial visits—must be performed and documented in the patient's record to substantiate a particular level of service.

The four remaining components are called "contributory components" and are: nature of the presenting problem, counseling, coordination of care, and time.

The various levels of service for each component are described on the following pages and include requirements under both the 1995 and 1997 E/M guidelines.

Some of the confusion experienced when first approaching E/M is likely the way that each description of a code component or element seems to have yet another layer of description beneath. Each of the three key components—history, examination, and decision making—comprises elements that combine to create varying levels of that component.

For example, an expanded problem focused history includes the chief complaint, a brief history of the present illness, and a system review focusing on the patient's problems. The level of exam is not made up of different elements but rather distinguished by the extent of exam across body areas or organ systems.

Perhaps the single largest source of confusion is the "labels" or names applied to the varying degrees of history, exam, and decision making. Terms such as expanded problem focused, detailed, and comprehensive are somewhat meaningless unless you know their definition. The lack of explanation in the CPT® book relative to these terms was precisely what caused the first set of federal guidelines to be developed back in 1994 and 1995.

COMPONENT SEQUENCE AND CODE SELECTION

The general format for the original guidelines followed the manner in which providers are taught to approach and address clinical problems. The SOAP note—subjective, objective, assessment, and plan—maps directly to history, exam, and decision making. This is constant through all versions and will be given further attention in the next chapter.

The 1995 guidelines placed great emphasis on the history and exam portions of the encounter. Of 49 pages of text in the original guidelines, 45 were

KEY POINT

Both 1995 and 1997 guidelines state that a notation of "normal" is acceptable for normal aspects of the exam. Abnormal or unexpected findings require notation of the abnormalities.

devoted to these areas. Medical decision making received only four pages. This focus led many providers and coders to become mired in the detail of history and exam elements and, in essence, miss the big picture when it comes to true code selection.

To further complicate matters, various subspecialty societies objected to the breadth of the physical exam required at higher levels of service. They asked for revised guidelines that allowed the specialist to focus the physical exam within the systems related to their specialty. What followed were the 1997 guidelines, whose changes were focused within the physical exam section. This version entailed even more "counting," or quantification of the exam, and led to an AMA protest that ultimately forestalled the implementation of the 1997 version as the sole set of guidelines. Providers may use either set of E/M documentation guidelines.

Without going into great detail, the 1995 guidelines were generous in that they asked only for a notation of "normal" on systems with normal findings. The only narrative required was for abnormal findings. The 1997 version calls for much greater detail, or an "elemental" or "bullet-point" approach to organ systems, although again a notation of normal was sufficient when addressing the elements within a system. This later version lent itself well to templates for recording E/M services.

The sequence in which the guidelines are presented, as well as the sequence of the E/M components in the CPT book—history, exam, and medical decision making—has led to a somewhat misleading focus when both coding and documenting these services.

The order of a SOAP note is descriptive of how an encounter usually unfolds in terms of real time. The subjective component is the history that the patient offers the provider related to the problem plus other questions the provider may ask of the patient. The objective portion is the provider's own physical examination of the patient. And lastly, after the previous two elements are performed as needed, the assessment and plan is determined. It is this last component that indicates the level of medical decision making involved. This order matches the CPT guidelines and the normal sequence of components as *written* in the chart.

However, there is an important aspect of most encounters that can change the way a provider views coding E/M services. In almost every case the patient will tell the healthcare provider why he or she is there—the chief complaint. In many cases the complexity of the encounter suggested by this will point directly at the level of medical decision making. The subjective, nature of presenting problem, objective, counseling and/or coordination of care, assessment, medical decision making, and plan [SNOCAMP] format, discussed in the next chapter, does an excellent job of bringing this consideration to the forefront and clearly detailing the sequence of provider thought processes, not just the visible elements of the encounter.

One of the two tracks that the CMS announced it is pursuing in terms of finalizing guidelines is one that weighs the decision making component more than history or exam. The reason for this is simple: patients go to a provider to have their health problem or problems dealt with, not to have some degree of history or exam performed. The history and exam components are only the ways that providers gather data to arrive at some decision making relative to the problem. *It is the decision making component that will most often determine the true complexity of the management involved. The history and exam are best viewed as supporting components in terms of both work performed and documented.* (**Note:** Changes to CPT by the CPT Editorial Panel, as well as CMS CY2020 Physician Fee Schedule Final Rule, state that **effective January 1, 2021,** providers will base selection of new (99202–99205) or established (99212–99215) office/other outpatient E/M codes on the level of MDM or total time. These changes were reiterated in the CY2021 Physician Fee Schedule Proposed Rule. Refer to page 23 for more details on these upcoming changes.)

In most cases, when decision making at a certain level is required or occurs, the degree of history and exam will follow. *Providers take only as much history as they need, and perform as much physical exam as they need, to address the problem. In a sense these elements are governed somewhat by the nature of the presenting problem or problems.* Again, we might turn to the SNOCAMP format here for clear documentation of this process. This format is preferred by many providers over SOAP notes as it outlines the very considerations that will drive the breadth and depth of the encounter at the component level.

Most traditional efforts used to teach providers both coding and documentation rules are weakened by the emphasis on history and exam precisely because physicians already know they will do as much of these things as are needed. The documentation guidelines are often perceived to be an effort to "make them do more than they need to." Medical necessity dictates that one would never do more than one needs, and responsible clinicians will stick with what is needed or pertinent. The emphasis on documentation is directed at documenting all that you do—for both general medical record keeping reasons and to support the E/M work performed and coded.

In terms of correct coding with the emphasis on decision making, providers should be encouraged to essentially determine the level of service *in the first few moments of the encounter when possible.* When we review the elements of decision making later in this section you will see how descriptors from the decision making matrices will help in this. In effect, these matrices give a range of acuity from uncomplicated through complex episodic presentations. They also list a quantitative progression of chronic conditions and a hierarchy of treatment options.

The provider will usually know early in the encounter what types of problems are being presented. Even when confronted with an unknown new problem, this is clearly earmarked as at least moderate level decision making. Of course, some encounters may take a dramatic turn after the initial presentation, but most do not.

If providers can sense the level of service that presenting problems require, they can then be certain to document the history and exam elements required to support the service. *If you don't know what the code is, you don't know what needs to be documented.* This is not to say that a code should be selected, and then various amounts of history or exam performed to support it. Rather, the point is that if the level of decision making describes the real effort in terms of identifying and managing a problem, and, as is almost always the case especially with established patients, either the history or exam performed will support that level of decision making—be sure to document these supporting elements.

Consider the alternative. Many coding texts will suggest that the provider perform the service, document what he or she did, and then look back to review the documentation to see what the supported code is. Does this sound like the way that most providers approach coding?

Most providers select the code at the end of the face-to-face portion of the encounter. There needs to be at least some sense of the level provided right away, whether notes are completed or not. Documentation, even with electronic medical records (EMR), may not be completed until after the patient has left the practice. During the actual visit, many providers may complete part of the documentation with brief notes to enable completion of the record later. This is true of electronic medical records as well as handwritten and dictated documentation.

This does not allow for review of notes prior to code assignment. These practices can cause compliance problems related to documentation often because by the time the note is dictated many particulars of the encounter, nonpertinent ROS negatives and normal exam findings for example, are lost to memory and not recorded.

One reason that there is safety in coding by decision making is that this component is the one most closely linked to medical necessity. The management of the problem or problems, the number and/or acuity of diagnoses, diagnostics ordered and/or performed, and any planned follow-up will support medical necessity as well as the level of decision making. The number and severity of problems will also dictate to some degree the amount of history and/or physical required.

The following section will review each component as it appears in the CPT book and the guidelines. This should familiarize the reader with the particular elements of each component of E/M coding. However, subsequent sections of this guide will take a different approach to describing the codes in the code type section. The level of decision making will be reviewed first, then the required levels of history and exam will be provided. This should be useful when reviewing charts to get a sense immediately of whether the level of decision making is correct. The other components can then be reviewed for support.

KEY COMPONENTS

Effective January 1, 2021, the AMA and CMS have adopted new guidelines and code descriptions for reporting E/M codes for new and established office or other outpatient services (99202–99215). The history and physical exam elements are not required for code level selection for office and other outpatient services. However, a medically appropriate history and/or physical examination should still be documented. The nature and degree of the history and/or physical examination will be determined by the treating physician or other qualified healthcare professional reporting the service. Therefore, the following guidelines section does not apply to new and established office or other outpatient services (99202–99215).

History

The history is the first of three key components described in the CPT book. While not always a supporting component of documentation, virtually all records contain some degree of history. The areas of history are:

- Chief complaint (CC)
- History of present illness (HPI)
- Review of systems (ROS)
- Past medical history, family medical history, social history (PFSH)

Within each area of history, there is basic information that makes up the elements of that history area. Once performed and documented, the elements are then quantified to substantiate the level of history. These elements are described below in detail:

Chief complaint: A concise statement, usually in the patient's own words, describing symptoms, problems, conditions, diagnoses, or reason for the patient encounter.

- Each note must always include a chief complaint. Even if the chief complaint describes that the patient is presenting for follow-up of a previous problem, the reason for the visit must be clear.
- With the implementation of ICD-10-CM, additional details, such as the severity of pain, which side of the body is affected (i.e., right or left), as well as determining if the condition or injury is a new problem or a late effect (sequela) and how many times the patient has been seen at the practice for this problem, all become critical elements of information about the patient encounter.

Examples of chief complaints, along with the corresponding diagnosis code description and/or additional information needed to determine code selection based on which code set is used are shown in the following table.

Problem	ICD-10-CM
My foot hurts.	Right or left foot?
I'm having trouble seeing.	Right, left, or both eyes? Occurs primarily during the day, night, or all the time?
I think I broke my ankle.	Right or left ankle? Is this a new injury? Cause of fracture is pathological or traumatic? Open or closed?
I have breast cancer.	Primary, secondary, or in situ malignancy? Location? Gender (i.e., male or female)?
My stump hurts.	Involving upper or lower extremity? Right or left side? Amputation resulted from acquired or congenital condition or traumatic injury? What type of injury (e.g., MVA, machinery accident) and where did it occur (e.g., work, highway, farm)? Is this a new problem?

 KEY POINT

Chief complaint is required and identifies the condition that precipitated the visit. The chief complaint can be a separate element of the documentation or clearly stated in other portions of the history.

History of present illness: Includes information described by the patient about the current condition including:

- Location
- Severity
- Timing
- Modifying factors
- Quality
- Duration
- Context
- Associated signs and symptoms

An explanation of each of these elements follows:

- **Location:** Refers to a specific location of the problem (e.g., pain in the groin area, elbow pain, headache)
- **Severity:** Description of the severity of the presenting problem (e.g., mild, severe, 5 on a scale of 10)
- **Timing:** Refers to the interval of the pain or suffering (e.g., every night, in the middle of the night, constant pain, comes and goes, intermittently)
- **Modifying factors:** Information about how the pain is modified by other factors (e.g., "pain is relieved by standing erect," "headache somewhat better after taking aspirin")
- **Quality:** Description of the sensation, such as dull, sharp, aching, stinging, etc.
- **Duration:** The patient will describe an approximate duration of the symptoms (e.g., "for the last week," "since yesterday," "it began when I fell this morning")
- **Context:** Describes how the symptoms began or occur (e.g., "after the auto accident," "after eating out at a restaurant," "after bumping my head," "when I sit down")
- **Associated signs and symptoms:** These are significant signs or symptoms that the patient feels are related to or part of their injury or illness (e.g., some dizziness with nausea, swelling with an ankle injury, double vision with headache)

There is frequently a wide degree of interpretation when reviewing or evaluating this area. Although the definitions of each element may seem clear, there is often disagreement among coders and auditors as to what type of comments fits in which element. Context is related to the context of the problem, for example, not the context of the visit, which is more properly the chief complaint. Associated signs and symptoms are generally regarded as more detailed information than the chief complaint itself.

According to CMS, there are two types of HPI: brief and extended. It further defines a brief HPI as including one to three of the HPI elements and an extended HPI as including at least four HPI elements.

These descriptors are not the only way to address HPI. For the extended level of HPI, another approach is described in the 1997 guidelines. If the status of three or more chronic illnesses is discussed, the HPI also qualifies for an expanded HPI. A FAQ published by CMS states, "For services performed

---

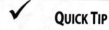

QUICK TIP

Providers may document the status of three chronic or inactive conditions for an extended HPI, even when using the 1995 guidelines for the patient encounter.

after September 10, 2013, physicians may use the 1997 guideline for an extended HPI in combination with the 1995 guidelines to document an E/M service. This means providers may document the status of three chronic or inactive conditions for an extended HPI, even if using the 1995 guidelines for the rest of the encounter."

Providers frequently fall short in documenting HPI by simply stating "here for follow-up or recheck" when following chronic problems. Often the "duration" or "severity" elements are missed even though they were discussed. Some E/M services, such as preventive services, will not have an HPI as there is no "I" (illness) in that type of service.

The CY 2019 Medicare Physician Fee Schedule (MPFS) Final Rule changed the policy for office/outpatient E/M encounters. Effective January 1, 2019, the chief compliant and history, including HPI, PFSH, and ROS, documented in the medical record by ancillary staff does not have to be re-documented by the provider. The provider must review the information, make changes or supplement the information as necessary, and document in the medical record that he or she has done so.

Many practices have already established a convention where a nurse or medical assistant will record this information. If the provider indicates "HPI as above significant for xxxx" this should serve to indicate first-hand knowledge of this information. Practices should verify other payers' policies to see if they require additional documentation, because if an audit arises, CMS's documentation policies may not suffice for all payers.

HPI Elements Quiz

Find and label the HPI elements in the following scenarios using the eight HPI elements just discussed.

The answer key is located at the end of the "History" section, page 43.

1. Patient has had a sore throat for two days. States it is "burning" and she can hardly swallow. She has tried otc throat spray but it has not controlled her symptoms.

2. The patient's nasal congestion has significantly improved with steroid nasal spray and is now described as "mild" in severity.

3. The patient is a 55-year-old male who developed sudden onset of shortness of breath, which began last night. He has also experienced some dizziness and lightheadedness.

4. A 19-year-old patient presents with abdominal pain of two-day duration not relieved by otc medicine, including sharp RLQ pain today. Patient does admit to N&V for the past 24 hours and a fever today of 102 degrees.

5. A 56-year-old male presents with persistent, moderately severe proteinuria, which has been present for four months and has been associated with lower extremity edema.

6. The patient complains of chest pain, which began two hours ago. Pain has been off and on since that time with each episode lasting two to three minutes. The pain is described as "crushing" and at times is rated as a seven on a scale of one to 10. The pain occurs with minimal exertion

and is associated with nausea and shortness of breath. The pain was relieved with sublingual NTG in the ambulance.

Review of systems: Includes the patient's inventory of signs and/or symptoms of body systems. Health history forms completed by the patient, or that portion of the electronic medical record (EMR), allows the staff to ask more pointed questions, have the patient elaborate on points of concern, and further describe signs and symptoms related to the current problem or problems the physician will be addressing. These are most often the result of questions asked by the provider in an effort to establish a working diagnosis. These questions assist the provider in narrowing the range of differential (or potential) diagnoses.

The systems are described as:

- Constitutional (e.g., weight loss, fever, chills, malaise, etc.)
- Ear, nose, throat, and mouth (e.g., hearing loss, sinusitis, sore throat, oral cavities, ulcers)
- Gastrointestinal (e.g., nausea, vomiting, diarrhea, constipation, ulcer)
- Integumentary (e.g., skin rashes, moles, dryness, lumps, pigmentation)
- Endocrine (e.g., polyuria, polydipsia, cold/heat intolerance, diabetes)
- Genitourinary (e.g., hematuria, nocturia, menopause, hernia)
- Hematologic/lymphatic (e.g., anemia, bruising, bleeding, lymph node enlargement)
- Eyes (e.g., diplopia, blurred vision)
- Cardiovascular (e.g., chest pain or pressure, palpitations, murmur, hypertension)
- Musculoskeletal (e.g., arthritis, joint stiffness, joint pain, swelling, myalgias, gout)
- Neurologic (e.g., dizziness, syncope, seizures, vertigo, weakness, tremor)
- Allergic/immunologic (e.g., allergies to medicine, food, dye; hepatitis, HIV)
- Respiratory (e.g., cough, hemoptysis, pleuritic chest pain, wheezing, asthma)
- Psychiatric (e.g., depression, agitation, panic-anxiety, memory disturbance)

Examples of questions/topics appropriate to ask on the forms or in direct questioning of the patient include, but are not limited to:

Body System	Topic for Patient Questions
Constitutional	Unexplained weight loss or gain
Ears, nose, throat	Nasal congestion/nose bleeds/earaches/sore or strep throat
Gastrointestinal	Abdominal pain/constipation/diarrhea/blood in stool/nausea and/or vomiting
Integumentary	Itching/rash/change in skin lesion or skin color/new or recurrent lesion
Endocrine	Sudden gain or loss of weight/excessive thirst
Genitourinary	Frequency/urgency/pain/unable to urinate/blood in urine/urinary tract infection (UTI)
Hematologic/lymphatic	Bruising/excessive bleeding/swollen lymph nodes

Body System	Topic for Patient Questions
Eyes	Redness/irritation/swelling/blurry vision
Cardiovascular	Chest pain/palpitations/tightness, heart racing
Musculoskeletal	Neck pain, stiffness, swelling/pain in extremity, upper or lower
Neurological	Weakness/dizziness/headaches/numbness, tingling
Respiratory	Shortness of breath/cough, sputum
Psychiatric	Irritability/behavioral issues/depression, anxiety, or suicidal thoughts

Additional detail under the history component also helps to ensure correct ICD-10-CM code assignment as illustrated in the following example.

Sample Documentation

The patient presents for evaluation of continued arm pain resulting from a recent motor vehicle accident (MVA). The arm was splinted to keep it immobile, but the patient continues to C/O "unbearable pain" despite taking pain medication. There are no prior surgeries on this arm and no family history of delayed healing issues. Otherwise, the patient has no other complaints. All superficial abrasions are healing. The patient lives alone and is employed as a secretary.

HPI:
Location: arm
Context: MVA
Modifying factor: splinted, pain medication
Severity: "unbearable"
Past History: no surgeries
Family History: no delayed healing
Social history: lives alone/employed as a secretary
ROS:
Musculoskeletal: arm pain
Integumentary: abrasions, healed
History level for patient encounter: Established patient: detailed history

In order to correctly assign the ICD-10-CM codes, additional information is needed. For example, the documentation does not specify exactly when the patient returned to the clinic or which arm (e.g., left or right) was injured. In fact, there is no further information available to indicate what type of injury the patient sustained (e.g., fracture, dislocation, and sprain/strain). Further, there are no details regarding the MVA.

- Was the patient the driver or a passenger or was the patient a pedestrian?
- Did the vehicle strike another vehicle or a stationary object?

In addition, the documentation does not indicate whether the patient is taking over-the-counter (OTC) or prescription pain medicine and there is no description as to the location of the abrasions.

The following shows the same scenario with the missing information included and the ICD-10-CM codes assigned.

Sample Documentation

The patient returns for evaluation of continued left arm pain one week after she crashed The patient presents for evaluation of continued left arm pain one week after she crashed her vehicle into a pole on October 24. When she was seen in the emergency room, her arm was splinted due to the severe bruising, to keep it immobile. At that time, she was told to see her primary care physician if she had any problems. The patient continues to C/O "unbearable pain" despite taking prescription pain medication (Vicodin). Since that time, her primary care physician has decided that he would like her to see an orthopedic physician for a consultation. There are no prior surgeries on this arm and no family history of delayed healing issues. Otherwise, the patient has no other complaints. The superficial abrasions on her face, right arm, and left leg are healing nicely. The patient lives alone and is employed as a secretary.

HPI:
Location: arm
Context: MVA
Modifying factor: splinted, pain medication
Severity: "unbearable"
Past history: no surgeries
Family history: no delayed healing
Social history: lives alone/employed as a secretary
ROS:
Musculoskeletal: left arm pain
Integumentary: abrasions, healed
History level for patient encounter:
New patient: detailed history (99243)
ICD-10-CM:

M79.622	Pain in upper left arm
S00.81XD	Abrasion of other part of head, subsequent encounter
S40.811D	Abrasion of right upper arm, subsequent encounter
S70.312D	Abrasion of left thigh, subsequent encounter
V47.0XXD	Car driver injured in collision with fixed or stationary object in non-traffic accident

Review of systems: An area often comingled with the HPI area in the note. The ROS is in fact an extension of the HPI as a rule. They do not have to be separate or clearly labeled as HPI and ROS, but would obviously be useful for review purposes. However, it is important that items not be counted twice as both HPI and ROS. An item would be counted only once, either as an HPI element or an ROS element. Regarding the ROS, the documentation guidelines state that this information can be obtained by ancillary personnel or provided by the patient. Frequently, forms filled out by the patient or checklists addressed by the provider are used to obtain a complete ROS. If the form is separate from the encounter note it is suggested this be dated and initialed by the provider with pertinent comments noted.

The provider will usually elaborate on any positive responses by obtaining further information from the patient. This can be a very problematic area in terms of documentation. Nonpertinent (after the question is asked and the answer is provided) responses are often not recorded. Some categories of codes require a complete ROS, 10 or more systems, and this requirement is generally viewed by the medical establishment as unreasonable.

In an effort to alleviate some of the documentation burden, CMS finalized new guidelines on documenting office and other outpatient E/M encounters. Beginning January 1, 2019, providers are no longer required to re-document elements of the ROS recorded by ancillary staff for Medicare beneficiaries. The provider must review the information, make necessary changes or supplement the information and indicate in the medical record

 KEY POINT

The complete ROS taken by the provider may be documented by noting the pertinent positives and negatives and then a notation of "all other ROS negative."

that he or she has done so. This new rule should help alleviate some deficiencies in documentation related to the ROS for these services.

Both the 1995 and 1997 guidelines state that "in the absence of a notation for each of ten systems, a notation of otherwise normal or negative is sufficient." In the past, providers have indicated "ROS negative." This is not acceptable. A notation of "all other ROS negative" meets this criterion as long as the pertinent positive system is specified and other systems are reviewed.

CMS defines the three levels of ROS as problem pertinent, extended, and complete. The problem-pertinent level requires the review of only one system that is directly related to the patient's problem. The next level, extended ROS, requires that the physician inquire about two to nine systems that include those directly related to the patient's problems and additional systems. The highest level, complete, requires that the physician inquire about at least 10 systems, including those directly related to the patient's problem.

Past, family, and social history: The final elements of the history. They are described as:

> **Past medical history:** Adult and childhood illnesses or trauma; vaccinations and screenings, and past surgical history, past and present medications
>
> **Family history:** Describes parents, siblings, children, genetic diseases of the family or other familial history
>
> **Social history:** Descriptive information about the patient's habits and circumstances. For example, smoking, alcohol consumption, drug use, sexual orientation, marital status (married, widowed, divorced, and so forth), place of birth, residence, occupation, education level, religion, recent travel destinations, and military history

CMS identifies two levels of past, family and social history (PFSH). The first level, pertinent PFSH, requires that the provider document at least one item from any of the three areas. A complete PFSH requires that two or three areas are documented depending on the category of E/M code that is reported.

Two PFSH elements are required for a comprehensive type for:

- Established patient office or other outpatient services
- Subsequent nursing facility care
- Emergency department services
- Established domiciliary care patient
- Established home care patient

Three PFSH elements are required for a comprehensive type for:

- New patient office or other outpatient services
- Hospital observation services
- Initial care hospital inpatient services
- Consultation services
- Comprehensive assessments of nursing facility patients

- New patient domiciliary care services
- New patient home care services

Recording PFSH information can also be useful if the providers are currently, or will be, participating in the reporting of quality measures. Other questions that should be considered when querying the patient regarding PFSH include smoking history, diabetes control, if applicable, and, particularly for elderly patients, fall history, and safety precautions in the home.

These areas may also be reviewed by having the patient complete a questionnaire regarding past, family, and social histories. A complete health history form ensures that this information is readily available for the provider to review and verify with the patient for accuracy and completeness, as well as to document details with respect to any positive responses. If the form is separate from the note it is suggested this be dated and initialed by the provider. Remember, if the physician appropriately references this information, it can then be factored in to guide selection of the medically appropriate level of service.

ICD-10-CM and the Past, Family and Social History Elements

In reviewing the patient information contained in the health history forms, gathering the pertinent details also helps ensure the most accurate, most specific ICD-10-CM code is assigned for the patient encounter. For example, if the provider documented a previous broken leg, it would be important to note which leg (i.e., laterality), which bone, even which part of the bone was broken (anatomic site, body part), if the fracture was open or closed, the type of fracture (i.e., comminuted), and whether or not this injury is relevant to the issues being addressed in the current visit as the increased granularity inherent in ICD-10-CM allows reporting of all of these specific details.

Sample Documentation

A patient with a history of a broken left tibia presents to the office with a C/O of pain and swelling in the left lower extremity.

Clearly, this information is relevant to the current patient encounter and describes a sequela event that would be needed in the selection of an ICD-10-CM code to identify this injury as pertinent to the patient's current ongoing pain and swelling.
ICD-10-CM:
S82.202S Unspecified fracture of shaft of left tibia, sequela

---

Quantifying the History

The extent to which history elements are addressed will determine the "type" of history performed (and hopefully documented). This is where the "labels" come into play. We have added the more detailed information with each level that the federal guidelines provide but that are not found in the CPT book. There are four types described in the levels of E/M codes:

Problem focused: Chief complaint, brief HPI (one to three elements)

Expanded problem focused: Chief complaint, brief HPI (one to three elements), problem-pertinent system review (one system)

Detailed: Chief complaint, extended HPI (four or more elements or the status of three or more chronic problems [1995 or 1997]), problem-pertinent system review extended to include a review of a limited number of additional systems (two to nine systems), and pertinent past, family, and/or social history directly related to the patient's problems (one of these history areas)

Comprehensive: Chief complaint, extended HPI (four or more elements or the status of three or more chronic problems [1995 or 1997]), review of systems that are directly related to the problems identified in the history of present illness, plus a review of all additional body systems (10 or more), and complete past, family, and social history (two or three depending on code type)

When billing Medicare, a provider may choose either version (1995 or 1997) of the documentation guidelines, not a combination of the two, to document a patient encounter.

Answers to HPI Elements Quiz

1. Patient has had a sore throat for two days. States it is "burning" and she can hardly swallow. She has tried otc throat spray but it has not controlled her symptoms.
    Location: throat

    Modifying factors: throat spray

    Quality: burning

    Duration: 2 days

    AS&S: hardly swallow

2. The patient's nasal congestion has significantly improved with steroid nasal spray and is now described as "mild" in severity.
    Location: nose

    Severity: mild

    Modifying factors: steroid nasal spray

3. The patient is a 55-year-old male who developed sudden onset of shortness of breath, which began last night. He has also experienced some dizziness and lightheadedness.
    Location: respiratory (lungs)

    Duration: since "last night"

    AS&S: dizziness and lightheadedness

4. A 19-year-old patient presents with abdominal pain of two-day duration not relieved by otc medicine, including sharp RLQ pain today. Patient does admit to N&V for the past 24 hours and a fever today of 102 degrees.
    Location: abdomen, RLQ

    Modifying factors: not relieved by otc medicine

    Quality: sharp

    Duration: two days

    AS&S: N&V, fever

5. A 56-year-old male presents with persistent, moderately severe proteinuria, which has been present for four months and has been associated with lower extremity edema.

Location: urinary

Severity: moderately severe

Timing: persistent

Duration: four months

AS&S: lower extremity edema

6. The patient complains of chest pain (location), which began two hours ago (duration). Pain has been off and on since that time with each episode lasting two to three minutes (timing). The pain is described as "crushing" (quality) and at times is rated as a seven on a scale of one to 10 (severity). The pain occurs with minimal exertion (context) and is associated with nausea and shortness of breath (associated signs and symptoms). The pain was relieved with sublingual NTG in the ambulance (modifying factors).

Location: chest pain

Severity: rated as a seven

Timing: off and on since that time with each episode lasting two to three minutes

Modifying factors: sublingual NTG

Quality: "crushing"

Duration: began two hours ago

Context: minimal exertion

AS&S: associated with nausea and SOB

Physical Examination

The physical examination, the second of the three key components for evaluation and management, is documented by the physician/physician extender and is then quantified. Beginning January 1, 2019, providers are no longer required to re-document elements of a physical examination, for an established Medicare patient, that have not changed since the previous encounter when seen for an office or other outpatient E/M encounter. Providers need only to indicate in the medical record that the information was reviewed and updated as necessary. The following body areas and organ systems comprise the range of the physical examination:

- **Body areas:**
  - head, including face (normocephalic; scalp)
  - chest, including breasts and axillae (symmetry, skin changes, dimpling, nipple area)
  - neck (trachea-larynx, thyroid [goiter, nodules, mass, tenderness, bruit], crepitus)
  - abdomen (rebound, scars, distension, palpate liver, spleen, tenderness)
  - genitalia, groin, buttocks (visual inspection, nodes)
  - back, including spine (contour, tenderness, swelling)
  - each extremity (clubbing, edema, asymmetry)
- **Organ systems:**
  - constitutional (general appearance, vital signs: blood pressure, pulse, temperature, respiration, height, weight)

- eyes (pupils equal, round, reactive to light and accommodation; discs; retinal vessels; extraocular movements)
- ears, nose, throat (pinnae, external auditory canal, tympanic membrane; mucosa, septum, polyps, turbinate; lips, gingiva, posterior pharynx, tonsils, gag reflex)
- cardiovascular (murmur, rub, gallop, hypertension, peripheral vascular pulses, varicose veins)
- respiratory (breath sounds [wheezes, rales, rhonchi], resonance, contour)
- gastrointestinal (bowel sounds, soft abdominal bruits, ascites, fluid waves)
- genitourinary (male: penis, scrotum, hydrocele, hernia; female: external genitalia, Bartholin's glands, cervix, uterus)
- musculoskeletal (range of motion, strength, atrophy, swelling, tenderness, tone)
- skin (cyanosis, pigmentation, turgor, lesions, ulcers, petechiae, purpura)
- neurological (Romberg, tremor, tic, ataxia, aphasia, reflexes)
- psychiatric (alertness, orientation, memory, calculation, abstract concepts, speech, cortical integration)
- hematologic/immunologic/lymphatic (blood specimens, immunoassays, lymph nodes)

Note: The examples in parentheses above are not an exhaustive or complete list of elements under the 1997 guidelines.

Quantifying the Examination

There are four types of exams indicated in the levels of E/M codes. Although the descriptors or labels are the same under 1995 and 1997 guidelines, the degree of detail required is different. The complete multisystem and single system specialty exams under the 1997 guidelines can be found in appendix D. The levels under each set of guidelines are:

- **1995 guidelines:**
  - *Problem focused:* one body area or system
  - *Expanded problem focused:* two to seven systems (of which one may be a body area[s])
  - *Detailed:* two to seven systems (of which one may be a body area[s]) with one organ system being examined and documented in detail
  - *Comprehensive:* eight or more organ systems, or a complete single system examination

Note: Some Medicare auditors have looked for the higher end of the range of two to seven systems in the detailed exam. Although this is not spelled out in any regulation, this seems to be the expectation by some regulators. Many practices have divided the range of two to seven systems into "safe harbor" ranges for the expanded problem focused and detailed exam requirements. For example, many providers document two to four systems for the expanded problem focused exam and five to seven for the detailed exam. This approach is often consistent with the actual exam required by the problems that either low or moderate level decision making might require.

 QUICK TIP

The *Medicare Physician Guide: A Resource for Residents, Practicing Physicians, and Other Healthcare Professionals* states: "Providers may use either the 1995 or 1997 *Documentation Guidelines for Evaluation and Management Services.* Medicare contractors must conduct reviews using both the 1995 and the 1997 guidelines and apply the guidelines that are most advantageous to the provider."

When using the 1997 E/M guidelines, there are two types of examinations that can be performed and documented. The first is a general multisystem examination. This exam identifies bulleted elements in every body area or organ system. Alternately, a provider may perform a single organ system examination. A single organ system is a more extensive review of a specific organ system and will include examination of related elements from other organ systems.

- **1997 guidelines:**
  - *Problem focused:* perform and document examination of one to five bullet elements in one or more organ systems/body areas from the **general multisystem examination**
    OR
    examination of one to five bullet point elements from one of the 10 **single-organ-system examinations**, shaded or unshaded boxes
  - *Expanded problem focused:* perform and document examination of *at least six* bullet elements in one or more organ systems from the **general multisystem examination**
    OR
    perform and document examination of at least six bullet point elements from one of the 10 **single-organ-system examinations**, shaded or unshaded boxes
  - *Detailed:* perform and document examination of *at least* six organ systems or body areas, including *at least two* bullet elements for each organ system or body area from the **general multisystem examination**
    OR
    perform and document examination of *at least* 12 elements in two or more organ systems or body areas from the **general multisystem examination**
    OR
    perform and document examination of *at least* 12 bullet elements from one of the **single-organ-system examinations**, shaded or unshaded boxes,
    EXCEPT
    eye and psychiatric single-system examinations: perform and document *at least* nine bullet elements, shaded or unshaded boxes
  - *Comprehensive:* perform and document examination of *at least* nine organ systems or body areas, with *all bullet elements* for each organ system or body area (unless specific instructions are expected to limit examination content with at least two bullet elements for each organ system or body area) from the **general multisystem examination**
    OR
    perform and document examination of *all* bullet point elements from one of the 10 **single-organ system examinations** with documentation of every element in shaded boxes and at least one element in each unshaded box from the **single-organ-system examination**.

The complexity, breadth, and depth of the 1997 exam criteria are the primary reasons this approach was never adopted formally. Although these criteria work well for certain specialists using the single system specialty exams, other specialists and generalists do not fare as well.

Additionally, from an ICD-10-CM perspective, it is extremely important for the clinician to clearly denote laterality, severity, additional symptoms, and any other applicable information as it pertains to the patient's chief complaint. Without these details in the documentation, assignment of the most specific ICD-10-CM code will not be possible.

Examples from the musculoskeletal section of ICD-10 are commonly shown because this section requires a significant amount of detail in order to code the greatest degree of specificity.

Previously, coding for the condition rheumatoid arthritis (RA), noting the type, indicating chronic or acute, as well as the body area affected was sufficient for code selection. However, in ICD-10-CM, the medical record documentation must identify other factors before a code can be assigned.

The table below contains some ICD-10-CM rheumatoid arthritis codes and their associated descriptors.

ICD-10-CM Code	Description
M06.062	Rheumatoid arthritis without rheumatoid factor, left knee
M05.761	Rheumatoid arthritis with rheumatoid factor of right knee without organ or systems involvement
M05.822	Other rheumatoid arthritis with rheumatoid factor of left elbow
M05.611	Rheumatoid arthritis of right shoulder with involvement of other organs and systems

Keep in mind that while this small sample of codes represents only one specialty, it serves to illustrate the degree of detail required of the provider and staff when documenting the encounter.

Paper and electronic forms should function as a reminder to document details and, thereby, allow reporting of the most appropriate encounter code as well as the diagnoses for the patient's condition. Using time with the patient throughout the course of the encounter and capturing all necessary information will significantly reduce the number of physician queries at the end of the day; but even more importantly, will help to minimize claims rejections and requests for additional information from the payers.

Note that though the basic requirements for each of the four levels of physical examination remain the same, the ICD-10-CM code selected as being the reason for the specific encounter may require the inclusion of additional details. While the provider is required to follow applicable coding guidelines as well as document accordingly, further notations should be incorporated into those findings in order to assist with ICD-10-CM code selection. Observations and findings should be thorough and include items such as laterality (right or left side), the specific area with an organ system or body area, depth, size, degree, stage (when known), and other specific details of the patient's condition.

An examination of the patient focuses on the area described by the patient as the chief complaint based on the history and issues identified during the course of the exam. As such, the clinician may also evaluate other organ systems or body areas as they relate to the current issue or the comorbid conditions. For example, if the patient is being seen for a preoperative clearance, it may be necessary for the provider to conduct a full body examination. Conversely, if the patient presents with flu-like symptoms, a more targeted examination of one or two organ systems is all that may be warranted. Remember, only the physician determines this and not which form, template, or EHR is used.

In the example of the exam portion in an E/M encounter note shown below, the additional documentation needed for ICD-10-CM code assignment is noted with italicized text in parentheses.

Sample Documentation

Physical Examination:
Vitals signs are stable.
Pupils are equal, round, reactive to light and accommodation (PERRLA).
Slight edema on (*the left*) one leg.
The other leg has a pressure ulcer on the patient's (*right*) thigh (*with necrosis of*) and is down to bone; about 6 cm. in diameter. (*Stage IV*).
Slight diminished sensation in both lower limbs.
Exam level:
Expanded Problem Focused (99242)
ICD-10-CM:

L89.894	Pressure ulcer of other site, stage 4
R20.8	Other disturbances of skin sensation
R60.0	Localized edema

Medical Decision Making

Medical decision making is the third key component of determining the level of an evaluation and management service. This guide book takes the position that of all of the key components, this one most often plays the primary role in determining the correct level of service or E/M code. The CPT book provides the three basic subcomponents, or elements, of medical decision making, but does not provide much in the way of detail as to how to identify the different elements, and for each element, what makes up the different degrees within them.

For a true understanding of this critical component one must reference the documentation guidelines. Going further, to develop a real sense of what the guidelines are trying to describe, it is useful to look at several versions of the decision making matrices or tables as they have appeared since the introduction of the E/M codes.

In 1995 the original federal documentation guidelines included a set of tables to define the various attributes or elements that defined the different levels of decision making (see tables I, II and III on pages 37 and 38). In 1997 the AMA produced a version of one of these tables known as the Table of Risk, which differed somewhat from the original CMS version. In 1999 the AMA further revised its own table of risk. Although the AMA proposals have physician backing, they have not been adopted by CMS. Only the CMS 1995 and 1997 guidelines are officially recognized for selecting E/M codes.

KEY POINT

Effective January 1, 2021, providers may base the level of office/other outpatient visits (99202–99205 and 99212–99215) solely on the level of medical decision making. For these specific services, revisions will be made to the three elements of MDM, as well as utilization of a new MDM table developed by the CPT Editorial Panel. Refer to page 23 for more details on these upcoming changes.

KEY POINT

Tables I, II, and III may be used when selecting a level of medical decision making. The Table of Risk (table III) is found in this format only in the official CMS guidelines.

The basics of decision making as outlined in the CPT book and the federal guidelines apply across all sets of tables. There are three areas to consider when determining the level of medical decision making:

- **Number of diagnosis(es) or management options:** The following should be considered:
  - all known diagnoses that are being treated or affect treatment
  - undiagnosed conditions that are being evaluated
  - treatments being used, considered, or planned
  - complexity of establishing a diagnosis

Additional guidelines from CMS state that each encounter should have an assessment, clinical impression, or diagnosis documented. This may be explicitly stated or implied within the document. A presenting problem with an established diagnosis should also state if the problem is improved, well controlled, resolving, or resolved as opposed to inadequately controlled, worsening, or failing to change as expected. A presenting problem without an established diagnosis should include differential diagnoses. A differential or unsubstantiated diagnosis can be described as possible, probable, or rule out.

Management options should be documented, including initiation or changes to a treatment plan. This also includes patient instructions, instructions to ancillary healthcare providers, therapy ordered, and medications, as well as discussion with other care givers. The E/M guidelines by CMS indicate that the provider should also document any referrals or consultation orders, including "to whom or where the referral or consultation is made or from whom advice is requested."

- **Amount and/or complexity of data to be reviewed:** The following can be considered:
  - orders and review of all tests—lab, radiology, and medical
  - discussion of test results with performing physician
  - independent review of image, tracing or specimen
  - decision to obtain and review of old records
  - history obtained from someone other than the patient

Documentation should demonstrate review of laboratory, radiology, and other diagnostic tests. According to CMS guidelines, the provider may initial and date the report reviewed or include a simple notation noting the findings are acceptable. Relevant findings from a record review should also be documented; just noting that old records are reviewed is considered insufficient. The provider should elaborate on the findings. Documentation should also summarize discussion with performing providers or personal visualization and report of diagnostic services.

Risk of complications and/or morbidity or mortality (the table of risk): Look for documentation of the following:

- presenting problem(s) or the number of diagnoses and/or risk of complications
- diagnostic procedures ordered
- management options selected

When using the table of risk, the assessment of presenting problem risk is "based on the risk related to the disease process anticipated between the present encounter and the next encounter," according to CMS guidelines. This is different from the risk of diagnostic procedures or management options, which is considered to be during and immediately following any procedures or treatment.

Quantifying Medical Decision Making

Other factors that increase the decision making and risk should be documented in the patient record. Some of these include comorbidities, underlying diseases, and other factors that increase the risk of complications, morbidity, or mortality. Documentation should also indicate any diagnostic or therapeutic procedures that are ordered, planned, or scheduled during or as a result of the encounter. Documentation should note services or procedures provided on an urgent basis, including the nature of the urgency.

The original set of decision making tables provided by CMS contained a point system associated with medical decision making much like those in the history and examination components. The point system for calculating the decision making was removed from the 1997 version of the official CMS guidelines; however, many of the contractors continue to use the "point system" format in their audit procedures. The original tables are printed here to clearly illustrate the elements so that it's easier to objectively determine the component levels for determining a final level of decision making complexity.

The ultimate determination of the level of medical decision making performed is based on two of three of the medical decision making areas either meeting or exceeding the definitions of that level of decision making within the tables. There are currently four levels of decision making whose definitions are listed below:

Straightforward: Minimal number of possible diagnoses or management options; minimal, if any, amount and complexity of data to be reviewed; and minimal risk of complications and/or morbidity or mortality.

Low complexity: Limited number of possible diagnoses or management options, limited amount and complexity of data to be reviewed, and low risk of complications and/or morbidity or mortality.

Moderate complexity: Multiple numbers of possible diagnoses or management options, moderate amount and complexity of data to be reviewed, and moderate risk of complications and/or morbidity or mortality.

High complexity: Extensive number of possible diagnoses or management options, extensive amount and complexity of data to be reviewed, and high risk of complications and/or morbidity or mortality.

Part of what has historically made the decision making area hard to decipher is the fact that, to arrive at a particular level, one had to consider three tables, and within the last table, the Table of Risk, three sections within it. The three tables issued by CMS follow.

Table I. Number of Diagnosis or Management Options (Number x Points = Result)

	Number	Points	Points
Self-limited or minor (stable, improved, or worsening)	Max = 2	1	
Est. problem (to examiner); stable, improved		1	
Est. problem (to examiner); worsening		2	
New problem (to examiner); no additional work-up planned	Max = 1	3	
New problem (to examiner); additional work-up planned		4	
Transfer total to line A of Final Result for MDM table		**TOTAL**	
1–minimal 2–limited 3–multiple 4+ –extensive			

Table II. Amount and/or Complexity of Data to Be Reviewed

	Points
Review and/or order of clinical lab tests	1
Review and/or order of tests in radiology section of CPT	1
Review and/or order of tests in the medicine section of CPT	1
Discussion of test results with performing physician	1
Decision to obtain old records and/or obtaining history from someone other than patient	1
Review and summarization of old records and/or obtaining history from someone other than patient and/or discussion of case with another healthcare provider	2
Independent visualization of image, tracing, or specimen itself (not simply review of report)	2
Transfer total to line B of Final Result for MDM table	**Total**
1–minimal 2–limited 3–moderate 4+ –extensive	

Table III. Table of Risk of Complication and/or Morbidity or Mortality

	Presenting Problem(s)	Diagnostic Procedure(s) Ordered	Management Options Selected
MINIMAL	• One self-limited or minor problem; e.g., cold, insect bite, tinea corporis	• Laboratory tests requiring venipuncture • Chest x-rays • EKG/EEG • Urinalysis • Ultrasound; e.g., echo • KOH prep	• Rest • Gargles • Elastic bandages • Superficial dressings
LOW	• Two or more self-limited or minor problems • One stable chronic illness; e.g., well controlled hypertension or non-insulin dependent diabetes, cataract, BPH • Acute uncomplicated illness or injury; e.g., cystitis, allergic rhinitis, simple sprain	• Physiological tests not under stress; e.g., pulmonary function tests • Non-cardiovascular imaging studies with contrast; e.g., barium enema • Superficial needle biopsies • Clinical laboratory tests requiring arterial puncture • Skin biopsies	• Over-the-counter drugs • Minor surgery with no identified risk factors • Physical therapy • Occupational therapy • IV fluids without additives
MODERATE	• One or more chronic illnesses with mild exacerbation, progression, or side effects of treatment • Two or more stable chronic illnesses • Undiagnosed new problem with uncertain prognosis; e.g., lump in breast • Acute illness with systemic symptoms; e.g., pyelonephritis, pneumonitis, colitis • Acute complicated injury; e.g., head injury with brief loss of consciousness	• Physiologic tests under stress; e.g., cardiac stress test, fetal contraction stress test • Diagnostic endoscopies with no identified risk factors • Deep needle or incisional biopsy • Cardiovascular imaging studies w/ contrast and no identified risk factors; e.g., arteriogram, cardiac catheterization • Obtain fluid from body cavity; e.g., lumbar puncture, thoracentesis, culdocentesis	• Minor surgery w/ identified risk factors • Elective major surgery (open, percutaneous or endoscopic) w/ no identified risk factors • Prescription drug management • Therapeutic nuclear medicine • IV fluids with additives • Closed treatment of fracture or dislocation w/o manipulation
HIGH	• One or more chronic illnesses with severe exacerbation, progression, or side effects of treatment • Acute or chronic illnesses or injuries that pose a threat to life or bodily function; e.g., multiple trauma, acute MI, pulmonary embolus, severe respiratory distress, progressive severe rheumatoid arthritis, psychiatric illness with potential threat to self or others, peritonitis, ARF • An abrupt change in neurologic status; e.g., seizure, TIA, weakness or sensory loss	• Cardiovascular imaging studies with contrast with identified risk factors • Cardiac electrophysiological tests • Diagnostic endoscopies w/identified risk factors • Discography	• Elective major surgery (open, percutaneous or endoscopic) w/ identified risk factors • Emergency major surgery (open, percutaneous, endoscopic) • Parenteral controlled substances • Drug therapy requiring intensive monitoring for toxicity • Decision not to resuscitate or to de-escalate care because of poor prognosis

Within this last table, the highest level of risk in any of the three columns determines the overall level of risk. This applies only to table III.

To determine the overall level of decision making, two of the three tables (I, II, or III) must agree to establish the level.

Final Result for Complexity of Medical Decision Making: 2 of 3 required

Table I	Number of diagnoses or management options	1 (point) Minimal	2 (points) Limited	3 (points) Multiple	4 (points) Extensive
Table II	Amount and complexity of data to be reviewed	1 (point) Minimal	2 (points) Limited	3 (points) Moderate	4 (points) Extensive
Table III	Risk of complications &/or morbidity or mortality	Minimal	Low	Moderate	High
Type of Decision Making		Straight-forward	Low Complexity	Moderate Complexity	High Complexity

ICD-10-CM and Medical Decision Making

The medical decision making component of E/M code assignment is also influenced by the level of detail required for ICD-10-CM code assignment.

Below is a sample of the medical decision making portion of an E/M encounter with italicized text in parentheses identifying the additional documentation requirements needed to assign the ICD-10-CM code.

Sample Documentation

Assessment and Plan (A/P)
Patient is an active teenager with acne (*vulgaris*) and (*left upper quadrant*) abdominal pain. He won an eating contest at the local fast food restaurant last night.
DX: acne, abdominal pain
Level of MDM: Low
ICD-10-CM:

L70.Ø	Acne vulgaris
R1Ø.12	Left upper quadrant pain
R63.8	Other symptoms and signs concerning food and fluid intake
Y92.511	Restaurant or café as the place of occurrence of the external cause

Medical decision making (MDM): moderate

Summary of Decision Making

Probably the most important indicator of the nature of the presenting problem and the likely level of decision making that will be coded is found in the first and last tables. To a certain extent, the information contained in table I is also found in the Table of Risk, first column. Both of these areas address the number and complexity of the problem or problems facing the provider.

The inclusion of table II to indicate complexity based on the performance of diagnostic tests, studies, or reference to other records or providers is useful when these types of activities are performed, but clearly the moderate and high levels can be present without them.

CONTRIBUTORY COMPONENTS

Effective January 1, 2021, the AMA and CMS have adopted new guidelines and code descriptions for reporting E/M codes for new and established office or other outpatient services (99202–99215). Therefore, the following guidelines section does not apply to new and established office or other outpatient services (99202–99215).

The following section further discusses the four remaining contributory components of E/M service levels mentioned previously.

Nature of the Presenting Problem

The nature of the presenting problem should be used by the provider to determine the amount and complexity of the three key elements that will be required to appropriately treat the patient. The nature of presenting problem is listed as one of the following five levels:

- **Minimal:** Problem that may not require the presence of the physician or other qualified healthcare professional, but service is provided under the physician's or other qualified healthcare professional's supervision
- **Self-limited or minor:** Transient problem, and low probability of permanently altered state; or good prognosis with management/compliance
- **Low severity:** Problem that has a low risk of morbidity or little, if any, risk of mortality without treatment; full recovery is expected without functional impairment
- **Moderate severity:** Problem that carries a moderate risk of morbidity or mortality without treatment, uncertain outcome or increased probability of prolonged functional impairment
- **High severity:** Problem that has a high to extreme risk of morbidity, moderate to high risk of mortality without treatment, or high probability of severe, prolonged functional impairment

The first two categories, minimal and self-limited, are most often associated with the straightforward level of decision making. Remember that a provider is generally afforded the risk associated with the morbidity/mortality of differential diagnoses, not just what is ruled in. This is a key principle when addressing provider cognitive work: the condition or problem need not ultimately be found for it to be considered as the basis for the work-up—or the complexity of that work.

Some documentation systems indicate that based upon the nature of the presenting problem the provider knows the level of history and exam that must be performed to appropriately treat the patient. Although a contributing component, the nature of the presenting problem is closely related to medical necessity. The provider can ascertain the medically necessary level of service to render and document based upon the nature of the presenting problem. Providers who use the nature of the presenting problem as a basis for treatment are less likely to overperform or overdocument and more likely to understand medical necessity.

QUICK TIP

Contributory components are secondary and should help to direct the provider or coder to the correct code.

KEY POINT

The nature of presenting illness component is based on the five types of presenting problems—minimal, self-limited or minor, and low, moderate, and high—as defined in the CPT book.

CODING AXIOM

The nature of the presenting problem component plays a critical role in determining the appropriate level of E/M service code by providing documentation to support medical necessity of the services provided.

> **Sample Documentation**
>
> **Nature of Presenting Problem**
> • Patient's asthma is stable on present medications
> The patient is a chronic asthmatic with severe exacerbation.

The level of the severity of the presenting problem may vary during the encounter, usually based on the presence or development of differential diagnoses. Chart documentation should clearly define the findings and reflect the thought process of the provider in ordering diagnostic or therapeutic services to support medical necessity for those services. This component is the foundation for establishing the level of service based on medical necessity and is also somewhat inherent in the decision making process described above.

The presenting problem reflects the patient's chief complaint and can be a disease, condition, illness, injury, symptom, sign, finding, or other reason for the encounter. The physician's subjective perception of the nature of presenting illness can influence the extent of history obtained, the extent of examination performed, and the complexity of medical decision making as previously described. The nature of the presenting problem may range between two levels, such as a problem that is of low to moderate severity. A mention of the initial evaluation of the risk will later support the details in the assessment and decision making areas.

> **Sample Documentation**
>
> **Meets Expected Requirements:**
> Longstanding hypertension, uncontrolled, with probable end organ changes. The patient indicates that lightheadedness and impotence are the most bothersome residuals. Exam indicates no real emergency; therefore, will treat as outpatient.
> **Does NOT Meet Expected Requirements:**
> Hypertension with probable end organ changes.

Counseling and Coordination of Care

Counseling is defined in the CPT book as a discussion with a patient and/or family concerning one or more of the following areas:

- Diagnostic results, impressions, or recommended diagnostic studies
- Prognosis
- Risks and benefits of management (treatment) options
- Instructions for management (treatment) or follow-up
- Importance of compliance with chosen management (treatment) options
- Risk factor reduction
- Patient and family education

 QUICK TIP

Counseling and coordination of care should be documented even if it takes less than half of the encounter time.

Sample Documentation

Meets Expected Requirements:
I had a discussion with the patient about his hypertension. The patient has a good understanding about the potential side effects of the various drugs used to treat his disease. I apprised the patient in detail of the potential side effects of not treating his condition. The patient expressed an understanding of the high risks of noncompliance, stating no one had "spelled it out before." I firmly explained to the patient that I would be willing to help him explore alternative therapy for hypertension, but only if he were to strictly adhere to a conventional regimen of therapy until his hypertension was well controlled and stable.

Does NOT Meet Expected Requirements:
I apprised the patient in detail of the potential side effects of not treating his condition.

Additional criteria for code selection revolve around coordination of care, which includes contact with other physicians or healthcare practitioners. Counseling, coordination of care, and the nature of the presenting problem are not major considerations in most encounters, so they generally provide contributory information to the code selection process. The exception arises when counseling or coordination of care dominates the encounter (more than 50 percent of the time spent).

Sample Documentation

Meets Expected Requirements:
After evaluating the patient in recovery from a stroke, I spoke at length (approximately 30 minutes) with the hospital's rehabilitation service to coordinate an appropriate physical therapy plan.

Does NOT Meet Expected Requirements:
Discussed physical therapy plan with hospital's rehabilitation service.

When coordination of care does not include a patient encounter on that day, the services should be reported using the case management codes. However, it should be noted that case management codes are not covered by many third-party payers.

Time

Time is only used in selecting an E/M code when counseling and/or coordination of care represents more than 50 percent of the time the physician/qualified healthcare professional spent face to face (outpatient) or bedside and on the floor or unit with the patient or family (inpatient); *both time elements*—total length of time for the visit and total length of time involved in counseling or coordination of care—as well as the nature of the counseling and coordination of care must be documented explicitly in the medical record. Family, as used above with regard to inpatient visits, includes not just family members but also other parties that have assumed responsibility for the care of and/or decision making for the patient, whether or not they are family (e.g., foster parents, person acting in locum parentis, legal guardian).

It should also be noted that times contained within code descriptors are averages, and as such signify a range of times that may be greater or less than the stated time contingent on the circumstances of the actual visit. Further, time is not considered a component of the emergency department codes because these types of services are usually offered on a changing basis that can involve more than one encounter with more than one patient over a long

---

 DEFINITIONS

coordination of care. Often provided concurrently with counseling and includes treatment instructions to the patient or caregiver, special accommodations for home, work, school, vacation, or other locations, coordination with other providers, agencies, and living arrangements.

counseling. Discussion with a patient and/or family concerning one or more of the following areas: diagnostic results, impressions, and/or recommended diagnostic studies; prognosis; risks and benefits of management (treatment) options; instructions for management (treatment) and/or follow-up; importance of compliance with chosen management (treatment) options; risk factor reduction; and patient and family education.

☞ **KEY POINT**

Effective January 1, 2021, providers may base the level of office/other outpatient visits (99202–99205 and 99212–99215) solely on total time on the date of the encounter. For these specific services, time may be used regardless of whether or not counseling and/or coordination of care dominate the service. Refer to page 23 for more details on these upcoming changes.

---

period of time. As such, it can prove challenging to establish accurate time estimates.

MODIFIERS USED WITH E/M CODES

The following modifiers apply to E/M codes; other modifiers may apply in some situations.

24 Unrelated Evaluation and Management Service by the Same Physician or Other Qualified Healthcare Professional During a Postoperative Period
The physician or other qualified healthcare professional may need to indicate that an evaluation and management service was performed during a postoperative period for a reason(s) unrelated to the original procedure. This circumstance may be reported by adding modifier 24 to the appropriate level of E/M service.

25 Significant, Separately Identifiable Evaluation and Management Service by the Same Physician or Other Qualified Healthcare Professional on the Same Day of a Procedure or Other Service
It may be necessary to indicate that on the day a procedure or service identified by a CPT code was performed, the patient's condition required a significant, separately identifiable E/M service above and beyond the other service provided or beyond the usual preoperative and postoperative care associated with the procedure that was performed. A significant, separately identifiable E/M service is defined or substantiated by documentation that satisfies the relevant criteria for the respective E/M service to be reported (see Evaluation and Management Services Guidelines for instructions on determining level of E/M service). The E/M service may be prompted by the symptom or condition for which the procedure and/or service was provided. As such, different diagnoses are not required for reporting of the E/M services on the same date. This circumstance may be reported by adding modifier 25 to the appropriate level of E/M service. **Note:** This modifier is not used to report an E/M service that resulted in a decision to perform surgery. See modifier 57. For significant, separately identifiable non-E/M services, see modifier 59.

Optum360 Note: This modifier is used to identify the E/M service when provided with another service reported with a CPT or HCPCS code.

27 Multiple Outpatient Hospital E/M Encounters on the Same Date
For hospital outpatient reporting purposes, utilization of hospital resources related to separate and distinct E/M encounters performed in multiple outpatient hospital settings on the same date may be reported by adding modifier 27 to each appropriate level outpatient and/or emergency department E/M code(s). This modifier provides a means of reporting circumstances involving evaluation and management services provided by physician(s) in more than one (multiple) outpatient hospital setting(s) (eg, hospital emergency department, clinic). **Note:** This modifier is not to be used for physician reporting of multiple E/M services performed by the same physician on the same date. For physician reporting of all outpatient evaluation and management services provided by the same physician on the same date and performed in multiple outpatient setting(s) (eg, hospital emergency department, clinic), see Evaluation and Management, Emergency Department, or Preventive Medicine Services codes.

 KEY POINT

Modifier 25 is appended to the E/M code and not to codes for other procedures or services performed.

32 Mandated Services
Services related to mandated consultation and/or related services (eg, third-party payer, governmental, legislative, or regulatory requirement) may be identified by adding modifier 32 to the basic procedure.

52 Reduced Services
Under certain circumstances a service or procedure is partially reduced or eliminated at the discretion of the physician or other qualified healthcare professional. Under these circumstances the service provided can be identified by its usual procedure number and the addition of modifier 52, signifying that the service is reduced. This provides a means of reporting reduced services without disturbing the identification of the basic service.
Note: For hospital outpatient reporting of a previously scheduled procedure/service that is partially reduced or cancelled as a result of extenuating circumstances or those that threaten the well-being of the patient prior to or after administration of anesthesia, see modifiers 73 and 74 (see modifiers approved for ASC hospital outpatient use).

Optum360 Note: This modifier cannot be appended to an E/M code for Medicare.

57 Decision for Surgery
An evaluation and management service that resulted in the initial decision to perform the surgery may be identified by adding modifier 57 to the appropriate level of E/M service.

Optum360 Note: Medicare recognizes modifier 57 only for major procedures, those with 90 follow-up days.

95 Synchronous Telemedicine Service Rendered Via a Real-Time Interactive Audio and Video Telecommunications System
Synchronous telemedicine service is defined as a real-time interaction between a physician or other qualified healthcare professional and a patient who is located at a distant site from the physician or other qualified healthcare professional. The totality of the communication of information exchanged between the physician or other qualified healthcare professional and the patient during the course of the synchronous telemedicine service must be of an amount and nature that would be sufficient to meet the key components and/or requirements of the same service when rendered via a face-to-face interaction. Modifier 95 may only be appended to the services listed in Appendix P. Appendix P is the list of CPT codes for services that are typically performed face-to-face, but may be rendered via a real-time (synchronous) interactive audio and video telecommunications system.

AI Principle Physician of Record
Modifier AI identifies the principal physician of record—that is, the admitting or attending physician who is overseeing the patient's care while in an inpatient or nursing facility setting. Only the admitting physician should report this modifier. The use of this modifier is subject to individual commercial payers' policies regarding inpatient admissions and consultative services; therefore, it is advised to always check with individual payers for specific guidelines regarding the use of this modifier.

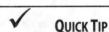

QUICK TIP

Do not use modifier 52 to report a reduced fee. It is specific to a service that was less than that described by the CPT code but not described by another available code.

SELECTING AN E/M CODE

To select the appropriate level of service, one should take the following steps:

- Identify the place of service (e.g., office, inpatient hospital, emergency room visit) or type of service (e.g., consultation) provided, and select the appropriate category and subcategory from the CPT book.

- Read the guidelines at the beginning of the category and subcategory to determine what special instructions, if any, apply to that subcategory of E/M codes.

- From the medical record documentation, determine the complexity of the medical decision making, the extent of the history, and the examination performed and documented.

- Review the code narratives in the appropriate category and subcategory. Each narrative includes the specific criteria that must be met or exceeded if the code is to be assigned correctly.

- For billing purposes, select the code that matches the levels of medical decision making, history, and examination documented. When reviewing charts for coding and documentation accuracy, carefully review the decision making area and see if this is either higher or lower than both other components. If it is usually higher, chances are that the provider is under-documenting the history or exam. If it is lower, the provider may be providing "stock" history or exams that bolster service levels. Both conditions address documentation habits or conventions. (If chart documentation indicates that counseling and coordination of care take up more than 50 percent of the time spent on the face-to-face encounter between the physician and patient and/or family or the time the physician spent bedside and on the floor or unit, use time as the determining factor.)

- Apply appropriate E/M modifiers, as needed.

KNOWLEDGE ASSESSMENT CHAPTER 2

See chapter 19 for answers and rationale.

1. History, exam, and medical decision making are the key components in an E/M service.
   a. True
   b. False

2. Time is connected only to counseling and coordination of care and is not the only consideration in code selection.
   a. True
   b. False

3. Why is the medical decision making component so important?
   a. The medical decision making component is the only component completed entirely by the physician or other qualified healthcare provider, alone
   b. The medical decision making component is the only key component that is required for every E/M service
   c. The medical decision making component will most often determine the true complexity of the management involved. The history and exam are best viewed as supporting components in terms of work performed and documented
   d. None of the above

4. When can you use time as a controlling factor for selecting the appropriate level of E/M code?
   a. When the provider has spent at least 50 percent of the time counseling the patient and coordinating care
   b. When the provider has spent the specified time in face-to-face contact with the patient
   c. When the provider has documented that face-to-face counseling was provided to the patient
   d. When the provider documents 100 percent of the time spent with the patient and that some counseling was given

5. What are the areas defined in CPT guidelines that are considered counseling services?
   a. Diagnostic results, impressions, prognosis, risks and benefits, patient and family education
   b. Diagnostic results, impressions, medication list, problem list
   c. Instruction for treatment and follow-up, determination of diagnosis codes
   d. Both a and c

6. Although it is not considered a key component, what role does the nature of presenting problem play in determining the level of E/M code?
   a. It determines the chief complaint
   b. It helps the provider determine the amount of history, exam, and decision making required to treat the patient
   c. It determines the diagnosis codes and decision making
   d. It does not factor into determining the level of E/M service

7. Which is an example of additional information to determine ICD-10-CM code selection for the chief complaint of "my foot hurts"?
   a. What caused the pain?
   b. Do other body parts hurt?
   c. Which foot?
   d. Is the injury weather related?

8. Of all the body areas/organ systems reviewed during an E/M encounter, which body system requires the greatest level of specificity in terms of documentation as it relates to ICD-10-CM?

    a. Neurological

    b. Respiratory

    c. Ears, nose, throat

    d. Musculoskeletal

9. In the medical decision making (MDM) example seen on page 39, where a teenager with acne is also evaluated for a complaint of abdominal pain, why does the inclusion of clinical detail required for ICD-10-CM diagnosis assignment raise the MDM level potential from low to moderate?

    a. Acne is always a very serious medical condition

    b. Seeing the patient for acne and abdominal pain is very unusual

    c. Most E/M services require moderate decision making

    d. The abdominal pain complaint required additional clinical detail

Chapter 3: The Elements of Medical Documentation

Medical documentation furnishes the pertinent facts and observations about a patient's health, including past and present history, tests, treatment and medications, and outcomes. The primary purpose of the medical chart is continuity of patient care. An accurate and complete medical chart protects the patient by providing complete information about the patient's history, current health status, and the effectiveness of past and current therapy. An accurate and comprehensive medical chart can also protect the physician, when necessary, in liability actions.

The medical chart also provides the information that supports the ICD-10-CM and CPT®/HCPCS codes used to report the services provided and submitted to various payers for reimbursement. Therefore, it is absolutely essential that the medical record—whether office, emergency department, or hospital—is complete and concise and contains all information regarding the following:

- Reason for the encounter
- Complete details of the information provided by the patient and by the clinician's evaluation of the patient
- Results of diagnostic, consultative, and/or therapeutic services provided to the patient
- Assessment of the patient's conditions
- Plan of care for the patient, including advice from other physician specialists
- Other services, procedures, and supplies provided to the patient
- Time spent with the patient for counseling and/or coordination of care, if applicable

The style and form of medical documentation depends on the provider, as demonstrated by the samples of documentation included in this book. However, it is important that any reader of the medical record be able to understand, from the documentation, the service rendered and medical necessity for the service.

In addition, the medical documentation must be legible and understandable for all providers who care for the patient. If the handwriting of the provider cannot be read, Medicare auditors, as well as other payers, consider the service to be unbillable.

Abbreviations or shorthand used in medical record documentation should be listed on an identification key accessible to all who read the documentation. Abbreviation lists should be specific to the facility or practice and identify abbreviations that have more than one applicable definition.

All entries should be dated and legibly signed according to the *Evaluation and Management Services Guide*, revised by CMS in December 2010. It is recommended that the signature also include credentials (e.g., MD, DO,

 OBJECTIVES

This chapter discusses:
- The principles of documentation
- SOAP and SNOCAMP formats
- Common documentation deficiencies
- Electronic health records (EHR) and documentation

 QUICK TIP

Documentation should contain only commonly accepted abbreviations. Specialty-specific abbreviations should be approved by the facility HIM department before they are used in documentation.

 KEY POINT

Authentication of documentation is the key to identifying the author, credential, and date of service. Addendums should be dated when written and refer to the date they are modifying.

DC, etc.). Moreover, medical documentation should be completed during or immediately following the services provided.

Note that the work involved in charting and dictation of medical records is included in all CPT codes.

PRINCIPLES OF DOCUMENTATION

To provide a basis for maintaining adequate medical record information, follow the official medical record documentation standards listed below. The following principles were developed jointly by representatives of the American Health Information Management Association, the American Hospital Association, the American Managed Care and Review Association, the American Medical Association, American Health Quality Association, the Blue Cross and Blue Shield Association, and the Health Insurance Association of America:

- The medical record should be complete and legible
- The documentation of each patient encounter should include the date; the reason for the encounter; appropriate history and physical examination; review of lab, x-ray data, and other ancillary services, where appropriate; assessment; and plan for care (including discharge plan, if appropriate)
- Past and present diagnoses should be accessible to the treating and/or consulting provider
- The reasons for and results of x-rays, lab tests, and other ancillary services should be documented or included in the medical record
- Relevant health risk factors should be identified
- The patient's progress, including response to treatment, change in treatment, change in diagnosis, and patient noncompliance, should be documented
- The written plan for care should include, when appropriate, treatments and medications, specifying frequency and dosage; any referrals and consultations; patient/family education; and specific instructions for follow-up
- The documentation should support the intensity of the patient's evaluation and/or treatment, including thought processes and the complexity of medical decision making
- All entries to the medical record should be dated and authenticated

Documentation guidelines in the *Evaluation and Management Services Guide* also indicate that the documentation should be able to validate where the services were rendered and that the services were medically necessary and appropriate.

The CPT/ICD-10-CM codes reported on the health insurance electronic or paper claim form or billing statement should be supported by the documentation in the medical record.

Both the history areas and medical decision making areas frequently suffer from lack of detail as described above. It is quite common to see the words "patient here for f/u" as both the chief complaint and the HPI. This is insufficient. Likewise with decision making, the notations "continue present

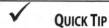

QUICK TIP

CMS documentation guidelines state that the reason for tests and procedures should be indicated in the documentation or "easily inferred."

meds" and "f/u 3 months" tell us little or nothing of the problem(s), the status of the problem, and the treatment or management of the problem(s).

EVALUATING YOUR DOCUMENTATION

If you answer "yes" to all of the following questions, your documentation contains the information necessary to correctly assign and/or support evaluation and management codes.

- Is the reason for the patient encounter documented in the medical record?
- Are all services that were provided correctly documented?
- Does the medical record clearly explain the medical necessity of the level of E/M service, diagnostic and therapeutic procedures, support services and supplies provided?
- Is the assessment of the patient's condition apparent in the medical record?
- Does the medical record contain information about the patient's progress, as well as the results of treatment?
- Does the medical record include the patient's plan for care?
- Does the information in the medical record describing the patient's condition provide reasonable medical rationale for the services and the choice of setting in which the services were provided?
- Does the information in the medical record support the care given, especially when another health care professional must assume care or perform medical review?
- Is the medical record legible and comprehensible to the other health care personnel?

THE SOAP FORMAT

Many medical school and residency programs advocate a method of problem-oriented medical record (POMR) documentation. In this system, known by its acronym SOAP, the provider's notes concerning a patient's health and treatment are divided into four parts (the bolded and italicized terms identify where the components of the E/M levels of service can be found in the SOAP format):

- **(S)ubjective:** This component summarizes the patient's complaints, generally using the patient's own words or a synopsis (e.g., chest pain or sore throat). It should include the nature and duration of the patient's symptoms, the time the patient first noticed the symptoms, the patient's opinion as to the possible causes of the illness or condition, any remedies that the patient may have tried, or other medical treatment previously received for the same illness or condition, any contributory factors that may influence the patient's health or response to treatment.

  In the SOAP format, the subjective (S) component documents the *chief complaint* and the *history of the present illness, review of systems*, and relevant *past, family, and or social history*.

- **(O)bjective:** This section gives the measurable, pertinent findings of the provider's actual examination, as well as the results of diagnostic tests

QUICK TIP

The SOAP format is the most commonly used documentation tool used by providers and ancillary staff.

(e.g., laboratory tests or x-rays), which are recorded or referenced in this portion of the medical documentation.

In the SOAP format, the objective (O) component documents the *physical examination* and the *diagnostic evaluation*.

- **(A)ssessment:** This component of the documentation defines the provider's determination of the cause of the patient's condition, based on the information recorded in the subjective and objective components, and includes the provider's differential diagnoses, diagnostic and therapeutic options, and potential for complications.

- **(P)lan:** This part of the medical record documentation states the agreed-upon treatment plans for the patient.

In the SOAP format, the assessment (A) and plan (P) document the *complexity of medical decision making*.

The POMR generally incorporates a baseline database of information that includes the patient's past, family, and social history, as well as a chronological problem list. In this format, the provider identifies each problem being addressed from the patient's problem list and then documents each individual problem addressed during an encounter within the SOAP note. Past, family, and social history database information should be updated at appropriate intervals, annually in most cases.

As we reviewed in the previous chapter, this approach is a sequential record of how information was obtained, analyzed, and acted upon in the order in which it appeared. But remember, that for ease of identifying the general level of decision making, much of the nature of the encounter can be determined very early on. If the reason for the visit is follow-up of hypertension, diabetes, hyperlipidemia, and obesity there is a reasonable certainty that this encounter may be a level four established patient visit.

The reason we continue to make this point is that when the provider recognizes early on what the general tenor of the encounter is, he/she can be certain to *document* those ROS or exam elements that may be performed but not turn out to be particularly relevant. Remember that the nature of the presenting problem is not just a contributing component; it will most often drive the breadth and depth of the components within the SOAP format.

THE SNOCAMP FORMAT

The SNOCAMP format, developed by Walter L. Larimore, MD, of Kissimmee, FL., allows the provider to identify specifically the subjective elements of an E/M service code. In this alternative method of medical documentation, the provider's opinions of the patient's nature of presenting problem, medical decision making, and/or counseling are specified by the provider. These elements are then combined with the components of the SOAP format—subjective, objective, assessment, and plan. This approach supports the general thesis that the nature of the problem drives the encounter components and makes an effort to address this part of decision making early in the note.

- **(S)ubjective:** The first component in the SNOCAMP format, as in the SOAP format of medical documentation, is subjective and includes the patient's chief complaint, all pertinent information regarding the history of present illness, system review as well as the past, family, and social history.

- **(N)ature of presenting problem:** The presenting problem reflects the patient's chief complaint and can be a disease, condition, illness, injury, symptom, sign, finding, or other reason for the encounter. The provider's subjective perception of the nature of presenting illness can influence the extent of history obtained, the extent of examination performed and the complexity of medical decision making as we have previously described. Thus, this component plays a critical role in determining the appropriate level of E/M service code by providing documentation to support medical necessity of the services provided. The nature of presenting illness component is based on the five types of presenting problems—minimal, self-limited or minor, and low, moderate, and high severity—as defined in the CPT book. The nature of the presenting problem may range between two levels, such as a problem that is of low to moderate severity. A mention of the initial evaluation of the risk will later support the details in the assessment and decision making areas.

- **(O)bjective:** The third component of the SNOCAMP format contains the discernible findings of the physical examination. Each organ system or element should be itemized in the record, and pertinent conclusions about each system as well as abnormal findings should be detailed.

- **(C)ounseling and/or coordination of care:** When counseling and/or coordination of care takes up more than 50 percent of the total visit time, the element of time is the key or controlling factor for selecting the appropriate level of E/M code and must be documented in the record. Often this element is difficult to determine from the standard documentation. Specifically designating what was discussed, as well as documenting the time involved providing this service, helps substantiate and guides when selecting a level of E/M service code.

  Moreover, documenting this component—whether or not it takes up most of the time spent with the patient—may help support the provider's position during a malpractice suit. It can also be helpful to show that the provider discussed diagnosis and management options with the patient or family.

- **(A)ssessment:** The assessment component is the provider's determination of the patient's problem. Documentation in this section should include any differential diagnoses, management, and treatment options and the potential for complications or morbidity and/or mortality.

  To document this aspect of the encounter completely and without any possibility of misinterpretation, we suggest that the provider use the words found in either the tables of risk or the descriptions of the nature of the presenting problem. There will be little doubt left in the mind of any auditor or reviewer what is meant when the provider states "high risk of morbidity without treatment" or "uncertain prognosis" or "full recovery without impairment is expected." Use the words the regulators provide.

- **(M)edical decision making:** For this component, the provider must specify the complexity of establishing a diagnosis and/or selecting a management option as described in the assessment and plan components of documentation. Because the medical decision making

 KEY POINT

Effective January 1, 2021, providers may base the level of office/other outpatient visits (99202–99205 and 99212–99215) solely on total time on the date of the encounter. For these specific services, time may be used regardless of whether or not counseling and/or coordination of care dominate the service. Refer to page 23 for more details on these upcoming changes.

 KEY POINT

When reporting "low complexity" or "moderate complexity," be sure that the documentation supports these summary statements.

component is subjective and determining the appropriate level depends on several factors—number of diagnoses or management options, amount and/or complexity of data to be reviewed, and risk of complications and/or morbidity or mortality—the provider rendering the service is the best qualified to assess the type of decision making provided. The types—straightforward, low complexity, moderate complexity, and high complexity—defined in the CPT book, should be specified in this section of the documentation. Again, use the words provided by stating "low complexity" or "moderate complexity." Why make an auditor guess?

- **(P)lan:** The final section of SNOCAMP format involves the treatment options the provider considers for managing the patient's problem. This area also should include the rationale for recommending or changing a previously designated therapy or ordering diagnostic tests.

  Remember that selecting an appropriate level of E/M service code depends on those components documented as well as performed. The history and exam areas are fairly easy to count as the elements can be easily learned. Using the SNOCAMP format, however, as compared with the SOAP format, better clarifies those elements of decision making and the nature of the presenting problem which will cause the levels of the other E/M service components to be performed. This format makes it much easier to see what code is most appropriate assuming the history and exam are well documented. There is no requirement to use this method of documentation. It is simply another option available to physicians and nonphysician practitioners in documenting their E/M services.

AUDIT CONSIDERATIONS IN DOCUMENTATION

A major concern related to documentation and reimbursement for services is "under-documentation." Government regulators call a service that is not supported by documentation "over-coded." This would be considered by most to be, to some degree, semantics, with this guide taking the position that there is a difference between over-coding and a lack of documentation. If one assumes that the level of decision making generally points towards the correct code level, and is supported in the chart, then it is either history or exam, or both, that fail to support that level based on code type. This encounter is more accurately described as under-documented. In most cases it is these areas that are under-documented.

When the level of decision making is below the level required by a code, in many cases these are the charts that are over-coded. Medical decision making, if properly documented, is very closely linked to medical necessity and truly acts as the anchor for the real complexity of services performed. Some payers have endorsed the idea that when dealing with established patient visits, where only two of three of history, exam, and decision making are required, that one of those should be decision making. It is hard to imagine an encounter, other than preventive services, where higher level history and exams would be required without at least some differential diagnosis or suspected condition that warranted the more extended services.

Over-coding is likely linked to a lack of medical necessity and decision making, not a missing element or two from either history or exam.

Keeping in mind that the **encounter note for each individual date of service is a stand-alone entry**, the medical chart notes for a given date of service must substantiate all services billed for that date, including the level of E/M service, as well as the medical necessity for the services. If the stand-alone entry for a specific date does not support the codes submitted for payment, the service may be considered "under-documented/over-coded" on review or audit, **despite the severity of the patient's illness, injury, or condition.** *In other words, from a compliance perspective, even if the true level of work based on decision making is higher than the other supporting components, the code cannot be billed.*

Many payers may also use background edits that will evaluate the reported diagnoses with the level of E/M service reported. This is not an invitation to over-diagnose the patient as manual review of the documentation will not support a higher level of care. During a chart audit, many payers as previously stated will require the decision making to be one of the required elements to help meet medical necessity guidelines.

True over-coding is likely linked to a lack of medical necessity and decision making, not a missing element or two from either history or exam.

The medically necessary level of complexity of medical decision making is generally reflected by the history and/or physical examination documentation for the specific date of service being reviewed, in addition to the number of diagnoses and management options recorded, the complexity of data to be obtained, analyzed, and reviewed, and the overall risks of the presenting condition, as well as comorbidities and complicating conditions.

In an effort to reduce the amount of documentation physicians are tasked with, CMS has finalized new guidelines applicable to office/outpatient visits (99202–99215). Effective January 1, 2019, ancillary staff, and/or the patient, may document the chief complaint and history in the medical record (including the history of present illness), eliminating the need for providers to document or re-document the information. Also, for established patient encounters providers may choose to document only the parts of the history and physical exam that have changed since the last encounter, instead of re-recording a list of defined elements. The provider must only indicate in the medical record that he or she has verified and/or updated these elements.

OVER-DOCUMENTING THE ENCOUNTER

Many providers, who are new to using a documentation template or have been trained to overdocument, may report higher levels of E/M than will meet the medical necessity.

When the E/M codes and the documentation guidelines were first released, there were providers who determined that all of their services had to be the highest levels and documented to meet the higher levels even without the medical necessity. Many also misinterpreted the Table of Risk to increase the level of decision making.

For example, a patient who is seen by the oncologist for a follow-up exam after completion of chemotherapy may not meet the guidelines for the highest level of risk. Cancer can pose a "threat to life or bodily function" but

 KEY POINT

The level of risk from the Table of Risk is determined based on the patient's current conditions at this encounter. A stable patient with a long term illness that may eventually result in death is not an automatic high level of risk.

when the patient is stable and not in imminent danger of dying, the level of risk will be moderate.

Remember that the risk assessment is based on the risk anticipated between the current patient encounter and the subsequent encounter.

Another example is the post myocardial patient who is now stable and under ongoing treatment, is not an "acute MI," and, therefore, not considered high risk.

Providers who are unfamiliar with EHR templates or are not fully trained may consider the template to be a "mandatory" list of check boxes that all must be completed. The documentation templates need to be completed so that the higher level of E/M service can be captured and documented. However, providers should perform only as much history, exam, and decision making as is necessary for appropriate treatment of the presenting problem. Over-documenting on a template uses provider time performing and documenting unnecessary components of the history and exam.

This is reiterated by CMS in the *Medicare Claims Processing Manual,* Pub. 100-04, chapter 12, sections 30.6 and 30.6.10:

- Medical necessity of a service is the "overarching criterion" for payment in addition to the individual requirements as defined by the CPT code nomenclature
- It is not medically necessary or appropriate to bill a higher level of evaluation and management service when a lower level of service is warranted
- Sheer volume of documentation is not a factor for selecting a specific level of service

When providers are comfortable with templates, both paper and electronic, they will be used appropriately as prompt sheets to remind them to document the elements of the exam that were performed.

Some providers have also been taught that just because a patient has a new complaint that it automatically increases the level of E/M service. Nevertheless, there needs to be history, exam, and decision making documented at the level reported or, in the absence of increased levels of key components, there needs to be significant counseling and coordination of care that is appropriately documented.

Over-documenting the level of E/M continues to be an ongoing problem that is under greater scrutiny by Medicare and other payers. Over-performing and over-documenting should be closely monitored in the practice.

The distinction between under-documentation and over-coding is most useful when reviewing internal chart audit results with providers. It is quite effective when it is pointed out that the correct code is likely 99233 for example, but because of the two-system exam and one ROS documented, the provider cannot bill that code. Chances are the provider will volunteer that he or she in fact performed some of the missing data, but just did not document the data.

In some states, more than 30 percent of the patient encounters submitted for payment to Medicare are deemed over-coded by two to three levels of service

KEY POINT

The E/M guidelines state: "The extent of examinations performed and documented is dependent upon clinical judgment and the nature of the presenting problem(s)."

KEY POINT

Medicare payment policy does not recognize or allow the use of rubber stamps to authenticate documentation. Other payers may also disallow the use of rubber-stamp signatures.

when compared to the chart documentation. Some Medicare contractors have found that more than two-thirds of all encounters are "over-coded" by at least one level of service.

The greatest numbers of deficiencies are generally found in documentation for review of systems as part of the patient's history. Family and social history information is also often omitted. But, do these deficiencies really diminish the value of the overall encounter? From a billing and compliance perspective, yes they do. From a correct coding perspective—the code was most likely correct, just under-documented.

Specialty and subspecialty providers seem to have more documentation errors than primary care providers. Although there are "single-organ system" definitions for the physical examination component of an E/M service, the history of the present illness, review of systems, and past family and social history requirements are the **same for all providers**, specialists as well as primary care. Primary care providers on the other hand seem to have a bad habit of under-coding their services.

Specific Documentation Pitfalls

There are only two levels of history of present illness (HPI), brief and extended. According to the documentation guidelines for brief and extended history, documentation must be explicit as to the condition being treated, or the actual signs and symptoms and the differential diagnoses as appropriate for the encounter, as well as for any conditions the patient has that may complicate or change medical care. A chart reviewer should never have to guess as to the nature of the illness.

Only a problem focused history level does not require a review of systems. An expanded problem focused history requires only a problem-pertinent review of systems. Detailed and comprehensive-level new patient encounters, emergency room visits, hospital admissions, and consultations codes cannot be assigned unless the provider clearly documents the required components of these history elements, regardless of the specialty of the provider.

The extent of the physical examination should be determined by the nature of the presenting problem, the documented HPI and additional history components. Detailed and comprehensive levels of physical examinations are not necessary for every patient encounter unless the chart clearly supports the medical necessity for that level of physical examination. Auditing of charts often reveals inadequate data supporting the medical necessity for detailed and comprehensive levels of physical examinations. For specialists, often an effort is made to follow the single-system specialty exams and great detail is provided in one or two organ systems. However, these frequently miss one of the elements or other related organ systems and thereby fail to meet single-system exam criteria. Often it would be easier for these specialists to follow the 1995 general exam guidelines and simply review eight organ systems. For some specialties, that eighth system is a bit of a stretch.

The medically necessary level of complexity of medical decision making is generally reflected by the history and/or physical examination documentation for the specific date of service being reviewed, in addition to the number of diagnoses and management options recorded, the complexity of data to be obtained, analyzed, and reviewed, and the overall risks of the presenting condition as well as comorbidities and complicating conditions.

 QUICK TIP

CY 2019 Medicare Physician Fee Schedule (MPFS) Final Rule indicates, effective January 1, 2019, the chief complaint and all history elements may be documented by the patient or ancillary staff. For office/outpatient visits, the documentation must then be reviewed by the provider and pertinent comments added.

The presenting condition is the diagnosis or the medical signs and symptoms combined with the appropriate differential diagnoses responsible for the patient's chief complaint or the reason the patient scheduled the visit for the date of service.

Remember that each individual encounter note is a "snapshot" of medical care that must clearly document the medical necessity of all the services provided on that particular date of service. Documentation deficiencies that combine to support the level of E/M service charged to the patient may be considered "over-coded" upon chart audit and review, **despite the severity of the patient's illness, injury, or condition.** Although we have referred to history and exam as less than primary and often supporting elements, they are in fact required to support the overall code.

Signatures

Complying with payers' signature guidelines is vital, especially when a practice is audited. CMS has modified its signature guidelines several times over the years. These guidelines not only apply to providers, but they serve as a reference for medical reviewers when reviewing medical records and claim documentation.

If a signature is illegible, practices may choose to use a signature log (a list of the typed or printed name of the author associated with initials or illegible signatures) or an attestation statement to determine the identity of the author of a medical record entry.

If a signature is missing from the medical record, an attestation statement may be completed. Below is an example of a CMS approved attestation statement:

"I, _____[**print full name of the physician/practitioner**], hereby attest that the medical record entry for _____[**date of service**] accurately reflects signatures/notations that I made in my capacity as _____[**insert provider credentials, e.g., M.D.**] when I treated/diagnosed the above-listed Medicare beneficiary. I do hereby attest that this information is true, accurate, and complete to the best of my knowledge and that I understand that any falsification, omission, or concealment of material fact may subject me to administrative, civil, or criminal liability."

Providers should avoid adding late signatures to the medical record (beyond the short delay that occurs during transcription) but instead use the signature attestation. The signature attestation can also be used for illegible signatures.

ELECTRONIC HEALTH RECORDS

Great emphasis has been placed on the adoption of electronic health records (EHR) in both the hospital and outpatient clinical settings. Some of the obvious benefits include legibility, portability within a clinic or facility, and improved quality of care.

Before screening for or selecting an EHR system, the provider and staff should review what is considered an EHR. The Office of the National Coordinator for Health Information Technology (ONC), a division of HHS, defines an EHR as: "An electronic record of health-related information on an individual that conforms to nationally recognized interoperability standards and that can be created, managed, and consulted by authorized clinicians and staff across more than one healthcare organization."

The EHR should be a compilation of patient-centered records that can be securely accessed by the appropriate care providers. It is hoped that eventually the health-related information of the patient from "cradle to grave" will be available to assist in the care of current conditions and managing long-term conditions. It is hoped that the longitudinal record will also aid in the concept of patient wellness by monitoring change over time and appropriate health counseling. A good way of thinking about an EHR is that it functions as the portal to manage and control patient information and appropriate access.

The EHR will also aid in the promotion of telehealth applications such as remote monitoring of devices. Telehealth encounters can be documented and recordings of vital signs, monitoring, and testing can be immediately available.

EHR Documentation of Encounters

One benefit to adopting an EHR is the increase in legibility of provider documentation. When determining which EHR system to adopt, the ability to create and define documentation templates is an important consideration.

When determining which evaluation and management (E/M) code to report for an encounter, the documentation of the key components will drive the code selection. There are some EHR systems that include counting systems, or encoders, with the provider templates that will help the professional determine the specific code to document. Although these systems are of great help, they should not be the final determination of code selection. As valuable as encoders are, they cannot evaluate the real level of medical necessity.

When professionals use templates, many mistakenly use the template as a mandatory checklist of history and exam elements that must be completed regardless of medical necessity. Professionals should instead use the template as a prompter to document the necessary elements performed.

Because of the misunderstanding of how to effectively use EHR templates, there is often a significant increase in the levels of codes reported without an increase in the severity of patients seen. This may trigger a payer audit to determine why there is such a shift in billing practices. For this reason, it is suggested that internal audits be performed to verify understanding and completion of templates with consideration of medical necessity.

Other common errors associated with the adoption of an EHR include the copy function. Instead of considering each encounter with the patient as a separate item, there is a commonly adopted habit of copying over history and exam elements. This has resulted in incorrect reporting of services, especially when compared to the patient's account of the encounter. This is often identified by auditors and payers when every chart note appears to be exactly the same.

What is important, with regard to the use of templates, is that only the elements of the exam *actually* performed are documented on the template. This is important not only from a coding and billing compliance standpoint

✓	QUICK TIP

Each encounter should be a snapshot of that visit documenting the unique nature of the patient and service provided.

KEY POINT

Beginning January 1, 2019, providers are not required to redocument elements of a physical examination, for an established Medicare patient, that haven't changed since the previous encounter when seen for an office/other outpatient E/M encounter (99212-99215). Providers need only to indicate in the medical record that the information was reviewed and updated as necessary.

but also from a legal and liability standpoint. It is easy to start clicking and select elements that a provider did not actually perform.

Providers must remember that each encounter is a unique document. Just as there is variation from patient to patient, there should be variances, even with templates, in the documentation of the patient encounter. Even when treating the same patient for chronic conditions there are variations in the necessity of exam elements or review of history. This type of documentation is often called cloning and is a common problem with EHR systems.

Lack of narration is another problem often seen when using an EHR. Many of the templates are very good at identifying the history and exam elements and providing fill-in-the-blank areas for the decision making or pick lists to select diagnostic tests and procedures. These same templates may also lack appropriate places to provide additional narration. For example the chief complaint should be a descriptive statement taken from the patient account of the illness or injury that occasioned the encounter. Choosing a chief complaint from a pick list is inappropriate.

Another example of narration is elaboration of negative or unexpected results of the physical exam. For example, a skin lesion should include documentation of the size, color, shape, and location. A heart murmur should describe the quality, loudness, and nature of the murmur. It is appropriate to include a check box for tympanic membrane's red, but bleeding, abrasions, and other abnormalities may need to be elaborated in a narrative manner.

Documentation as a diagnostic tool and record for continuity of care has become secondary to documenting for code selection and reimbursement. By learning how to use an EHR template, the routine portions of history and exam can be completed quickly leaving time for the provider to document meaningful narrative regarding the patient and his or her condition.

Electronic Health Record Templates

Another key benefit of an EHR is that documenting a patient encounter can be standardized. While almost all EHR systems have parts that require manual entry of text, there are other portions that can be streamlined through the use of templates to help expedite documentation.

In order for documentation to serve its designated purpose, it should summarize the provider's thought sequence that led to the specific orders as well as function as clear communication to other providers involved with the patient's care and convey the diagnosis and plan of treatment.

Accurate templates designed in an intuitive manner will also help to increase provider productivity, reduce denials, and help to increase the accuracy of documentation and ultimately code selection. Workflow can be evaluated, streamlined, and coordinated between providers.

Customized templates with prompts can help to achieve consistent care opportunities for all patients. Templates enable consistent documentation. Information can be captured and relayed to other care providers and printed for patient use. Templates can also remind the provider to check for health maintenance milestones.

Quality in healthcare is increasing in importance and more and more carriers are moving towards proactive preventive and wellness medicine to treat conditions and injuries before they become more serious and chronic. The emphasis is now on helping patients to be more actively involved in managing their own health and wellness. Templates can serve as reminders to the provider of age- and sex-appropriate screenings for patients. It may also be tied to the results of the last screening or even vaccinations. Additionally, templates help ensure documentation contains important and necessary information such as a problem list or reconciling the patient's medication list. Lastly, templates aid in providing complete data regarding the patient encounter.

With all the types of templates that are available, it is critical that the practice develop and use templates that will enhance documentation and aid in the correct code selection. The templates also need to be flexible enough to allow for patient-focused entries. One of the most common errors when using a template is the "cookie cutter" appearance of many chart notes without patient-specific documentation.

> Examples of the different types of templates, include, but are not limited to:
>
> - Chart documentation of encounter procedures, phone calls, medication lists, and problem lists
> - Prescriptions and refills, including e-prescribing
> - Referral to other provider forms
> - Requests for ancillary services such as x-rays, lab services, or physical therapy
> - Patient instruction sheets
>
> Templates can be customized to the specialty of the practice; for example, a pediatric practice would have age–appropriate, well-child visit templates as well as common pediatric condition templates such as those for an ear ache (otitis media), sore throat (e.g., strep throat), and respiratory issues (e.g., croup, RSV, asthma) as well as injury templates.
>
> A number of methods are available for help in determining template types for a practice. The use of a frequency report of the diagnosis codes reported offers guidance to determine what type of preventive, injury or illnesses are most common to the practice and can serve as the basis for a solid, general all-purpose template that can be modified as needed.

EHR Encoders

Many EHR systems offer an encoder option. In the truest sense an encoder is a set of algorithms and computer code that takes the documented medical record and selects codes for the encounter. Some encoders will select the E/M codes based upon the completed check marks in a template. Other encoders will provide guidance and the provider determines the final code selection.

On the surface it is appealing to use an encoder to select the codes to be reported on a claim. However, providers should carefully consider certain issues prior to selecting and using an encoder system. The auto selection program is most often the defining feature of an encoder. An auto selection encoder does not consider medical necessity. These systems consider that if

 DEFINITIONS

encoder. Computer application that assists in the assignment of a diagnosis or procedure code and may also assign reimbursement categories and values.

the documentation is in the chart, the level of history, exam, or decision making was necessary. When compared to the presenting problem or final diagnosis, this may not hold true.

When using an auto-selection encoder, the provider must be careful not to over perform and document an encounter. If the majority of established patient encounters are coded based upon the history and exam components and not the decision making, there is a high probability that a chart audit for medical necessity would find discrepancies.

A provider should also be able to override the auto selection recommendation of an encoder system. The trained provider can determine the code selection for those cases where the documentation may overstate complexity of the visit.

Coder Verification

Although the provider may select the E/M or other codes to be reported or may use an auto-selection system to provide an initial recommendation, some practices choose to have the codes verified by a coder. This practice prevents over and under reporting of services. The coder can also detect errors in correlation between the procedure codes and diagnosis codes. However, final code assignment should be made by the clinician.

Even when using an auto-selection encoder, the biller should verify any questionable code assignments. The practice may choose, for example, to have all high-level E/M codes verified before the bills are submitted. The coder could review all codes selected based upon history and exam components only and not include the decision-making component. The coder could also verify any diagnosis codes that are not on the template. Lastly, the coder could verify the documentation for a code selected based upon time to ensure that the nature and extent of counseling or coordination of care were adequately noted.

Once an EHR system has been implemented and providers and staff have become comfortable with the system, it is imperative that billing patterns be evaluated and monitored by performing a month-by-month comparison of codes billed over the prior year. In doing so, practices will be able to determine any potential shift in coding patterns, such as changes in levels of E/M encounters reported or frequency of services reported.

KNOWLEDGE ASSESSMENT CHAPTER 3

See chapter 19 for answers and rationale.

1. Abbreviations can have multiple meanings and can confuse those who need to review the medical record documentation.
   a. True
   b. False

2. Why is legibility a key requirement of documentation?
   a. Patient care and treatment may be delayed and/or compromised
   b. If the handwriting of the provider cannot be read, Medicare auditors, as well as other payers, consider the service as not billable or reimbursable
   c. Legibility is not a key requirement of documentation at the present time
   d. None of the above

3. The benefits of the SOAP and SNOCAMP formats of documentation are that the SOAP format is a sequential record of how information is obtained, analyzed, and acted upon during the encounter and the "N" in the SNOCAMP format provides a place to document the nature of the presenting problem, which most often drives the depth of the components within the SOAP format.
   a. True
   b. False

4. Define over-coding and under-documenting.
   a. Over-coding is selecting the same code for every encounter and under-documenting is not completing a template
   b. Over-coding is selecting the highest code for every encounter and under-documenting is completing only the exam and decision making portions
   c. Over-coding is reporting a higher level code than documented and under-documenting is having a lower level of history and exam than decision making
   d. Over-coding is reporting a code based solely on the history and exam components and under-documenting is reporting a code based solely on the decision making

5. What is a common reason a provider might over-document an encounter?
   a. Using a template as a documentation mandate and completing all fields regardless of the presenting problem and misinterpretation of the Table of Risk
   b. Using a template as a prompter to record the history and exam completed
   c. Using nursing and ancillary staff as scribes
   d. Using the Table of Risk for the final level of E/M service

6. What is an advantage to using templates with an electronic health record?
   a. Templates are used to document all necessary elements for a specific level of E/M service
   b Templates help provide consistent format and tools for electronic documentation
   c. Templates allow other staff to fill in blank data
   d. Templates are mandated by the EHR legislation

7. Why should billing patterns be evaluated after implementing an EHR?
   a. To penalize providers not using an EHR
   b. To verify any shift in coding patterns
   c. To keep the coders busy
   d. Both a and b

Chapter 4: Adjudication of Claims by Third-Party Payers and Medicare

The following are medical documentation guidelines many third-party payers use when reviewing claims for accuracy of payment or when performing an audit. Many commercial reviews are geared more towards medical necessity than evaluation and management (E/M) documentation guidelines, as many of the third-party payers have not formally adopted federal documentation guidelines. If they have done so, this should be clear in any contracting language relative to chart or service audit activity. Also, be sure you thoroughly examine your provider's manual, as provided by your third-party payers. Often, if a payer requires one set of documentation guidelines over another, the provider manual is where you will find that information. Your contract with that payer typically binds your practice to follow the rules as set forth in the provider's manual.

Although the specific federal guidelines may not be required by any given payer, it is a prudent policy to have providers document to the level of the highest requirements. Some facilities and practices bill E/M codes based on payer type, and have lesser documentation standards for nongovernmental payers. Though legal at this time, because contractual arrangement supersedes general conventions, this may not be the wisest course. Providers should likely be taught one set of coding and documentation requirements for all patients for at least two reasons: 1) Does the practice truly always know what coverage is in effect on a given day, and who secondary payers might be? and 2) It is hard enough for providers to remember one set of rules much less different rules for different payers. Following a single set of coding and documentation requirements is much safer for practices from a compliance perspective.

MEDICALLY NECESSARY SERVICES

Appropriate documentation is important to substantiate services as medically necessary. For a service to be deemed medically necessary, most third-party payers expect the service to be medically required and appropriate for diagnosing and treating the patient's condition and consistent with professionally recognized standards of medical care.

Claims reviewed for medical necessity are usually reimbursed based on the medical documentation supporting the level of service selected. If the documentation does not verify the level of service code reported, the third-party payer, upon review of the documentation, may assign a lesser level of service code and pay accordingly.

Many payers may also use background edits that will evaluate the reported diagnoses with the level of E/M service reported. This is not an invitation to over-diagnose the patient as manual review of the documentation will not support a higher level of care. During a chart audit, many payers, as previously stated, will require the decision making to be one of the required elements to help meet medical necessity guidelines.

The medically necessary level of complexity of medical decision making is generally reflected by the history and/or physical examination documentation for the specific date of service being reviewed, in addition to the number of diagnoses and management options recorded, the complexity of data to be obtained, analyzed, and reviewed, and the overall risks of the presenting condition as well as comorbidities and complicating conditions.

The following sections outline the contents of the medical record documentation that are necessary to substantiate and validate the medical necessity of services provided to patients. Various types of services (e.g., office visit, consultation) and medical settings (e.g., medical office, inpatient hospital) are illustrated.

Office or Other Outpatient Services

For the initial E/M visit, the medical record should include specific documentation for the level of E/M services provided.

- Medically appropriate history, as well as the reason the patient sought medical care
- Medically appropriate physical/psychological examination
- Results of diagnostic tests
- Elements of medical decision making
- Allergy status
- Diagnostic assessment
- Treatment plan and rationale
- Immunization record (for pediatric patients)
- Time, if time is used for code selection

For subsequent visits, the medical record should include specific documentation for the level of E/M of ongoing medical care provided.

- Interval history, including current symptoms and the patient's response to therapy
- Results of any further diagnostic testing
- Elements of medical decision making
- Clinical findings on reexamination
- Diagnostic assessment
- Therapy plan and rationale (including specific documentation of any treatment or procedure performed or prescribed)
- Time, if time is used for code selection

Inpatient Hospital Care

For initial hospital care, the medical record should include specific documentation for the level of E/M services provided. The three key components must be documented and should include:

- Current and past medical, family, and social history
- Clinical findings
- Results of diagnostic tests

- Diagnostic assessment including a statement regarding the primary reason for admission
- Therapy plan and rationale

According to the hospital's conditions of participation, a complete history and physical (H&P) should be dictated or written within 48 hours of admission, including comprehensive documentation of the elements outlined above.

For scheduled admissions, if a complete H&P has been performed within 30 days prior to the hospital admission and there are no major changes in the patient's conditions, a repeat H&P need not be performed. A legible copy of the original H&P with additional documentation to update the record in the event of changes in the patient's condition should be filed in the medical record.

If the current hospitalization is a readmission within 30 days for the same or related problems, an interval H&P documenting any changes in the patient's condition may substitute for a new, complete H&P as long as a legible copy of the original H&P is included with the interval H&P in the medical record for the current hospitalization.

For subsequent hospital care, the medical record should include specific documentation for the level of E/M services provided. Two of the three key components must be documented and should include the patient's:

- Interval history, including current symptoms and reference to patient's response to therapy
- Clinical findings on reexamination
- Interpretation of results of diagnostic tests
- Diagnostic assessment
- Medical decision making
- Changes in the therapy plan and rationale (including specific documentation of any treatment or procedure performed or prescribed)

Progress notes should be written daily, with time of the encounter noted. Unit or floor time is defined as the time the provider is on the patient's hospital unit and at the bedside providing services for that patient. This includes the time spent establishing and reviewing the patient's chart, examining the patient, writing notes, and communicating with other professionals and the patient's family.

The patient's medical record should show that the provider's orders were acted on in a timely manner and that the physician's action was consistent with the working diagnoses and therapeutic rationale as documented in the progress notes. In addition, a physician's or other qualified healthcare professional's orders should be dated and signed and countersigned by the provider within 24 hours if given orally in person or by phone.

Subsequent hospital care is often one of the least well documented levels of care which may open it up for review. Often there is little change in history and minimal change in the physical exam. Decision making is often split between order sheets and documentation forms. Some electronic records are easier to review as they may "link" the components from a single encounter or day together.

 QUICK TIP

Completion of the H&P is not usually reported separately to the payer when the purpose of the admission is for a scheduled procedure.

Wisconsin Physician Services (WPS), a Medicare contractor, routinely performs a targeted probe and educational review process. These service-specific probes with E/M codes have become quite common as documentation is unfortunately not improving across the industry. Currently WPS has specific probes targeted around initial hospital care services reported with 99223 and critical care services reported with 99291 and 99292.

On December 19, 2019, the Centers for Medicare and Medicaid Services (CMS) released the Medicare Fee-for-Service 2019 Improper Payments report, which revealed that E/M services had an unadjusted improper payment rate of 11.3 percent, accounting for 12.8 percent of the overall Medicare FFS improper payment rate. In terms of a dollar amount, E/M services accounted for approximately $3.8 billion in improper payments during 2019. The report stated that E/M services comprised a significant portion of the improper payments in 2019 and were more than half as likely to have errors as compared to other Medicare Part B services.

The report also indicated that the majority of improper payments for subsequent hospital visits were due to incorrect coding with the servicing provider specialty internal medicine comprising 40.6 percent of improper payments for subsequent hospital visits. For initial hospital services, Comprehensive Error Rate Testing (CERT) identified that the majority of improper payments for initial hospital visits were due to incorrect coding due to insufficient documentation and noted that the servicing provider specialties of internal medicine and cardiology comprised over 42 percent of improper payments for initial hospital visits.

Another interesting finding was related to E/M services provided by nonphysician practitioners (NPP). The CERT program identified a number of improper payments for E/M services billed using physicians' national provider identifiers (NPI) but provided exclusively by an NPP. For certain E/M visits and settings, if a physician and a qualified NPP each perform and document a substantive part of an E/M visit face-to-face with the same patient on the same date of service, then the physician can bill this visit under his or her NPI. However, NPPs must bill under their own NPIs if they provide an E/M service (in person) for a physician's patient in a hospital and the physician does not also perform and document a substantive part of an E/M visit face-to-face with the same beneficiary on the same date of service.

The majority of E/M services paid in error were attributed to incorrect coding and insufficient documentation. Incorrect coding errors were typically identified in cases where the provider documentation was not sufficient to support the code billed. The report emphasizes that this continues to be a problematic area for providers. Specifically, submitted records lacked physician authentication or the provider failed to obtain the records for the billed E/M services that were performed in other place of service sites other than their office (e.g., hospital, ASC, etc.).

Consultations

The medical documentation of consultations should contain complete information for the level of E/M services provided. Three key components are required for new and established patients for office and inpatient consultation services and should include:

- Name of the requesting provider
- Reason for the consultation
- Date the consultant was notified
- Date and time the consultation was completed
- History
- Evidence of a physical examination, system review of the affected body areas or organ systems
- Consultant's findings, diagnostic impressions, and recommendations
- Signature of the consultant
- Copy of the letter or report sent by the consultant to the provider who requested the consultation detailing findings and recommendations (in outpatient records)
- A self/family referral is not a consult and should be reported with the appropriate code from the office visit, home service, or domiciliary/rest home care codes
- Subsequent care is reported using an established patient or subsequent inpatient care in the instructional notes for this subsection
- Instructional notes clarify what an appropriate source is to request a consult. The guidelines indicate that an appropriate source includes:
  - another physician
  - physician assistant
  - nurse practitioner
  - doctor of chiropractic
  - physical therapist or occupational therapist
  - speech-language pathologist
  - psychologist or social worker
  - lawyer
  - insurance company

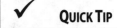

QUICK TIP

Medicare does not cover consultations. The appropriate inpatient or outpatient service should be reported.

DOCUMENTATION POLICY UNDER THE MEDICARE PROGRAM

Below are the documentation policies that the Medicare program uses.

- **Use of the highest levels of E/M codes by a single-system specialist**

  Physicians and practitioners such as physician assistants and nurse practitioners, including single-system specialists (such as ophthalmologists), may use the highest levels of E/M codes if the services they provide meet the definition of the code (e.g., to bill the level 99205 new patient visit, the documented history must meet the CPT® code book definition of a comprehensive history).

  The comprehensive history must include the chief complaint, extended history of the present illness, a review of all the systems and a complete past (medical and surgical), family, and social history. In the case of an established patient, it is acceptable for a provider to update the existing record to reflect only the changes in the patient's medical, family and/or social history from the last encounter as long as the physician makes reference to the updated data in his/her documentation for the current encounter. For safety here, reference the date of the previously obtained data in the current note, or sign and date the original as reviewed.

The comprehensive examination may be a complete single-system exam, such as a cardiac, respiratory, or psychiatric exam, or a complete multisystem examination.

- **Request for specialty consultation from the attending physician**

  In an inpatient setting, the request may be documented as part of a plan written in the requesting physician's progress note, an order in a hospital record or a specific written request for the consultation.

  In the office setting, the requirement may be met by a specific written request for the consultation from the requesting physician, or the consultant's records should show a specific reference to the request.

- **Documentation of time for counseling and coordination of care**

  The medical record should reflect the nature and extent of counseling and coordination of care.

  In the office and other outpatient setting, counseling and coordination of care must be provided in the presence of the patient if the time spent providing the service is used to determine the level of service reported.

  In an inpatient setting, the counseling and coordination of care must be provided at the bedside or on the patient's hospital floor or unit.

  Time spent counseling the patient or coordinating the patient's care after the patient has left the office or the provider has left the patient's floor should not be considered when selecting the level of service to be reported.

  The duration of counseling and coordination of care provided face to face or on the hospital floor may be estimated but that estimate, along with the total duration of the visit, must be recorded in the medical record when time is used to select a code for a visit that predominantly involves coordination of care or counseling.

- **Documentation for reporting the extent of the history obtained and physical examination performed**

  Each progress note should stand by itself; it should not be necessary to search earlier notes to determine the reason for the visit.

  The SOAP system of recordkeeping is satisfactory, but rigid adherence to the formal SOAP format is not required.

TEACHING PHYSICIAN DOCUMENTATION

Medicare will cover professional services provided by attending physicians when they deliver personal direction to interns or residents participating in the care of their patients in teaching hospitals and in skilled nursing facilities with teaching programs. Payment is based on the physician fee schedule and is subject to strict guidelines. Conditions for eligibility for Part B reimbursement by the attending physician were first published in intermediary letter (IL) 372, entitled "Part B Payments for Services of

Supervising Physicians in a Teaching Setting," dated April 1969. In 1996, teaching physician reimbursement guidelines were revised and clarified.

Medicare guidelines of payment of physician services provided in a teaching setting require that the teaching physician be present during any services involving a resident for which payment will be sought under the Medicare program. Under Medicare's teaching physician reimbursement guidelines, the services provided by the teaching physician must be of the same character (in terms of responsibilities to the patient that are assumed and fulfilled) as the services rendered to other paying patients. These responsibilities by the teaching physician are demonstrated by:

- Reviewing the patient's history and conducting a physical examination
- Personally examining the patient within a reasonable period of time after admission
- Confirming or revising the diagnosis
- Determining the course of treatment to follow
- Assuring that any supervision needed by the interns and residents is furnished
- Making frequent review of the patient's progress

Teaching physicians and residents may both chart on the same patient. However, a teaching physician who is billing Medicare must personally document "his or her participation in the management of the patient." This includes managing the patient or being present during the critical or key portions of the patient care (*Guidelines for Teaching Physicians, Interns, and Residents*, December 2011, ICN: 006347, pages 2–3). A statement by the resident that the attending physician was present is not sufficient.

Students may document in the medical record. However, the teaching physician must verify all portionsof the medical record, including history, physical examination, and medical decision making. The teaching physician must personally perform or re-perform the physical examination and medical decision making activities. However, these elements do not have to be re-documented by the teaching physician, verification of the students' documentation is sufficient.

Fellows and the Teaching Physician Guidelines

Since the term "fellow" can be applied to individuals for different reasons, understanding the relationship between services provided by fellows and the teaching physician guidelines can be confusing. This term may be used for either an individual who:

- Has completed a basic residency program and is now in a formally organized and approved subspecialty program, which may or may not be recognized as an approved residency program under Medicare
- Has completed all residency programs but is staying at the teaching hospital/medical school complex for a variety of reasons, such as a faculty appointment or the opportunity to develop or refine his or her skills outside the context of the residency program

Medicare law has clearly established direct graduate medical education (GME) payments as the payment mechanism for services provided in a hospital by individuals in an approved residency training program that leads to certification in a specialty or subspecialty. However, fees for some

 DEFINITIONS

key portion. Part (or parts) of a service determined by the teaching physician to be a critical or key portion.

physically present. Teaching physicians must be in the same room, or partitioned or curtained area as the patient and resident and/or perform a face-to-face service.

resident. Individual participating in an approved graduate medical education (GME) program or a physician who is not in an approved GME program but who is authorized to practice only in a hospital setting. Including interns and fellows but does not include medical students.

teaching physician. Physician, other than another resident, who involves residents in the care of his or her patients.

 KEY POINT

The notes recorded in a patient's medical record by the resident, teaching physician, or others regarding the service provided may be dictated and typed, hand-written, or computer generated. They must be dated and include a legible signature or identity. In the very least, they must describe the service rendered, the participation of the teaching physician, and whether the teaching physician was physically present.

physicians who are designated as fellows may also be appropriately billed as physician services.

According to the CMS instructions for billing the services of supervising physicians in a teaching setting, Medicare will pay for physician services furnished in a teaching setting under the physician fee schedule only if:

- Services are provided personally by a physician who is not a resident
- The teaching physician was physically present during the critical or key portions of the service performed by the resident
- The teaching physician provides care under the exception for E/M services furnished in certain primary care centers

Under the circumstances listed above, the services rendered by the resident are paid by Medicare through the direct GME payment or on a reasonable cost basis.

Exception: E/M Services Furnished in Certain Primary Care Centers

Physician claims for services furnished by residents without the presence of the teaching physician may be paid when furnished in primary care centers that were granted the primary care exception. These centers must attest in writing that they meet specific criteria for a particular residency program. The E/M codes that may be billed in these cases are 99202–99203 (new patient) and 99211–99213 (established patient). Code G0402 Initial preventive physical examination; face-to-face visit, services limited to new beneficiary during the first 12 months of Medicare enrollment, is also included under the primary care exception.

For this exception to be applicable, the center must attest in writing that all of the following conditions are met:

- The services must be furnished in a center located in the outpatient department of a hospital or another ambulatory care entity in which the time spent by residents in patient care activities is included in determining direct GME payments to a teaching hospital. This requirement is not met when the resident is assigned to a physician's office away from the center or makes home visits.
- Any resident furnishing the service without the presence of a teaching physician must have completed more than six months of an approved residency program.
- The teaching physician must not supervise more than four residents at a given time and must direct the care from such proximity as to constitute immediate availability. The teaching physician must:
  - have no other responsibilities at the time of the service for which payment is sought
  - have the primary medical responsibility for those patients seen by the residents and ensure that the services furnished are appropriate
  - review with each resident during or immediately after each visit the patient's medical history, physical examination, diagnosis, and record of tests and therapies
  - document the extent of his or her own participation in the review and direction of the services furnished to each patient

- The patients seen must be an identifiable group of individuals who consider the center to be the continuing source of their healthcare and in which services are furnished by residents under the medical direction of teaching physicians. The residents must generally follow the same group of patients throughout the course of their residency program, but there is no requirement that the teaching physician remain the same over any period of time.
- The range of services furnished by residents includes all of the following:
  - acute care for undifferentiated problems or chronic care for ongoing conditions, including chronic mental illness
  - coordination of care furnished by other physicians and providers
  - comprehensive care not limited by organ system or diagnosis

Some state Medicaid programs also recognize the teaching physicians primary care exception guidelines. The state Medicaid programs also recognize the preventive medicine codes not recognized by Medicare. These include codes 99381–99397. It is important that you verify with your specific state whether they recognize these codes in addition to those recognized by CMS. As with other primary care exception guidelines, the supervising physician must be available to provide care if the resident encounters a problem requiring additional care or treatment during the provision of a preventive medicine service.

TEMPORARY EXPANSION OF THE PRIMARY CARE EXCEPTION DUE TO COVID-19 PUBLIC HEALTH EMERGENCY (PHE)

In the March 31 COVID-19 interim final rule with comment period (IFC) (85 FR 19230), CMS announced the emergent and temporary expansion of the primary care exception. It was stated that for the duration of the PHE, the primary care exception was expanded to include all five levels of an office/outpatient E/M service (99202–99205 and 99211–99215). Medicare will also allow payment for teaching physician services when a resident furnishes Medicare telehealth services under the primary care exception.

In the May 8, 2020 COVID-19 IFC, there were additional services added to the primary care exception. It now includes the following services: Telephone E/M Services (99441–99443), Transitional Care Management (99495–99496), and Communication Technology-Based Services (99421–99423 and 99452, HCPCS Level II codes G2010 and G2012).

In addition, revised supervision requirements have been implemented, which allow a teaching physician to review a visit furnished by a resident remotely using audio/video real time communications technology during the PHE.

Documentation requirements have temporarily been revised also. For office/outpatient E/M services provided via telehealth, the E/M level selection can be based on medical decision making (MDM) or time, with time defined as all the time associated with the E/M on the day of the encounter. CMS also eliminated the requirement of documenting a history and/or physical exam in the patient medical record.

Psychiatry

For psychiatry services furnished under an approved GME program, the requirement for the presence of the teaching physician during service may be met by concurrent observation of the service using one-way mirrors or video equipment. Audio-only equipment does not suffice, however. The Medicare teaching physician policy is not applicable to psychologists who supervise psychiatry residents in approved GME programs.

Although psychiatric intake evaluation and psychotherapy services are reported with codes 90785–90899, a psychiatrist may also report E/M services. It should be noted that physicians, NP's, and PA's may also report E/M services. However, other behavioral health providers are not licensed to provide diagnostic or prescriptive services not specific to psychiatric conditions and, therefore, may not report E/M services or psychotherapy with E/M codes such as 90832. Care should be taken when reporting codes from 90785–90838 that the licensure of the provider is also considered to appropriately report the service.

Time-Based Services

For procedures based on time, the teaching physician must be present for the period of time for which the claim is made. Time spent by the resident in the absence of the teaching physician cannot be added to the time spent by the resident and teaching physician or the teaching physician alone with the patient. For example, if a code specifically describes a service of from 20 to 30 minutes it should be billed only if the teaching physician is present for 20 to 30 minutes.

Examples of services in this category include the following:

- Individual medical psychotherapy
- Critical care services
- E/M codes in which counseling and/or coordination of care dominates (more than 50 percent of the encounter) and time are considered the key or controlling factor to qualify for a particular level of E/M service
- Prolonged services
- Care plan oversight services
- Hospital discharge day management

Services rendered by teaching physicians involving a resident in the care of their patients must be identified using one of the following modifiers. The modifiers are required only for teaching physicians in a teaching setting (a program receiving Part A graduate medical education funding). These modifiers were developed to assist CMS in its postpayment audits of Medicare Part B payments for services involving residents.

GC: This service has been performed in part by a resident under the direction of a teaching physician. This modifier is to be used with all services provided by a teaching physician except where modifier GE is applicable. It certifies that the physician was present during the key portion of the service and was immediately available during the other parts of the service.

GE: This service has been performed by a resident without the presence of a teaching physician under the primary care exception. This modifier is used to indicate that the teaching physician was not present during the E/M service being billed, but that the requirements for billing E/M services under the primary care exception have been met. Teaching physicians who seek to submit services with modifier GE must file an attestation with the carrier that their services meet the conditions for this exception.

Documenting Teaching E/M Services

For a given encounter, the selection of the appropriate level of E/M service should be based on the documentation guidelines for evaluation and management services developed by the AMA and CMS, and published by the AMA. When E/M services are billed by teaching physicians, the following must be personally documented:

- The teaching physician personally performed the service or was physically present during the key or critical portions of the service performed by the resident (resident documentation of the presence and participation of the teaching physician is inadequate)
- The teaching physician participated in the management of the patient

The documentation of these key elements may be satisfied by the combination of entries into the medical record made by the resident and the teaching physician.

Sample Documentation

Meets Expected Requirements:

Admitting note. "I performed a history and physical examination of the patient and discussed his management with the resident. I discussed the findings and plan of care with the resident and agree with the documented findings and plan of care."

Follow-up visit. "Hospital day 5. I saw and examined the patient. I agree with the resident's note except the heart murmur is louder, so I will obtain an echo to evaluate."

Does NOT Meet Expected Requirements:

Admitting or Follow-up visit.

A countersignature only or a countersignature with:

"Agree with above."

"Rounded, reviewed, agree."

"Discussed with resident. Agree."

"Seen and agree."

"Patient seen and evaluated."

All required elements are obtained by the resident in the presence of, or jointly with, the teaching physician and documented by the resident. In this situation, the teaching physician is required to document that he or she was present during the critical or key portions of the service and directly involved in the patient's management. In addition, the note of the teaching physician should reference the resident's note. For purposes of payment, the combination of the teaching physician's and the resident's documentation must reflect the medical necessity of the service provided as well as the level of service that is billed by the physician.

Sample Documentation

The teaching physician is required to document that he or she was present during the critical or key portions of the service and directly involved in the patient's management.

Meets Expected Requirements:
I was present with the resident during the history and examination. I discussed the case with the resident and agree with the findings and plan as documented in the resident's note."

Does NOT Meet Expected Requirements:
A countersignature only or countersignature with:

"Agree with above."

"Rounded, reviewed, agree."

"Seen and agree."

Some or all of the required elements of the service are performed independently by the resident and documented. The teaching physician then repeats the critical or key portions of the service, with or without the resident's presence, and discusses the case with the resident. The teaching physician is required to document that he or she personally saw the patient, performed the critical or key components of the service, and participated in the patient's management. The note from the teaching physician needs to reference the resident's note. The combined entries must be adequate to substantiate the medical necessity of the service provided as well as the level of service that was billed.

Sample Documentation

Meets Expected Requirements:
Initial visit. "I saw and evaluated the patient. I reviewed the resident's note and agree, except that the picture is more consistent with pericarditis than myocardial ischemia. Will begin NSAIDs."

Follow-up visit. "I saw and evaluated the patient. Discussed with resident and agree with resident's findings and plan as documented in the resident's note."

Does NOT Meet Expected Requirements:
A countersignature only or countersignature with:

"Discussed with resident. Agree."

"Patient seen and evaluated."

Documentation by Students

Any time a student participates in performing a billable service (other than the review of systems and/or past, family, or social history, which are part of an E/M service), it has to be performed in the physical presence of a teaching physician. Students are allowed to document services in the medical record. If the medical student documents E/M services, the teaching physician is required to verify the patient's history and perform or re-perform the physical exam and medical decision making portions of the service. The teaching physician's personal note can refer to a student's documentation of physical exam findings or medical decision making rather than redocumenting the work. To meet requirements, the teaching physician should sign and date the medical student's entry in the medical record.

INCIDENT-TO SERVICES

Incident-to Protocols

If the practice employs limited-licensed practitioners, it is advisable to periodically determine that the "incident-to" guidelines are being adhered to. Incident-to services are defined by CMS as "those services that are furnished incident to a physician professional services in the physician's office (whether located in a separate office suite or within an institution) or in a patient's home."

To qualify as incident-to, the services must be part of the patient's normal course of treatment, during which a physician personally performed an initial service and remains actively involved in the course of the patient's treatment. Auxiliary personnel performing these services must be employed by the physician or clinic and services must be performed under the direct supervision of the physician and billed by the physician. The physician does not have to be physically present in the treatment room while these services are provided but must be present in the office suite to render assistance, if necessary (direct supervision).

To be considered an employee, the nonphysician performing an incident-to service may be a part-time, full-time, or leased employee of the supervising physician, physician group, or the legal entity that employs the physician who provides the supervision. Under the provision that existed prior to January 1, 2002, the physician and the individual providing the incident-to service must be employed by the same employer. In other words, the physician is required to either employ the auxiliary personnel or also be an employee of the same entity for which the auxiliary personnel works. Although all auxiliary personnel will still be required to report to the physician according to the required level of supervision, the agency no longer feels that an employment relationship is important and has added independent contractors to those that may supervise auxiliary personnel.

Services provided by auxiliary personnel not in the employ of the physician, physician group, or other legal entity—even if provided on the physician's order or included in the physician's bill—are not covered as incident-to a physician's service since the law requires that the services be of the type commonly furnished in physicians' offices and typically either rendered without charge or included in physicians' bills. As with the physician's personal professional services, the patient's financial liability for the incidental services is to the physician, physician group, or other legal entity. Therefore, the incidental service must represent an expense incurred by the physician, physician group, or other legal entity responsible for providing the professional service. This does not mean, however, that to be considered incident-to each occasion of service by a nonphysician (or the furnishing of a supply) needs to also always be the occasion of the actual performance of a personal professional service by the physician. Such a service or supply could be considered to be incident-to when furnished during a course of treatment where the physician performs an initial service and subsequent services of a frequency that reflects his active participation in and management of the course of treatment. (However, the direct supervision requirement must still be met with respect to every nonphysician service.)

DEFINITIONS

auxiliary personnel. Individual acting under the supervision of a physician; may be an employee, leased employee, or independent contractor of the physician (or other practitioner) or of the same entity that employs or contracts with the physician (or other practitioner).

direct supervision. Physician must be present in the office suite and immediately available to provide assistance and direction throughout the procedure; however, the physician is not required to be present in the room when the procedure is performed.

independent contractor. Individual who performs full- or part-time work for which an IRS1099 form is required.

leased employee. Legal employment relationship established by a contract where an employer hires the services of an employee through another employer.

noninstitutional setting. All settings other than a hospital or skilled nursing facility.

practitioner. Physician or nonphysician practitioner authorized to receive payment for services or incident-to services he or she provides.

The patient record should document the essential requirements for incident-to services.

In other words, the medical records should document the following:

- The service was an integral part of the patient's treatment course.
- The service is commonly included in the physician's services.
- The service is furnished in a physician's office or clinic (not in an institutional setting).
- The service was an expense to the practice.

Commonly furnished services and supplies are those customarily considered incident-to physicians' personal services in the office or physician-directed clinic setting. The requirement could not be considered to be met where supplies are clearly of a type that a physician is not expected to have on hand in his or her office or where services are of a type not considered medically appropriate to provide in the office setting.

Examples of qualifying incident-to services include:

- Cardiac rehabilitation
- Providing non-self-administrable drugs and/or biologicals
- Supplies furnished by the physician in the course of performing his or her services:
  - gauze
  - ointments
  - bandages
  - oxygen

Remember, coverage of services and supplies incident-to the professional services of a physician in private practice is limited to situations in which there is direct physician supervision. This applies to services of auxiliary personnel employed by the physician and working under his or her supervision, such as nurses, nonphysician anesthetists, psychologists, technicians, therapists (including physical therapists), and other aides.

Nonphysician Services Furnished Incident-to Physician's Services

A physician may also have the services of certain nonphysician practitioners (NPP), who are licensed by the state under various programs to assist or act in the place of the physician, such as certified nurse midwives, certified registered nurse anesthetists, clinical psychologists, clinical social workers, physician assistants, nurse practitioners, and clinical nurse specialists.

Services performed by these nonphysician practitioners incident-to a physician's professional services include not only services ordinarily rendered by a physician's office staff person (e.g., medical services, such as taking blood pressures and temperatures, giving injections, and changing dressings), but also services ordinarily performed by the physician himself/herself, such as minor surgery, setting casts or simple fractures, x-ray interpretations, and other activities that involve evaluation or treatment of a patient's condition. An NPP such as a physician assistant (PA) or nurse practitioner (NP) may be licensed under state law to perform a specific medical procedure and may be able to perform the procedure without physician supervision and have the service separately covered and paid for by Medicare as a physician assistant's or nurse practitioner's service.

 KEY POINT

The incident-to provision requires that services and supplies must be:

- Provided in a noninstitutional setting to noninstitutional patients
- An integral, although incidental, part of the service of a physician (or other practitioner) provided during the course of diagnosis or treatment of an injury or illness
- Commonly furnished without charge or included in the bill of a physician (or other practitioner)
- Commonly provided in the office or clinic of a physician (or other practitioner)
- Provided under the direct supervision of the physician (or other practitioner)
- Furnished by the physician, practitioner with an incident-to benefit, or by auxiliary personnel

Sample Documentation

Meets Expected Requirements:
The patient presents for monthly blood pressure check; no new problems or complaints; BP: 145/85; Wt. 215 lbs, pulse 88, Resp. 20. Diet reviewed with patient. Scheduled an appointment with Dr. Jones next month; has enough meds to last until next appointment.

Dr. Jones (signature)

J. Smith, RN

Does NOT Meet Expected Requirements:
Monthly BP check; BP:145/85

J. Smith, RN

Under the incident-to provision, a nonphysician practitioner, such as a PA or an NP, can be reimbursed for services they provide in the physician's office. In order for these services to be covered as incident-to, the services must be:

- Of the type commonly furnished in physician offices or clinics
- An integral, although incidental, part of the physician's professional service
- Furnished under the physician's direct personal supervision

Nonphysician practitioners may bill for E/M services as long as the collaboration and general supervision rules are applied. In addition, the service provided is required to be medically necessary and provided within the scope of practice of the NPP. For services provided in the office or clinic setting, when the E/M service is shared by the physician and the NPP, the services may be paid as incident-to the physician's service, if those requirements are met, or it may be billed under the nonphysician practitioner's NPI.

For services provided in the hospital inpatient or outpatient settings as well as the emergency department, the service is billed under either the physician's or nonphysician practitioner's NPI if there is a face-to-face encounter between the physician and the patient. In the case that the physician does not have a face-to-face encounter with the patient, such as when the physician anticipates in his or her care by reviewing the medical record, then the service should be billed under the nonphysician practitioner's NPI.

 KEY POINT

For incidental services performed by a nonphysician practitioner, there must have been direct, personal, professional services furnished by the physician to initiate the course of treatment. There must also be documentation of subsequent services by the physician that reflects his/her continuing active participation in the management of the course of treatment.

Sample Documentation

Meets Expected Requirements:
Patient here for suture removal. Three sutures were placed in left index finger 10 days ago in the ED, following an accidental laceration from a broken glass. Tetanus booster given in ER.

Exam: Digit healing well. No erythema, exudate or tenderness.

Plan: All sutures removed without difficulty. Wound dressed.

Patient given instructions on wound care; instructed to call with any problems.

Susan Smith, PA

Does NOT Meet Expected Requirements:
Laceration left index finger, well healed. Three sutures removed and wound dressed. Wound care instructions given; instructed to call with any problems.

Susan Smith, PA

It is important to note that the Office of Inspector General (OIG) work plans have included reviews of incident-to services in recent years.

Split and Shared E/M Services Office and Clinic Setting

E/M services provided in the office or clinic setting by the physician must be billed using the physician's NPI. When the E/M service is shared or split between the physician and an NPP such as an NP, PA, clinical nurse specialist (CNS), or a certified nurse midwife (CNM) it may be reported in one of two ways:

- If the service is provided to an established patient, and the incident-to requirements are met, the service is billed using the physician's NPI.
- If the incident-to provisions are not met, the service must be billed using the NPI of the nonphysician practitioner.

Sample Documentation

Meets Expected Requirements:
Documentation indicates the NPP performed a portion of the encounter and the physician completed the E/M service.

Does NOT Meet Expected Requirements:
Notation by supervising MD that the he or she is actively participating in the patient's care.

Whenever an E/M service is shared by a physician and an NPP from the same group, and the physician provides any of the face-to-face portion of the service, the service may be reported using either the physician's or the nonphysician practitioner's NPI. In the situation in which there is no face-to-face visit between the patient and the physician (e.g., the physician reviewed the patient's medical record only), the service must be billed using the nonphysician practitioner's NPI.

 KEY POINT

For shared/split E/M services, each provider should document his or her portion of the E/M service. The documentation must support the face-to-face requirement and must clearly identify both providers involved in the service. Select the code for the level of E/M service based on the combined documentation.

 CODING AXIOM

In an office setting, the nonphysician practitioner performs a portion of an E/M encounter and the physician completes the E/M service. If the incident-to requirements are met, the physician reports the service. If the incident-to requirements are not met, the service must be reported using the nonphysician practitioner's NPI.

Sample Documentation

Emergency Department Setting
Patient is a 73-year-old white male who was brought to the emergency department by ambulance. He stated that he had vomited approximately 2000 cc of coffee ground vomitus in the morning. He was evaluated in the ED by the physician assistant who felt that the patient had an acute GI bleed. The PA contacts the physician to discuss the findings. The physician reviews the patient's electronic record and instructs the PA to admit the patient.

QUALITY PAYMENT PROGRAM

The Quality Payment Program (QPP) is a key piece of the Medicare Access and CHIP Reauthorization Act (MACRA) of 2015. MACRA is the legislation that ended the sustainable growth rate (SGR), which made Medicare Part B providers susceptible to the possibility of payment cliffs for 13 years. The focus of the QPP is to drive the payment system to reward high-value, patient-centered care and will continue to evolve over a number of years.

The QPP took effect on January 1, 2017 and eligible clinicians may participate through one of two tracks:

- Advanced alternative payment models (APM)
- Merit-based Incentive Payment System (MIPS)
    - comprises four performance categories:
        — quality (PQRS)
        — cost (VM)
        — improvement activities (new)
        — promoting interoperability (formerly, advancing care information)

MIPS

The following Year 4 criteria must be met in order to be considered an eligible clinician under MIPS:

- Clinician types:
    - physician
    - physician assistant (PA)
    - nurse practitioner (NP)
    - clinical nurse specialist (CNS)
    - certified registered nurse anesthetist (CRNA)
    - chiropractor
    - osteopathic practitioners
    - clinical psychologist
    - physical therapist
    - occupational therapist
    - speech-language pathologist
    - audiologist
    - registered dietitian or nutrition professional
- Medicare Part B billings exceeding $90,000/year

 FOR MORE INFO

Information regarding the requirements for QPP is available at the following website: https://qpp.cms.gov/about/resource-library.

- Rendering care to over 200 Medicare Part B beneficiaries/year
- Provide 200 or more covered professional services to Medicare Part B beneficiaries/year

The Year 4 reporting period begins on January 1, 2020, with the deadline to submit data being March 31, 2021. CMS will provide feedback to clinicians regarding their performance in 2020 then effective January 1, 2022, clinicians will receive a positive, negative, or neutral payment adjustment of up to 9 percent to their practice's Medicare payments based on participation results.

APM

An Alternative Payment Model (APM) is not simply an incentive, rather it is more of a fundamental change that CMS has made to how the agency pays for healthcare services. It may be helpful to think of an APM as a type of payment approach that factors in the quality of care rendered along with the total cost of that care into how CMS pays for healthcare as opposed to the typical fee-for-service model that has traditionally been used for reimbursement. MACRA states that APMs include:

- Any CMS Innovation Center model
- Medicare Shared Savings Program
- Demonstration or any other federal demonstration, under the Healthcare Quality Demonstration Program
- Other Demonstration required by federal law

For participating APM clinicians, CMS provides additional incentives when those clinicians render a high level of care while being efficient with costs. An APM can apply to a specific clinical condition, care episode or even a particular population of patients.

An Advanced APM is a subset of APMs. This is the second track of participation in the QPP because clinicians participating significantly in an Advanced APM are exempt from MIPS.

Proposed Changes to the QPP

In the CY2021 physician fee schedule proposed rule, CMS is proposing several significant changes to the QPP program including:

- Developing MIPS Value Pathways (MVPs)
- Introduction of the APM Performance Pathway (APP) for APM participant MIPS eligible clinicians to be able to report MIPS
- Updates to the MIPS performance measures and activities, and updates to cost and quality categories
- Elimination of the APM scoring standard
- Sunsetting the CMS Web Interface submission method for groups and virtual groups
- Incorporation of new measures, changes to existing measures, and removal of 14 quality measures
- A total of 206 quality measures proposed for 2021 performance year
- Inclusion of services provided via telehealth in quality and cost measures
- Changes in the percentage required for the cost performance category

- Establishing a performance period for the Promoting Interoperability category to a minimum of a continuous 90-day period within a certain timeframe
- Continuation of quality category scoring and bonus policies
- Increase in the maximum number of points available for the complex patient bonus
- Reduction to the performance threshold for the 2021 performance period
- Updated definitions of terms

The CY2021 physician fee schedule final rule was not available at the time of this publication. To verify which of the above changes were finalized and for more detail, refer to the CY2021 final rule at https://www.cms.gov/Medicare/Medicare-Fee-for-Service-Payment/PhysicianFeeSched or the QPP website at https://qpp.cms.gov/.

COMPREHENSIVE ERROR RATE TESTING (CERT) PROGRAM

CMS states that the aim of the CERT program is to "measure and improve the accuracy of Medicare claims submission, processing and payment." More than 40,000 claims are "randomly" selected for review each year. CMS released a list of overutilized codes identified by contractor. Overall, the estimated Medicare FFS improper payment for E/M services rate was 11.3 percent for a projected improper payment amount of $3.8 billion in 2019.

Incorrect coding and insufficient documentation are the two most common errors found in the CERT reviews. When reporting E/M codes it is critical that all the elements of the service be documented, especially when reporting a high-level E/M code. Often providers fail to document what is performed in a service, and others may overbill in error due to not knowing the code requirements.

Documentation of an E/M service is more than just the length of the progress note. The documentation must support all three key elements for new, initial, and consultation services and two of the three key elements at the levels defined for an established patient. For example, the key elements for code 99337 are:

- Comprehensive history
- Comprehensive examination
- Moderate to high complexity medical decision making

One of the most common deficiencies when reporting high-level E/M services is identifying high-complexity decision making. This is defined by the CPT book as two of these three components: extensive number of diagnoses or management options; extensive amount or complexity of data to be reviewed; and high risk to the patient of complications, morbidity, or mortality. Treatment of a problem-focused condition in a patient with a history of multiple comorbid conditions does not automatically make the decision making of high complexity. A visit with a patient with a problem-focused history would not normally include the ordering of multiple, complex diagnostic procedures.

QUICK TIP

The documentation guidelines state that ROS and PFSH information can be obtained by ancillary personnel or provided by the patient. Frequently, forms filled out by the patient or checklists addressed by the provider are used to obtain a complete ROS and PFSH. If the form is separate from the note, it is suggested this form be referenced in the chart note and be dated and initialed by the provider with pertinent comments noted as appropriate. When treating established patients, the provider may update a previous checklist and reference the original document, noting any changes that have occurred.

FOR MORE INFO

Information regarding the CERT program can be found at: http://www.cms.gov/cert/.

A review of the Table of Risk on page 38 indicates that the following conditions or circumstances are considered to be of high risk:

- One or more chronic illnesses with severe exacerbation, progression, or side effects of treatment
- Acute or chronic illness or injury that poses a threat to life or bodily function
- An abrupt change in neurological status
- Diagnostic studies that are invasive in nature and have identified risk factors
- Elective major surgery with identified risk factors
- Emergency major surgery
- Drug therapy requiring intensive monitoring for toxicity
- Decision not to resuscitate or to de-escalate care due to poor prognosis

There are several of these conditions that are frequently misused. The acute or chronic illness must pose an imminent threat to the patient. For example, a patient with a malignant neoplasm has a severe illness but when undergoing outpatient treatment does not usually face imminent threat to life or limb. There is also differing opinion as to which drugs require intensive monitoring, and the urgency of this monitoring should be documented.

CERT and Electronic Medical Records (EMR) Submission

Wisconsin Physician Services (WPS), a Medicare contractor, previously noted that providers have omitted key information from the electronic record documentation due to a failure to expand the electronic record subsections that collapse into larger sections of the encounter record when responding to a CERT contractor records request.

Providers and staff should verify that *all* portions of an e-record have been properly printed and include the complete record including, but not limited to, physician orders, provider signatures, test results, etc., prior to submitting to Medicare. Taking the extra time to ensure a complete Medicare record is submitted when responding to a CERT request will negate the need for additional requests or claim denials due to missing documentation.

Medical Necessity

Medical necessity is another factor used to determine if code assignment is appropriate. As previously discussed, a patient's presenting problems or conditions are a good barometer for helping to determine not only the appropriate level of decision making, but also the amount of history and exam that are required to treat the patient. Thus a patient with a problem-focused or detailed condition would not require a comprehensive history or exam.

Just because a service is "overdocumented" does not justify the assignment of a high-level E/M service code. In past audits by Medicare contractors, as part of the CERT program, E/M levels were apparently selected "based on the sheer volume of documentation rather than the level of service that was warranted based on the patient's condition."

It is important to note that all documentation must support the key elements. Default coding, or coding based upon high-risk specialties, does not meet the required guidelines.

Documentation Aids and Review Sheets

Templates

Given the seeming complexity of some of the documentation requirements, the concept of templates and other methods to assist in provider documentation have seen a recent increase. The move towards electronic medical records: typed, beamed, voice-recognized, or via hand-held device is well under way. In the interim, printed templates are often used to assist in documentation.

These methods are not intended to replace provider work; they are intended to make the documenting of work easier. As with any tool, these can be abused by providing "stock" or comprehensive pre-recorded histories or exams at the touch of a button or click of a mouse. The best guideline to follow when any of these systems are in use is to review the notes to be certain that the volume of history and exam stay consistent with the nature of the presenting problem or problems being evaluated.

As we have mentioned throughout—it is these supporting elements that are most often the source of under-documentation, and in regard to assisted documentation—these two components often go the other way and can become somewhat overblown or out of proportion. This result will ultimately be equally as disturbing to regulators as under documentation.

Documentation templates can be used by a provider to document services. These provide a sample roadmap of all elements that could be performed in the areas of history and exam. What is important with regard to the use of templates is that only the elements of the exam *actually* performed are documented on the template. This is important not only from a coding and billing compliance standpoint, but also from a legal and liability standpoint. It is easy to start "clicking" and select elements that a provider did not actually perform; it is crucial that this does not occur.

Specialty templates may differ in the physical exam areas only by substituting the individual single-system specialty exams in the exam area. The overall purpose of the template is to ease the burden associated with often repetitive ROS and exam elements. These can also be used during an encounter as an easy checklist that can be used later as a dictation guide.

Review Forms

Appendix A in this book provides forms that a practice can use to review completed documentation. These are set up much like a template in the history and exam areas, but also include an area to rate decision making. The only difference between specialty forms and review forms is the physical exam area.

The decision-making area lists the primary indicators from the federal guidelines Table of Risk. Optum360 has retained the straightforward level of decision making.

 QUICK TIP

Use of templates is permitted; however, the provider must still elaborate on any abnormal findings in the documentation.

 QUICK TIP

Review forms should include all the possible data to be scored and the final code selection made when the entire record is reviewed.

This decision making table is not a CMS-approved guide, but has been constructed and provided to present the most current body of thought on the real meaning of the various decision making levels.

For more information on electronic health records, see chapter 3.

KNOWLEDGE ASSESSMENT CHAPTER 4

See chapter 19 for answers and rationale.

1. Medical necessity is a critical element to medical record documentation because without it claims may be rejected or outright denied.
    a. True
    b. False

2. What is the description of "incident-to" services?
    a. Services provided by auxiliary personnel of a facility for a physician
    b. Services provided by a nurse practitioner using their own provider identification number
    c. Services provided by auxiliary personal under the supervision of and billed by the physician
    d. Services provided directly by the physician for secondary conditions

3. Where is the best place to find what set of documentation guidelines private payers are using?
    a. In the office or practice's policy and procedure manual
    b. Within the contract itself
    c. In the provider's manual issued by your third-party payers
    d. None of the above

4. What are the advantages to learning only one set of documentation guidelines?
    a. The practice may not always know what coverage is in effect for a given service and who secondary payers might be
    b. It can be very difficult for providers to remember different sets of rules for different payers
    c. There really are no distinct advantages; it is better to learn both sets of guidelines thoroughly
    d. Both a and b

5. What are the disadvantages of using documentation templates?
    a. They can be abused by providing "stock" or comprehensive prerecorded histories or exams
    b. No disadvantages; they are designed to replace provider work
    c. May not be used solely as a prompt to document elements performed
    d. Both a and c

6. The teaching physician does not need to be present for the key portion of an encounter if the resident relays all pertinent information in chart notes.
   a. True
   b. False

7. Which of the following is acceptable teaching physician documentation?
   a. Seen and agreed
   b. No changes
   c. Patient evaluated, care plan reviewed with resident and agreed with findings, no additional changes
   d. Signature and date

8. What is the responsibility of the teaching physician in a primary care exception program?
   a. Supervise residents in providing all E/M services
   b. Supervise up to four residents providing primary responsibility for the patient's care and review each case with the resident during or immediately after the encounter
   c. Have a full schedule of patients concurrent with the residents
   d. Cosign all resident notes

9. What is conveyed with modifier GC?
   a. The teaching physician completed the service without resident participation
   b. The teaching physician and the resident provided the service
   c. The resident provided the service under the primary care exception
   d. The resident acted as scribe for the teaching physician

10. What special criteria must a teaching physician utilize for psychiatric services?
    a. The resident service is concurrently monitored using one-way mirrors or video equipment and audio transmission
    b. The teaching physician records the audio transmission for review
    c. The teaching physician is not required to participate in the service due to patient privacy
    d. The teaching physician is only required to review medication changes

Chapter 5: Office or Other Outpatient Services (99202–99215)

New Patient (99202–99205)

QUICK COMPARISON

Office or Other Outpatient Services—New Patient

E/M Code	Medical Decision Making	History	Exam	Time Spent on Date of Encounter
99202	Straightforward	Medically appropriate	Medically appropriate	15–29 min.
99203	Low	Medically appropriate	Medically appropriate	30–44 min.
99204	Moderate	Medically appropriate	Medically appropriate	45–59 min.
99205	High	Medically appropriate	Medically appropriate	60–74 min.

GENERAL GUIDELINES

- Code selection is based on MDM or total time, including face-to-face and non-face-to-face time spent on the date of the encounter.
- History and physical examination elements are not required for code level selection for office and other outpatient services. However, a medically appropriate history and/or physical examination should still be documented. The nature and degree of the history and/or physical examination is determined by the treating physician or other qualified healthcare professional reporting the service.
- Clinical staff may collect information pertaining to the history and exam and the patient and/or caregiver may provide information directly (e.g., by electronic health record [EHR] portal or questionnaire) that is reviewed by the reporting provider.
- Total time for these services includes total face-to-face and non-face-to-face time personally spent by the physician or other qualified healthcare professional on the day of the encounter.
- Physician or other qualified healthcare professional time may include the following activities:
  - preparing to see the patient (e.g., review of tests)
  - obtaining and/or reviewing separately obtained history
  - performing a medically appropriate examination and/or evaluation
  - counseling and educating the patient/family/caregiver
  - ordering medications, tests, or procedures

> ✓ **QUICK TIP**
>
> Medical necessity is still the overarching criterion for selecting a level of service in addition to the individual requirements of the E/M code.

- referring and communicating with other healthcare professionals (when not separately reported)
- documenting clinical information in the electronic or other health record
- independently interpreting results (not separately reported) and communicating results to the patient/family/caregiver
- care coordination (not separately reported)

- Comorbidities or other underlying conditions should not be considered when selecting the level of service unless they are addressed during the encounter and their presence increases the amount and/or complexity of data to be reviewed and analyzed or the risk of complications and/or morbidity or mortality.

- Use these codes if the patient has not been seen or had a professional service provided by this physician/qualified healthcare professional or any other physician/qualified healthcare professional from the same practice and exact same specialty and subspecialty in the past three years.

- Consider using the appropriate critical care code instead of these codes if the physician/qualified healthcare professional provided constant care to a critically ill patient. Critical care codes are based on the patient's condition, not the site of service, and are selected according to time spent in attending the patient.

- Consider assigning the appropriate consultation code instead of these codes if the provider provided an opinion or advice about a specific problem at the request of another provider or other appropriate source.

- Report only the appropriate initial hospital care, hospital observation, or comprehensive nursing facility assessment code if the patient was admitted to the hospital or nursing facility on the same day as another visit.

- Do not include the time spent by any other staff (e.g.,nurse, nurse practitioner or physician assistant) toward the time thresholds. Face-to-face and non-face-to-face time is the time the treating provider spent on the date of the encounter.

- Use case management codes when coordination of care is provided on a date without a patient encounter. Case management codes are "bundled" according to Medicare and cannot be billed to the carrier. Other third-party payers may reimburse for these services.

- Report prolonged service code 99417 with 99205 when the service runs 15 minutes beyond the time specified in the CPT® code narrative. The time must be clearly documented in the medical record.

- Append modifier 25 to report that a separately identifiable E/M service was performed by the same provider on the same date as a minor procedure or other service. Only the content of the note documenting the separate E/M service should be used to determine the level of an additional E/M service.

- Append modifier 57 to report that the decision to perform surgery was made during this visit. For Medicare patients, modifier 57 is used to report the fact that the decision was made to perform major surgery (a procedure with a 90-day postoperative period).

- Append modifier 95 to indicate that the E/M service was rendered to a patient at a distant site via a real-time interactive audio and video telecommunications system. The communication between the

 KEY POINT

Modifiers 25 and 57 are to be appended to the E/M code and not to the codes for other procedures that may be performed.

physician or other qualified healthcare professional and the patient should be commensurate with the same key components or requirements of those that would be required if the service had been rendered in a face-to-face setting.

- Performance and/or interpretation of diagnostic tests or studies during an encounter are not included when determining the level of E/M service when reported separately. A separate code(s) for the diagnostic tests or studies performed in addition to the E/M codes may be reported.
- A test/study that is independently interpreted by the provider that is not separately reported but is part of the E/M service is considered part of MDM.

APC Note: Under the Medicare ambulatory payment classification (APC) system, the definition of a new patient is a patient who has not been registered as an inpatient or outpatient of the hospital within the three years prior to a visit.

Also, it is important to note that the use of the CPT evaluation and management codes in provider-based clinics and emergency departments for APC billing is not determined or reported the same as for a facility.

ISSUES IN THIS CODE RANGE

- When a patient has been seen or treated in the hospital within the last three years, as a consult or otherwise, he or she is no longer a new patient. Likewise, when moving to a new practice, and taking old patients along, they are best considered established.
- If a nonphysician practitioner is allowed to see new patients be certain the practitioner uses his or her own provider number.
- Codes for high-level E/M services have been targeted in the CERT program as being overutilized. Medical necessity and the level of medical decision making should be verified for all high-level E/M services.

99202

DOCUMENTATION REQUIREMENTS

Medical Decision Making: Straightforward
- Minimal number and complexity of problems addressed
- No or minimal amount and complexity of data reviewed and analyzed
- Minimal risk of complications and/or morbidity

History: Medically appropriate

Examination: Medically appropriate

Code Indicators (from the MDM table)

Number and Complexity of Problem(s)
- One self-limited or minor problem

Amount and/or Complexity of Data
- Minimal or none

Risk of Complications/Morbidity or Mortality
Minimal risk of morbidity from additional diagnostic tests or treatment

Time Spent on Date of the Encounter
- 15-29

KEY POINT

The redefined MDM guidelines were published by the AMA in the 2021 edition of CPT and adopted by CMS in the CY2020 Physician Fee Schedule Final Rule.

KEY POINT

The nature and extent of the patient history and physical examination are determined by the treating provider reporting the service.

QUICK TIP

CMS documentation guidelines indicate that it is appropriate to document normal findings without elaboration.

Sample Documentation—99202

Level II Initial Office Visit

S: This 20-year-old male patient, new to my practice, who presents with a three-day duration of painful right middle finger nail bed and surrounding area. Pt. denies trauma to the area. The fingernail discomfort has rapidly progressed to its present state. Pt. denies noticing suppuration/drainage. No self-treatment.

ROS: No arthralgias. All other joints without complaint.

O: Right hand—middle distal phalange with periungual induration. Skin with increased warmth and sensitivity. Joints WNL. Full ROM. Other right hand nail beds WNL. Remainder of upper extremity WNL. Neuro intact; sensory as stated.

A: Paronychia, right third digit.

P: Warm soaks q.4 to 6 hrs. Begin E-mycin 333 mg one every eight hours, #21. Protect digit. ASA/Tylenol PRN pain. Return as needed.

(General multisystem)

99203

DOCUMENTATION REQUIREMENTS

Medical Decision Making: Low
- Low number and complexity of problems addressed
- Limited amount and complexity of data reviewed and analyzed
- Low risk of complications and/or morbidity

History: Medically appropriate

Examination: Medically appropriate

Code Indicators (from the MDM table)

Number and Complexity of Problem(s)
- Two or more self-limited or minor problems
- One stable, chronic illness
- One acute, uncomplicated illness or injury

Amount and/or Complexity of Data
Each unique test, order, or document contributes to the combination of two or combination of three in Category 1 below.

- Limited
(Must meet the requirements of at least one of the two categories.)

Category 1: Tests and documents
- Any combination of two from the following:
  - review of prior external note(s) from each unique source*
  - review of the result(s) of each unique test*
  - ordering of each unique test*

or

Category 2: Assessment requiring an independent historian(s)
(For the categories of independent interpretation of tests and discussion of management or test interpretation, see moderate or high)

Risk of Complications/Morbidity or Mortality
Low risk of morbidity from additional diagnostic tests or treatment

Time Spent on Date of the Encounter
- 30–44

 KEY POINT

The redefined MDM guidelines were published by the AMA in the 2021 edition of CPT and adopted by CMS in the CY2020 Physician Fee Schedule Final Rule.

 KEY POINT

The nature and extent of the patient history and physical examination are determined by the treating provider reporting the service.

Sample Documentation—99203

Level III Initial Office Visit

Reason for visit: "Something is really wrong"

HPI: This 18-year-old white female complains of vaginal itching, burning, and pain for three days, getting "worse and worse." She tried an OTC preparation, but it provided little relief. She has never had a GYN exam before and is apprehensive. She has been sexually active for three years, has had four partners and "always" uses condoms for protection. Past history unremarkable. She denies use of tobacco, drugs, or alcohol except for a "beer or two" on weekends. She is a university student, lives in the dorms, works part time at the university. No known allergies. Menses regular, lasting three to four days, normal flow; LMP 10 days ago. No history of STD or previous GU infections. Review of systems otherwise within normal limits.

Physical exam: Vital signs: T: 97.8, R: 18, P: 76, BP: 116/78. Abdomen: no organomegaly, no masses or tenderness. External genitalia, red and irritated with a foul-smelling creamy discharge oozing from the vagina; no lesions noted. No adnexal tenderness or ovarian masses. Uterus 8 cm. Cervix firm, pink no discharge from os. Rectal negative. Pap smear deferred. Gram stain of vaginal discharge negative for GC. Wet mount + clue cells. KOH prep revealed no yeast or hyphae.

Impression: Bacterial vaginitis.

Plan: The patient was reassured, and her condition was explained. She was given an RX for metronidazole gel intravaginally BID x five days, and was also instructed that her partner should be treated concurrently. GC culture and VDRL sent.

(Single organ system—genitourinary-female)

Level III Initial Office Visit

History: A 41-year-old male complaining of pain, stiffness, "clicking" and swelling of both knees that is of gradual onset but seems to be getting worse. He cannot pinpoint when he first noticed a problem, but it was several months before his move here six months ago. He first noted pain in his knees after exercise but notes that exercise also makes the stiffness better. He occasionally gets nonradiating backache, especially after lifting and doing yard work, but sometimes it happens for no apparent reason. Over-the-counter preparations such as Advil with rest and heat help his back and used to make his knees feel better, but lately they seem worse. He notes no paresthesias from his back. Past history is otherwise noncontributory. He notes no problems with gait or stability.

Physical Exam: Well-developed, somewhat obese white male. Height 5'10", weight 205 pounds. BP 130/92. Gait and station are normal. Back appears normal; no kyphosis or scoliosis; no tenderness upon palpation of the lumbar area. Flexes to 90 degrees. Leg lengths even and joints symmetrical. Knees are nontender and are not erythemic or warm. Full range of motion. No back pain on straight leg raising. McMurray's negative. There is moderate crepitation noted on movement of the knees. Hip movement is normal and the patient reports no pain. Muscle strength, pulses and reflexes are all within normal limits. Babinski is negative. Normal response to touch and pinprick.

Impression:

1. Osteoarthritis, bilateral knees.
2. History of lumbago without evidence of sciatic nerve involvement.

Plan: Discussion with the patient regarding osteoarthritis, treatment options and nature of the condition. Patient instructed in the importance of daily exercise including stretching exercises to avoid further damage to the joints. Importance of weight reduction in management of DJD was also strongly stressed. Patient was instructed to use aspirin to relieve knee and back pain, and was given a referral for physical therapy evaluation and instructions on exercises and activities to help manage his condition. The patient was instructed to return in four months for follow-up and to call sooner if there are any problems. The patient was advised to contact his PCP for hypertension follow up.

(Single organ system—musculoskeletal)

99204

DOCUMENTATION REQUIREMENTS

Medical Decision Making: Moderate
- Moderate number and complexity of problems addressed
- Moderate amount and complexity of data reviewed and analyzed
- Moderate risk of complications and/or morbidity

History: Medically appropriate

Examination: Medically appropriate

Code Indicators (from the MDM table)

Number and Complexity of Problem(s)
- One or more chronic illnesses with exacerbation, progression, or side effects of treatment
- Two or more stable chronic illnesses
- One undiagnosed new problem with uncertain prognosis
- One acute illness with systemic symptoms
- One acute, complicated injury

Amount and/or Complexity of Data
Each unique test, order, or document contributes to the combination of two or combination of three in Category 1 below.

- Moderate

(Must meet the requirements of at least one of the three categories.)

Category 1: Tests, documents, or independent historian(s)
- Any combination of three from the following:
  - review of prior external note(s) from each unique source*
  - review of the result(s) of each unique test*
  - ordering of each unique test*
  - assessment requiring an independent historian(s)

or

Category 2: Independent interpretation of tests
- Independent interpretation of a test performed by another physician/other qualified healthcare professional (not separately reported)

or

Category 3: Discussion of management or test interpretation
- Discussion of management or test interpretation with external physician/other qualified healthcare professional/appropriate source (not separately reported)

Risk of Complications/Morbidity or Mortality
Moderate risk of morbidity from additional diagnostic testing or treatment

Examples only:

- Prescription drug management

KEY POINT

The redefined MDM guidelines were published by the AMA in the 2021 edition of CPT and adopted by CMS in the CY2020 Physician Fee Schedule Final Rule.

KEY POINT

The nature and extent of the patient history and physical examination are determined by the treating provider reporting the service.

- Decision regarding minor surgery with identified patient or procedure risk factors
- Decision regarding elective major surgery without identified patient or procedure risk factors
- Diagnosis or treatment significantly limited by social determinants of health

Time Spent on Date of the Encounter
- 45–59

 KEY POINT

The nature and extent of the patient history and physical examination are determined by the treating provider reporting the service.

Sample Documentation—99204

Level IV Initial Office Visit

This is a 44-year-old female new pt. who presents with fever/chills, headache, facial tenderness and swelling, and general malaise of two-day duration. Pt. reports feeling "like a Mack truck has run over me." Current symptoms began with a slight sore throat two days ago. The sore throat has diminished. Pt. does admit to rhinitis and nasal congestion. No cough. Appetite is diminished. Pt. does not want to report to work today and would like a sick certificate for same. Pt. does provide a history of sinusitis, treated in the past with antibiotics. Has never been to an ENT specialist. No sinus films taken in past.

ROS: HEENT: As above. No other significant factors. Headaches only with current symptomatology. No respiratory complaints. No GYN complaints; last menses three weeks ago. Otherwise negative.

PMH: T&A age 12. Sinusitis, as above.

FH: Unremarkable.

SH: Smokes cigarettes one pack/day; no ETOH. Works as a financial advisor.

O: T: 99.6. BP: 130/82; P: 88; R: 22. General: well-developed, well-nourished female appearing mild to moderately ill. HEENT: normocephalic. Eyes: sclerae sl. injected. PERRLA. Throat: sl. erythematous pharynx. No exudates. Tonsils absent. Tongue WNL. Dentition: good condition. Nose: mucosa pale. Yellowish exudates noted. Ears: TM's WNL, bilaterally. No sign middle ear fluid. Some cerumen debris noted in canals. Facial tenderness on palpation over ethmoid and maxillary sinuses. Chest: all fields clear; no rales/rhonchi. Heart: NSR; no murmur. Abdomen: benign. No mass; tenderness. No organomegaly. Neuro non-focal. Skin warm and dry.

A: Probable pansinusitis. Rule out sinus anomalies.

P: 1. Obtain sinus series from Community Radiology; order given.
2. Augmentin 500 mg one t.i.d. for 10 days with meals.
3. Encourage fluids; bedrest x 48 hours. Sick certificate given.
4. Can take OTC Sudafed PRN.
5. Acetaminophen for pain PRN.
6. Call for follow-up appt. if no improvement in a few days.

(Single organ system—ear, nose and throat)

(continued)

Sample Documentation—99204 (Continued)

Level IV Initial Office Visit

Reason for visit: "Mom and my school counselor say that I need to see you."

S: This 15-year-old white male high school tenth grader came in accompanied by his mother; she states that the counselor suggested an evaluation because he skipped school several times in the past three months, and they do not know why this has started. Prior to this time, the patient was a "model student" and an "all around good kid." His behavior and general attitude changed "for the worse—big time" about four months ago, and the mother is very concerned.

The patient was then interviewed privately, and initially stated that this interview is "a waste of time." He states that "people just don't understand" and he is "just being a normal kid," and that "everyone is overreacting all over the place." He also expressed concerns that if he talked with me, I would "tell everyone that he is depressed or nuts" and he'd have "even more problems" than he does now.

He is not currently dating, although he says he knows a girl he wants to ask out but she only goes out with "older guys." He tried to find part-time work but states that employers want him to wait till he is 16 so he won't need a work permit. He is not currently involved in any sports or school activities although he played football in middle school, and last year in ninth grade; he states that he "just didn't feel like doing it" this year. He states that he is just nervous all the time and that sometimes he thinks that "everyone is just trying to make me angry so I'll do something so really stupid that they can just lock me up and forget about me."

Past history, according to the form completed by his mother, is relatively unremarkable. Patient had a Colles fracture at age five, and otherwise has had no significant health problems. No hospitalizations, no other trauma and no surgery; no current medications. Family history is unremarkable. Patient denies use of alcohol, tobacco or drugs, although he does admit that he "smoked a joint" once. He states that he and his friend "borrowed" a joint from a third friend's older brother (apparently without the knowledge of either of the brothers) so they could "try it," but it "didn't do much."

Complete review of systems was generally within normal limits. The patient noted that his face "breaks out a lot" and that he gets "tension headaches" when his parents "bug" him, but otherwise no complaints.

Records from his family physician were unremarkable except for notations of "marked change in attitude, probably age-related" on his last visit three weeks ago.

O: BP 110/70, temperature 98.6, height 5'9", weight 150 lbs.; well-developed, well-nourished adolescent male, appropriate dress, defensive postures. Patient's speech was appropriate, a little reticent and flat initially but eventually became more animated and normal. Thought processes intact, well organized and logical; abstract reasoning and computative skills intact and normal, associations appropriate. Patient denies any suicidal ideation; says that he has "wondered what it would be like to be dead" but states that he certainly doesn't want to know about it "right now." Admits that he sometimes gets so "shaky" inside that he is afraid he will die. Patient's overall judgment and insight seem to be age appropriate. Patient is well oriented to time and place; attention span is age appropriate. The patient seems generally bewildered by what he is doing and by the reactions of his parents and school officials to his behavior.

I spent 50 minutes of face-to-face time with this young man today.

A: Depression.

P:
1. Administer the children's depression inventory; the children's depression scale and depression self-rating scale.
2. Psychotherapy twice weekly for now
3. Consider Desyrel or Prozac once testing is completed.

(Single organ system—psychiatric)

QUICK TIP

It may also be appropriate to report a psychiatric diagnostic interview examination if this service was performed by a psychologist and not a psychiatrist.

99205

DOCUMENTATION REQUIREMENTS

Medical Decision Making: High
- High number and complexity of problems addressed
- Extensive amount and complexity of data reviewed and analyzed
- High risk of complications and/or morbidity

History: Medically appropriate

Examination: Medically appropriate

Code Indicators (from the MDM table)

Number and Complexity of Problem(s)
- One or more chronic illness with severe exacerbation, progression, or side effects of treatment
- One acute or chronic illness or injury that poses a threat to life or bodily function

Amount and/or Complexity of Data
Each unique test, order, or document contributes to the combination of two or combination of three in Category 1 below.

- Extensive

(Must meet the requirements of at least two of the three categories.)

Category 1: Tests, documents, or independent historian(s)
- Any combination of three from the following:
  - review of prior external note(s) from each unique source*
  - review of the result(s) of each unique test*
  - ordering of each unique test*
  - assessment requiring an independent historian(s)

or

Category 2: Independent interpretation of tests
- Independent interpretation of a test performed by another physician/other qualified healthcare professional (not separately reported)

or

Category 3: Discussion of management or test interpretation
- Discussion of management or test interpretation with external physician/other qualified healthcare professional/appropriate source (not separately reported)

Risk of Complications/Morbidity or Mortality
High risk of morbidity from additional diagnostic testing or treatment

Examples only:

- Drug therapy requiring intensive monitoring for toxicity
- Decision regarding elective major surgery with identified patient or procedure risk factors

- Decision regarding emergency major surgery
- Decision regarding hospitalization
- Decision not to resuscitate or to de-escalate care because of poor prognosis

Time Spent on Date of the Encounter
- 60–74

Sample Documentation—99205

Level V Initial Office Visit

Reason for visit: "Need a new doctor."

History: This 47-year-old male states he "needs a new doctor" because he was discharged by his former physician about three months ago for noncompliance with hypertensive regimen. He has not seen anyone in the interim, and he takes his medications only sporadically when "it gets really bad." He uses a home BP monitor to check his blood pressure weekly. The patient sought treatment today following an episode of apparent amaurosis fugax last night, with vision returning to normal after about one hour. This was the first such episode for this patient who recognized the episode from his reading material. The patient also reports at least two episodes of probable TIA.

He was diagnosed with hypertension at age 38, and has been on a variety of hypertensive medications since then, with reportedly continual problems with various side effects of treatment. He has investigated a variety of alternative treatments for hypertension including various diets, herbs, and vitamins, acupuncture, various devices such as metal bracelets, prayer meetings, meditation, etc, in an attempt to control his disease without medications, with admitted limited success. He has not tried biofeedback training. He admits his blood pressure has not been well controlled.

Patient history is otherwise unremarkable. No surgery. Fractured ankle at age 24. No meds except antihypertensives and a variety of over-the-counter vitamins and herbal preparations.

His mother is alive and well at age 74, no known health problems except "her age." His father died of MI at the age of 57 and was hypertensive. He has one sister, age 50, who is overweight and hypertensive; he is divorced with two children ages 15 and 12 and apparently has little contact with the children but believes they are healthy. Grandparents apparently all died of "old age" at age 75 and older; his paternal grandfather died in an accident. Family history is otherwise unknown. He quit smoking about five years ago; was a one-pack a day smoker since age 16; drinks "four to five" beers three to four times a week; hard liquor rarely. Reports no illicit drug use; has lived with his girlfriend for the past four years; works as an executive for a manufacturing firm. Exercise includes walking "an hour or so" three to four times a week apparently depending on the weather. Otherwise the patient reports no other problems. Review of systems otherwise negative. See self-history form completed by patient.

Physical Examination:

BP supine 240/110 (left arm); P 80, BP (left leg) 254/118;

BP standing 226/112 (left); P 84; BP 222/110 (Right standing); R: 18, not labored; T: 98.8; weight 198 lbs.; Ht. 5'9"

Well-developed overweight white male in no acute distress.

Eyes—PERRL, EOMI, Fundi flat. + venous pulsations, arteriolar narrowing, copper wiring and A-V nicking. No hemorrhages or exudates.

ENT—good dentition, normal mucosa.

Neck supple, no masses or thyromegaly, no JVD

Respiratory—normal excursion, clear to percussion and auscultation.

Heart—regular rate and rhythm, S4 gallop and grade II non-radiating murmur at left sternal border. Normal carotid upstrokes with bruit on left.

Abdomen—rounded, soft, non tender, no masses or organomegaly. No aortic bruit or pulsation.

Rectal—normal tone, no masses, BPH Gr. I, heme neg.

(continued)

Sample Documentation—99205 (Continued)

Musculoskeletal back non tender, straight, motor + 4/4—all 4 extremities, no joint deformities.

Extremities—no clubbing, cyanosis, edema. Pulses +2 arms, +1 legs (no dorsalis pedis either foot).

Skin dry, normal turgor.

Neuro/Psychiatric—alert and oriented X3, normal gait and station, no focal defects. DTR's +2; affect defensive and anxious

Impression and plan:

1. Longstanding hypertension, uncontrolled, with probable end organ changes. Exam indicates no real emergency; therefore, will treat as outpatient. The patient indicates that lightheadedness and impotence are the most bothersome residuals.

2. Begin Moexipril 15 mgm qd.

3. UA, full chemistry panel, EKG, cholesterol today.

4. Return in three weeks, recheck orthostatics, K, and creatinine.

5. I had a discussion with this patient about his hypertension. The patient has a good understanding about the potential side effects of the various drugs used to treat his disease. I apprised the patient in detail of the potential side effects of not treating his condition. The patient expressed an understanding of the high risks of non-compliance, stating no one had "spelled it out before." I firmly explained to the patient that I would be willing to help him explore alternative therapy for hypertension, but only if he were to strictly adhere to a conventional regimen of therapy until his hypertension was well controlled and stable, and to explore the alternatives in addition to conventional therapy and not instead of it.

I spent 65 minutes with this patient today, including reviewing his previous records, examination, and a long discussion regarding the treatment of his uncontrolled hypertension.

(Single organ system—cardiovascular)

Level V Initial Office Visit

A 47 year-old white female presents to an OB/GYN on the advice of her primary care doctor. At her 'get established' visit there last week her hemoglobin was 6.3. He had wanted her to go to the hospital for transfusion. She refused and presents here today for evaluation.

This patient had a D/C four months ago in another state. Pathology was suggestive of perimenopause. She had been amenorrheic for the first two months following the D/C, then had a normal period menses last month. This month she has had an extremely heavy menses for 10 days. Her previous doctor started her on Climara .025 and Provera and she has not had a withdrawal period since. The plan was to have her stop her Provera, and expect a period, but he had doubled the dose up to 20 a day to try and keep her amenorrheic.

She has had some fatigue, occasional headache and dizziness. She states her heart feels like its beating fast. All other systems are negative by review with the patient.

Her past medical history is notable for the anemia, and her social history does not include alcohol, tobacco or social drug use. She has previously had three vaginal deliveries, G3, P3.

She is a well-developed, well-nourished pale white female in no acute distress. Her pulse is 92, BP 130/80 and weight is 190 lbs. A & O x 3, affect normal. Her neck and thyroid are normal. Her heart has regular rhythm with no murmur. Lungs clear. The abdomen is soft, non-tender, no masses, and the liver and spleen are non-palpable. No inguinal or axillary adenopathy. The vulva, vagina, periurethral, perirectal, periclitoral areas are normal. The cervix and uterus are normal and adnexa negative. Skin warm and dry.

Hurricane spray and a single-tooth tenaculum to the cervix result in its coming down moderately. Her uterus and vagina are well-supported.

Her diagnosis is menorrhagia with severe anemia. We discussed the complexity of the problem. She has tried a hormonal regimen in the past and it did not work. She tried a D & C and it did not work. There has been no anatomical problem found. I suggest a

(continued)

Sample Documentation—99205 (Continued)

hysterectomy as the only viable option. She understands this will make her infertile. We need to build up her hemoglobin and stop her period. The Hemocyte Plus bothers her stomach and she will be switched to a slow Iron. She is also taking Biaxin for upper respiratory problems and her chronic cough.

We need to keep her amenorrheic. We'll continue the Provera 20 mg per day. We'll give her Lupron 3.75 IM today. We discussed the risks and benefits of this. She will get a surge of estrogen in about 10–14 days. That is when she is likely to get a period. If the bleeding gets heavy, we can try switching her to Aygestin at that point. We will plan for surgery in about seven weeks. She should return in two weeks for a hemoglobin check. She will report any further bleeding in the meantime.

We also discussed Depo-Provera, but I am concerned that in about six weeks the lining may get too thin and she could bleed from that between the Depo-Provera and the Depo-Lupron. If there is any more significant bleeding she will need to be transfused. If this occurs in the next few days for any reason we will proceed with the hysterectomy much sooner to prevent another bleeding episode. One hour and 10 minutes was spent on the patient's case today, including review of records, documenting in the medical record, and face-to-face time with the patient.

(Single organ system—genitourinary female)

Established Patient (99211–99215)

QUICK COMPARISON

Office or Other Outpatient Services—Established Patient

E/M Code	Medical Decision Making	History	Exam	Time Spent on Date of Encounter
99211	Does not apply	N/A	N/A	N/A
99212	Straightforward	Medically appropriate	Medically appropriate	10–19 min.
99213	Low	Medically appropriate	Medically appropriate	20–29 min.
99214	Moderate	Medically appropriate	Medically appropriate	30–39 min.
99215	High	Medically appropriate	Medically appropriate	40–54 min.

☞ **KEY POINT**

Medical necessity is still the overarching criterion for selecting a level of service in addition to the individual requirements of the E/M code.

GENERAL GUIDELINES

The following guidelines apply to codes 99211–99215.

- Code selection is based on MDM or total time, including face-to-face and non-face-to-face time spent on the date of the encounter.
- History and physical examination elements are not required for code level selection for office and other outpatient services. However, a medically appropriate history and/or physical examination should still be documented. The nature and degree of the history and/or physical examination will be determined by the treating physician or other qualified healthcare professional reporting the service.
- Clinical staff may collect information pertaining to the history and exam and the patient and/or caregiver may provide information directly (e.g., by electronic health record [EHR] portal or questionnaire) that is reviewed by the reporting provider.
- Total time for these services includes total face-to-face and non-face-to-face time personally spent by the physician or other qualified healthcare professional on the day of the encounter.
- Physician or other qualified healthcare professional time may include the following activities:
  - preparing to see the patient (e.g., review of tests)
  - obtaining and/or reviewing separately obtained history
  - performing a medically appropriate examination and/or evaluation
  - counseling and educating the patient/family/caregiver
  - ordering medications, tests, or procedures
  - referring and communicating with other healthcare professionals (when not separately reported)
  - documenting clinical information in the electronic or other health record

- – independently interpreting results (not separately reported) and communicating results to the patient/family/caregiver
- – care coordination (not separately reported)
- Comorbidities or other underlying conditions should not be considered when selecting the level of service unless they are addressed during the encounter, their presence increases the amount and/or complexity of data to be reviewed and analyzed, or there is an increased risk of complications and/or morbidity or mortality.
- Use these codes if the patient has been seen by this physician/qualified healthcare professional or any other physician/qualified healthcare professional from the same practice and exact same specialty and subspecialty in the past three years.
- Consider using the appropriate critical care code instead of these codes if the physician provided constant care to a critically ill patient. Critical care codes are based on the patient's condition, not the site of service.
- Consider assigning the appropriate consultation code instead of these codes if the physician provided an opinion or advice about a specific problem at the request of another physician or other appropriate source.
- Report only the appropriate initial hospital care, hospital observation or comprehensive nursing facility assessment code if the patient was admitted to the hospital or nursing facility on the same day as another visit.
- Do not include the time spent by any other staff (nurse, nurse practitioner or physician assistant) towards the time threshold. Face-to-face and non-face-to-face time is the time the treating provider spent on the date of the encounter.
- Use case management codes when coordination of care is provided on a date without a patient encounter. Case management codes are "bundled" according to Medicare and cannot be billed to the carrier.
- Report prolonged services code 99417 with 99215, when the service runs 15 minutes beyond the time specified in the CPT® code narrative. The time must be clearly documented in the medical record.
- Append modifier 25 to report that a separately identifiable E/M service was performed by the same provider on the same date as a minor procedure or service. Only the content of the note documenting the separate E/M service should be used to determine the correct level of service code.
- Append modifier 57 to report that the decision to perform surgery was made during this visit. For Medicare patients, modifier 57 is used to report the fact that the decision was made to perform a major surgery (a procedure with a 90-day postoperative period).
- Append modifier 95 to indicate that the E/M service was rendered to a patient at a distant site via a real-time interactive audio and video telecommunications system. The communication between the physician or other qualified healthcare professional and the patient should be commensurate with the same key components or requirements of those that would be required if the service had been rendered in a face-to-face setting.
- Performance and/or interpretation of diagnostic tests or studies during an encounter are not included when determining the level of E/M service when reported separately. A separate code(s) for the diagnostic

 KEY POINT

Modifiers 25 and 57 are to be appended to the E/M code and not to the codes for other procedures that may be performed.

tests or studies performed in addition to the E/M codes may be reported.

- A test/study that is independently interpreted by the provider that is not separately reported but is part of the E/M service is considered part of MDM.
- CPT code 99211 is a nonphysician service and is usually performed as part of an "incident to" service as defined in the code descriptor. For more information on "incident to", see Chapter 4: Adjudication of Claims by Third-Party Payers and Medicare.

APC Note: Under the Medicare ambulatory payment classification (APC) system, the definition of an established patient is a patient who has been registered as an inpatient or outpatient of the hospital within the 3 years prior to a visit would be considered to be an established patient for that visit.

Also, it is important to note that the use of the CPT E/M codes in provider-based clinics and emergency departments for APC billing is not determined or reported the same as for a facility.

ISSUES IN THIS CODE RANGE

- Do not assign 99211 for a Medicare patient presenting for periodic surveillance unless the labs are drawn in the office.
- Codes for high-level E/M services have been targeted in the CERT program as being overutilized. Medical necessity and the level of medical decision making should be verified for all high-level E/M services.
- CPT code 99211 cannot be submitted to Medicare with a drug administration service (e.g., a therapeutic or diagnostic injection code, chemotherapy, or nonchemotherapy drug infusion code). However, if a medically necessary, significant, and separately identifiable E/M service that meets a higher complexity level than CPT code 99211 is performed in addition to one of these drug administration services, the appropriate E/M CPT code should be reported with modifier 25. Documentation should support the level of E/M service billed; a different diagnosis is not required. See Pub.100-04, *Medicare Claims Processing Manual*, chapter 12, section 30.6.

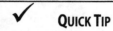

QUICK TIP

CPT Category II codes identify other health surveillance services considered part of the E/M service.

99211

DOCUMENTATION REQUIREMENTS

Problem Severity
- Problem not requiring the presence of the physician, but service provided under physician's supervision.

Special Coding and Documentation Considerations
- The concept of the level of MDM does not apply and time is not used in reporting this service.
- Report separately the codes for the diagnostic test or studies performed.
- Documentation of these nonphysician visits should be individualized to the patient, relevant to the problem present and include evidence of the evaluation and management of the patient and the presenting problem.
- The management documentation should clearly state the treatment or care plan related to the identified problem. It should also state who was involved in the development and initiation of the care plan and follow standard documentation guidelines, including date, patient name, and provider's signature with credentials. This documentation is to be part of the patient's permanent medical record.
- This code has been erroneously used to report nonphysician services that do not have an evaluation and/or a management component. Examples include:
  - taking of any or all of the routine vital signs (e.g., blood pressure check)
  - administering previously prescribed medication only
  - filling out forms
  - collecting blood or other specimens
  - dispensing educational material without further evaluation or management of the patient
- A blood pressure log alone is insufficient documentation. Appropriate documentation is important to substantiate services as medically necessary. For a service to be deemed medically necessary, most payers expect the service to be medically required and appropriate for diagnosing and treating the patient's condition and to be consistent with professionally recognized standards of medical care.
- Do not bill this code with any other E/M service provided on the same day.

Special Instructions for Code 99211

Wisconsin Physician Services (WPS), a Medicare contractor, released an updated article in September 2017 detailing findings from a CERT review indicating CPT code 99211 is an area of concern. As stated earlier in this section, the lack of supporting documentation continues to be an ongoing issue for providers. Oftentimes, an audit or medical records review will demonstrate documentation that simply indicates a lab service result or the type of service that was performed during the encounter such as "blood draw." However, reporting 99211-25 with a venipuncture code requires the documentation to demonstrate that a separately identifiable E/M service was performed. Clearly, noting "blood draw" does not substantiate a separate E/M service even if it is a low level encounter.

QUICK TIP

Code 99211 usually represents services provided by nursing staff when the provider does not see the patient.

Any E/M service should be considered medically necessary; that is, reasonable and required in order to make a diagnosis and treat an illness or injury. WPS has stated that a face-to-face encounter with the patient that includes the elements of an E/M service is necessary. Furthermore, WPS defines the evaluation portion of the service to be that "clinically relevant and necessary exchange of information between provider and patient" and the management portion to be the components that influence patient care such as medical decision making or patient education.

Sample Documentation—99211

Level I Established Patient Office Visit
The patient is here for monthly blood pressure check; no new problems or complaints; BP: 145/85; Wt. 215 lbs, pulse 88, Resp. 20. Scheduled an appointment with Dr. Jones next month; has enough meds to last until next appointment. Diet reviewed with patient.
Dr. Jones (signature)
J. Smith, RN
(General multisystem)

Level I Established Patient Office Visit
The patient is here for periodic lipid surveillance. Labs drawn. Results discussed with Dr. Underwood. Continue present regimen. Dr. Underwood has updated flow sheet.
(General multisystem)

Level I Established Patient Office Visit
Patient returns for blood pressure check after two weeks of current medication. Blood pressure remains at 160/98. Patient states compliance with medication and denies new or significant stress or other risk factors. Discussed the patient's response with the internist who requested the patient increase Vasotec from 10mg to 15mg daily and return to see him in one week. Patient to have blood pressure checked daily in the interim and bring log to appointment with internist.

99212

Documentation Requirements

Medical Decision Making: Straightforward
- Minimal number and complexity of problems addressed
- No or minimal amount and complexity of data reviewed and analyzed
- Minimal risk of complications and/or morbidity

History: Medically appropriate

Examination: Medically appropriate

Code Indicators (from the MDM table)

Number and Complexity of Problem(s)
- One self-limited or minor problem

Amount and/or Complexity of Data
- Minimal or none

Risk of Complications/Morbidity or Mortality
Minimal risk of morbidity from additional diagnostic tests or treatment

Time Spent on Date of the Encounter
- 10–19

Sample Documentation—99212

Level II Established Patient Office Visit
Patient comes in for suture removal; three sutures were placed in left index finger 10 days ago in the ED, following an accidental laceration from a broken glass. Tetanus booster given in ER.
Exam: Digit healing well. No erythema, exudate or tenderness.
Plan: All sutures removed without difficulty. Wound dressed. Patient given instructions on wound care; instructed to call with any problems.
(General multisystem)

Level II Established Office Visit
S: This 6-year-old male pt. returns today for follow up of left otitis media. Finished antibiotics three days ago.
O: Left TM clear, no signs of infection. Rest of ENT WNL.
A: Otitis resolved.
P: Return as needed.
(General multisystem)

 KEY POINT

The redefined MDM guidelines were published by the AMA in the 2021 edition of CPT and adopted by CMS in the CY2020 Physician Fee Schedule Final Rule.

 KEY POINT

The nature and extent of the patient history and physical examination are determined by the treating provider reporting the service.

99213

DOCUMENTATION REQUIREMENTS

Medical Decision Making: Low
- Low number and complexity of problems addressed
- Limited amount and complexity of data reviewed and analyzed
- Low risk of complications and/or morbidity

History: Medically appropriate

Examination: Medically appropriate

Code Indicators (from the MDM table)

Number and Complexity of Problem(s)
- Two or more self-limited or minor problems
- One stable, chronic illness
- One acute, uncomplicated illness or injury

Amount and/or Complexity of Data
Each unique test, order, or document contributes to the combination of two or combination of three in Category 1 below.

- Limited

(Must meet the requirements of at least one of the two categories.)

Category 1: Tests and documents
- Any combination of two from the following:
    - review of prior external note(s) from each unique source*
    - review of the result(s) of each unique test*
    - ordering of each unique test*

or

Category 2: Assessment requiring an independent historian(s)
(For the categories of independent interpretation of tests and discussion of management or test interpretation, see moderate or high)

Risk of Complications/Morbidity or Mortality
Low risk of morbidity from additional diagnostic tests or treatment

Time Spent on Date of the Encounter
- 20–29

Sample Documentation—99213

S: A 59-year-old male patient returning for recheck of prostatic hypertrophy discovered six months ago; he says Proscar has reduced the urgency and frequency and improved the diminished urinary stream and nocturia; he says urinary function is "not perfect but a lot better" than before. No dysuria; no other complaints except for seasonal allergies treated by his ENT physician. Medications sheet reviewed as well as health questionnaire.

O: Abdomen soft, no organomegaly, no masses. Bladder not percussible. Genitalia normal circumcised male penis; testes normal size; no masses; rectal sphincter tone normal; prostate enlarged, firm consistency. Rectal exam otherwise normal.

Labs: Urinalysis shows a few white cells, otherwise clear.

A: 1: BPH, stable at this time with improved urinary function on Proscar.
2. No indications of infection.

P: 1. Continue Proscar.
2. Recheck in six months; sooner if any change in urinary status or other problems.
3. Urinalysis on next visit.

How This Level of E/M Service Was Assigned

- **History:** Medically appropriate as deemed by the provider.
- **Physical Examination** Medically appropriate as deemed by the provider.
- **Medical Decision Making:** Diagnosis made by the physician is "BPH, stable—with improved urinary function on Proscar. Using the redefined MDM table published by the AMA and adopted by CMS, the note indicates that one stable but chronic condition was addressed, which equates to low number and complexity of problems addressed. A laboratory test (UA) is reviewed, which equates to a limited amount and/or complexity of data reviewed and analyzed. Level of MDM is based on two out of three elements; these two elements equate to Low MDM and code 99213.
- **Final E/M Level of Service:** CPT code 99213 is assigned.

Level III Established Patient Office Visit

A 48-year-old woman presents to her primary care physician complaining of a nine-day history of weakness, aching joints, cough and a sore throat. OTC meds provide temporary relief she reports on questioning. Fever to 102 on/off for five days, cough productive of thick green sputum.

Weight 290 lbs, Temp. 99.6, BP sitting 162/100. Obese WF in obvious discomfort. OP clear, no nodes, lungs clear w/upper airway mucus, CV RRR.

Imp. Bronchitis. Ceftin 25 mg, Muco-Fen 800.

(General multisystem)

99214

DOCUMENTATION REQUIREMENTS

Medical Decision Making: Moderate
- Moderate number and complexity of problems addressed
- Moderate amount and complexity of data reviewed and analyzed
- Moderate risk of complications and/or morbidity

History: Medically appropriate

Examination: Medically appropriate

Code Indicators (from the MDM table)

Number and Complexity of Problem(s)
- One or more chronic illnesses with exacerbation, progression, or side effects of treatment
- Two or more stable chronic illnesses
- One undiagnosed new problem with uncertain prognosis
- One acute illness with systemic symptoms
- One acute, complicated injury

Amount and/or Complexity of Data
Each unique test, order, or document contributes to the combination of two or combination of three in Category 1 below.

- Moderate

(Must meet the requirements of at least one of the three categories.)

Category 1: Tests, documents, or independent historian(s)
- Any combination of three from the following:
  - review of prior external note(s) from each unique source*
  - review of the result(s) of each unique test*
  - ordering of each unique test*
  - assessment requiring an independent historian(s)

or

Category 2: Independent interpretation of tests
- Independent interpretation of a test performed by another physician/other qualified healthcare professional (not separately reported)

or

Category 3: Discussion of management or test interpretation
- Discussion of management or test interpretation with external physician/other qualified healthcare professional/appropriate source (not separately reported)

Risk of Complications/Morbidity or Mortality
Moderate risk of morbidity from additional diagnostic testing or treatment.

Examples only:

- Prescription drug management

- Decision regarding minor surgery with identified patient or procedure risk factors
- Decision regarding elective major surgery without identified patient or procedure risk factors
- Diagnosis or treatment significantly limited by social determinants of health

Time Spent on Date of the Encounter
- 30–39

Sample Documentation—99214

Level IV Established Patient Office Visit

Chief complaint: One day history of left ear pain and discharge.

This 5-year-old female presents with left ear pain and discharge from the left ear canal. The mother reports the child awakened during the night complaining of pain in the left ear. The mother noted purulent discharge coming from the left ear canal which she states was increased this morning. The mother reports that the child was swimming in a lake at a family picnic two days prior to this visit. The child says she cannot hear well and appears to have difficulty in hearing questions. The mother says the child had a fever of 100 degrees this morning. The child indicates that her throat is sore; no G.I. complaints or other symptoms. She slept poorly last evening and refused to eat or drink. Immunizations are up to date. The child has had four prior episodes of serous otitis media associated with tonsillitis and pharyngitis; no prior episodes of otitis externa. She had chickenpox at age 16 months. No other pertinent history; no medications, no known allergies. Developmental milestones are within normal limits. No other family members are ill or have been within the past few weeks.

PE: Pulse 94 and regular, respirations 20 and unlabored, temperature 101.7; wt. 42. Well-developed, well-nourished child, appearing somewhat flushed, cranky and tired. HEENT normocephalic, no tenderness over the sinuses. Eyes clear, conjunctivae pink; nose, clear. Pharynx shows red, infected tonsils, +2 enlarged, no Koplik's spots on palate. Mouth otherwise normal. Left ear canal red, swollen with purulent material filling the canal and tenderness of the external ear. Right canal is clear—the TM is erythematous and slightly bulging. Fluid level noted retro-tympanically. The left TM was not visualized. Neck supple, minimal cervical lymphadenopathy present. Exam of the nose revealed yellow discharge. Chest is clear to P&A with no wheezes, rales or rhonchi. Heart regular rate and rhythm, no murmurs. Abdomen soft non-tender. No organomegaly. Skin: no rash, turgor good.

Impression:
1. Left otitis externa with possible tympanitis
2. Right otitis media
3. Acute tonsillopharyngitis

Plan:
1. 4 drops of Pedi-Otic were placed in the left canal, and the mother was given a prescription for same, three drops, TID x one week, both ears.
2. Amoxicillin Suspension 250 mgm TID x 10 days.
3. Recheck 10–14 days.
4. Consider ENT referral if no improvement.

Note: Decision making is moderate by the table of MDM, with an established problem worsening and a new problem and prescription management.

(Single organ system—ENT)

Sample Documentation—99214 (Continued)

Level IV Established Patient Office Visit

HX: A 55-year-old white female, hypertensive, here for follow-up; current meds atenolol 50 mg and HCTZ 25 mg daily. Complains of fatigue for the last few weeks , stating that she is tired and sleepy by the end of the day with trouble staying awake while watching TV. Fatigue is 7 on a scale of 10 compared to normal, No orthopnea, GU symptoms or palpitations. No other complaints.

PX: BP: 145/85, pulse 62, respirations 20, weight l58 lbs. HEENT: PERRLA; sclerae/conjunctiva clear. ENT normal; neck, no bruits, no JVD, or masses; lungs clear except for rare scattered high-pitched expiratory wheezes posteriorly; heart regular rhythm, no murmurs; gallops or rubs; abdomen is soft and non-tender. No hepatosplenomegaly. Extremities, no edema.

Labs: Hgb 12.4; potassium 3.2.

(continued)

Assessment:		
	1)	Hypertension controlled on present meds.
	2)	Mild hypokalemia due to diuretic.
	3)	Mild fatigue secondary to atenolol.
	4)	Mild bronchial constriction secondary to atenolol.
Plan:	1)	Continue atenolol and HCTZ as before.
	2)	Start potassium chloride tabs 8 mg TID with meals.
	3)	Explained cause of fatigue and assured patient that this is a common side effect of the medications that should improve with intake of potassium.
	4)	Recheck in two weeks and check potassium.

(General multisystem)

99215

Documentation Requirements

Medical Decision Making: High
- High number and complexity of problems addressed
- Extensive amount and complexity of data reviewed and analyzed
- High risk of complications and/or morbidity

History: Medically appropriate

Examination: Medically appropriate

Code Indicators (from the MDM table)

Number and Complexity of Problem(s)
- One or more chronic illness with severe exacerbation, progression, or side effects of treatment
- One acute or chronic illness or injury that poses a threat to life or bodily function

Amount and/or Complexity of Data
Each unique test, order, or document contributes to the combination of two or combination of three in Category 1 below.

- Extensive

(Must meet the requirements of at least two of the three categories.)

Category 1: Tests, documents, or independent historian(s)
- Any combination of three from the following:
  - review of prior external note(s) from each unique source*
  - review of the result(s) of each unique test*
  - ordering of each unique test*
  - assessment requiring an independent historian(s)

or

Category 2: Independent interpretation of tests
- Independent interpretation of a test performed by another physician/other qualified healthcare professional (not separately reported)

or

Category 3: Discussion of management or test interpretation
- Discussion of management or test interpretation with external physician/other qualified healthcare professional/appropriate source (not separately reported)

Risk of Complications/Morbidity or Mortality
High risk of morbidity from additional diagnostic testing or treatment.

Examples only:

- Drug therapy requiring intensive monitoring for toxicity
- Decision regarding elective major surgery with identified patient or procedure risk factors

KEY POINT

The redefined MDM guidelines were published by the AMA in the 2021 edition of CPT and adopted by CMS in the CY2020 Physician Fee Schedule Final Rule.

KEY POINT

The nature and extent of the patient history and physical examination are determined by the treating provider reporting the service.

- Decision regarding emergency major surgery
- Decision regarding hospitalization
- Decision not to resuscitate or to de-escalate care because of poor prognosis

Time Spent on Date of the Encounter
- 40–54

QUICK TIP

Although not in standard SOAP or SNOCAMP format, this note follows the flow of subjective, objective, assessment, and plan.

Sample Documentation—99215

Level V Established Patient Office Visit

Chief Complaint: A 61 y.o. white female with fever, weakness, weight loss and headaches x 3 weeks.

HPI: This patient reports fevers up to 102 degrees, no chills or sweats. Complains of bilateral headaches, worse in the morning. Denies having any of these symptoms prior to this illness. Has lost seven days of work in the past three weeks due to "just feeling bad." Notes anorexia, no dysphasia. Denies cough, rhinitis, ear pain or photophobia. Denies shortness of breath, sputum production, pleuritic or chest pain. Denies nausea, vomiting, diarrhea or abdominal pain. Denies flank pain, dysuria or urgency. Denies skin rashes.

Notes recent pain and stiffness in neck, shoulders and hips, not relieved by aspirin. Has had one episode of jaw pain while chewing. Admits to left-sided scalp tenderness.

Meds: Estrogen/Progesterone replacement, OTC multivitamins.

PMH: G4, P3, AB1, three children alive and well. Lives with her husband. No tobacco, uses alcohol socially, denies illicit drugs. Appendectomy age 15; fracture of right femur 20 years ago, no sequelae. No allergies. Prior to this illness, walked 5–7 miles a week and played tennis twice a week.

ROS: HEENT: Recent blurred vision such that she is afraid to drive. No dental problems. Pulmonary See HPI.

Cardiovascular: No pressure, pain, palpitations, syncope. No orthopnea, paroxysmal nocturnal dyspnea or dyspnea on exertion. O/W neg.

G.I.: See HPI.

GU: Menopause 10 Years ago. See HPI.

Musculoskeletal: No history of arthritis or joint problems. Now stiff and painful neck, shoulders, hips. Neurologic: See HPI. No focal weakness, numbness, paresthesias. No seizure history. Difficulty walking due to painful joints and weakness.

Physical Exam: Height 5'4". Weight 118 lbs. (-6 lbs. in 6 months). BP: 110/70 T: 100.5 P: 65 R: l8. General Appearance: Well developed, obviously fatigued white female in no acute distress.

HEENT: PERRLA, EOMI, conjunctiva and sclerae clear. TM's intact, nasal passages clear. Teeth in good repair without signs of infection. Swelling and tenderness over both temporal arteries. Artery on left no pulse is palpable. Bilateral temporal bruits 1/4.

Neck: Muscular stiffness noted. No bony tenderness, bilateral carotid bruits. No masses.

Lungs: Normal respiratory excursion, clear to percussion and auscultation.

Heart: Normal PMI, regular rate and rhythm; no gallops, murmurs or rubs. No neck vein distention. Abdomen flat, healed appendectomy scar RLQ, soft, no masses, organomegaly or tenderness.

Spine/Back: Non-tender, flexes to 90 degrees with effort, no CVA tenderness.

GU: Deferred to her gynecologist. Last exam 3 months ago reported as normal.

Musculoskeletal: Diffuse rigidity of hips and shoulders bilaterally. No redness, heat, effusions or focal deformities. Neck and deltoid areas markedly tender. No edema.

Skin: Warm, dry, no rashes, normal turgor.

Neurological: Alert, oriented to person, place and time. No focal defects, DTR's + 2 upper, + 1 lower.

(continued)

Sample Documentation—99215 (Continued)

Rectal: Normal tone, no masses; stool heme negative.

Impression: 1. Temporal Arteritis with Polymyalgia Rheumatica.
                 2. R/O occult infection, specifically UTI, abscess.

Plan: 1. CBC with Diff, ESR, UA.
           2. If ESR is elevated and CBC and UA do not show infection, start prednisone 60mg daily x 2 weeks and re-check. Clinical presentation precludes temporal biopsy at this time.

(General multisystem)

Level V Established Patient Office Visit

S: This 62-year-old female presents with a chief complaint of progressive weight loss, loss of appetite, fatigue, constipation associated with vague abdominal pain, vaginal itching and white discharge, occasional headaches and blurry vision. The patient reports these symptoms have been ongoing and steadily increasing over the past 6–8 months. The vaginal itching is severe at times and the constipation occurs at least once/week; she describes her stool as "rock hard." She occasionally notices blood on the toilet paper after defecating. The weight loss and decreased appetite are described as having been "noticed more by my family than me." The patient's diet consists of breakfast and lunch; no dinner is consumed. She snacks throughout the day consuming fruits, pastries and processed sweets. The patient states she has chronic hypertension and high cholesterol for which she takes medications. She has not modified her diet to accommodate the hypercholesterolemia because she says "the medicine makes up for it."

Past, Family and Social history reviewed and updated per chart entry September 18, 2003.

ROS: Blurry vision, especially noticeable while driving and watching TV. Headaches generally occur after these activities. Resp: no SOB. No cough. Cardio: no complaints except hypertension. GI: See HPI. GU: See HPI. Last Pap four years ago, normal. Pt. does report slight burning upon urination and reports this complaint for today at this time. Musculoskeletal: joints occasionally ache, more in the a.m. and subsiding as the day wears on. Neuro: no complaints. Endo: increased cholesterol, as noted. Denies diabetic history. General: fatigue, weight loss and decreased appetite as noted. Chronically cold. No fever, chills, diaphoresis. All other systems negative.

O: Weight: 155 lbs. Ht: 5'4". BP 140/110. Temp: 98.6. R: 16; P: 80. Slight gaunt appearance. Eyes: pupils round, reactive to light and accommodation. Sclerae/conjunctivae clear. Retinae: macular degeneration bilaterally. Fundi flat. Venous pulsations with arteriolar narrowing. Ears/EACs: WNL. Tympanic membranes WNL. Nose: nasal mucosa pink, healthy. No discharge. Throat: Tonsils absent. Posterior pharyngeal wall slightly erythematous. No exudate. Dentition poor; partially edentulous. Neck: no lymphadenopathy; thyroid nonpalpable. Heart: RRR; No murmur, gallop or rubs. Chest: normal breath sounds. No rales/rhonchi. Breasts: pedunculated; symmetrical; no mass/tenderness; nipples without discharge. Abdomen: soft, nontender. No organomegaly. Bowel sounds diminished. Musculoskeletal: normal gait. No tender joints. No muscle atrophy but pt. is extremely slender. Trace ankle pitting. Neuro: no deficits. Reflexes 2+. GU: vulva slightly erythematous. No gross discharge noted. Vagina: some whitish exudate noted—culture obtained. Mucosa slightly dry; no lesions. Cervical cuff WNL. Pap taken. No inguinale lymphadenopathy. Rectal: one external nonthrombosed hemorrhoid noted. Rectal vault: full, hard feces palpable. Several medium sized hemorrhoids noted. No visible blood. Hemoccult taken—positive.

LABS: UA—dipstick/microscopic: glucose +4; proteins 3+; ketones neg; all other neg. Micro: no WBCs. No RBCs or casts. No bacteria; rare candida albicans noted. Urine culture sent to outside lab. Fingerstick glucose—320 mg/dL. Hemoccult and Pap taken as noted. Vaginal culture/wet mount sent to lab. Blood/chemistry panel ordered via outside lab including thyroid profile. HgA1c pending. Creatinine clearance; 24-hour urine.

Review of medical records reveals hypertension and hypercholesterolemia, treated as noted previously. No elevated glucose at that time.

(continued)

Sample Documentation—99215 (Continued)

A: (1) New onset hyperglycemia; R/O diabetes mellitus. (2) Diastolic hypertension, uncontrolled on Monopril. (3) Proteinuria. R/O nephrotic syndrome; (4) Vulvovaginitis. (5) Weight loss. (6) Constipation. (7) Possible diabetic retinopathy with macular degeneration. (8) Internal/external hemorrhoids, bleeding occult. (9) Hypercholesterolemia, by history.

P: This patient had multiple issues that left untreated could be very dangerous to her well-being. My plan of treatment is as follows: (1) Hyperglycemia: patient counseled regarding proper diet and provided an ADA daily diet plan. The properties and progressive nature of NIDDM were discussed at length. HgA1c pending. Return for repeat glucose level when urine collection is complete. (2) Hypertension: add HCTZ 12.5 mg q.o.d. (3) Vulvovaginitis: Monistat vag cream, apply b.i.d. for five days. Add yogurt to diet. (4) Constipation/hemorrhoids: Colace 100 mg q.d. for 5 days; ProctoFoam: as directed. (5) Referral to ophthalmology for diabetic retinopathy consultation. (6) Nephrotic range proteinuria—testing as above. Will order renal US and/or refer to Nephrology as needed. (7) Make appointment with GYN physician for complete exam. Pap smear/vaginal culture info will be provided to pt. (8) Follow up in three weeks. Will discuss labs at that time and will determine efficacy of Mevacor. Will discuss ophthalmology findings with pt. when results are received.

(General multisystem)

KNOWLEDGE ASSESSMENT CHAPTER 5

See chapter 19 for answers and rationale.

1. History and physical examination elements are no longer used in selection of the level of office or other outpatient visits and therefore don't have to be documented in the medical record.
   a. True
   b. False

2. Total time on the date of the encounter includes non-face-to-face time. Which of the following activities personally performed by the treating provider may count toward the total time reported for purposes of code level selection? Select all that apply.
   a. Reviewing tests or other records
   b. Documenting clinical information in the medical record
   c. Ordering tests/procedures or medications
   d. Counseling and educating the patient or caregiver

3. Based on the time documented at the end of the sample documentation for 99205 that starts on page 114, code 99205 could be reported based on time alone.
   a. True
   b. False

4. A new patient presents to the office with two stable chronic illnesses. Limited data is reviewed, and changes are made to the patient's prescription drug regimen. Based on MDM elements, what level of service should be reported?
   a. 99203
   b. 99204
   c. 99214
   d. 99205

Chapter 6: Hospital Services (99217–99239)

Initial Hospital Observation and Discharge Services (99217–99220)

QUICK COMPARISON

Hospital Observation Services—Initial Care and Discharge

E/M Code	Medical Decision Making[1]	History[1]	Exam[1]	Counseling and/or Coordination of Care	Time Spent at Bedside and on Patient's Floor or Unit (avg.)
99217		Observation care discharge day management			N/A.
99218	Straightforward or low complexity	Detailed or comprehensive	Detailed or comprehensive	Consistent with problems and patient's or family's needs	30 min.
99219	Moderate complexity	Comprehensive	Comprehensive	Consistent with problems and patient's or family's needs	50 min.
99220	High complexity	Comprehensive	Comprehensive	Consistent with problems and patient's or family's needs	70 min.
1	Key component. All three components (history, exam, and medical decision making) are required for selecting the correct code.				

GENERAL GUIDELINES

- Hospital observation services codes are used to report services provided to patients designated as under "observation status" in a hospital.
- Three codes (99218, 99219 and 99220) describe "initial observation care, per day, with the evaluation and management of a patient." CPT® code selection depends on the level of complexity of the service, as defined by the three key components—history, examination and medical decision making.
- Code 99217 is used to discharge a patient from observation status when the discharge occurs on a date other than the initial date of observation. The patient does not need to be physically located in an observation unit, but does need to have a status of "observation" and not "inpatient." All of the observation codes describe "counseling and/or coordination of care with other providers or agencies"
- Codes 99218, 99219 and 99220 are appropriate for use by the supervising physician or other qualified healthcare professional whenever the patient has been designated as outpatient hospital

 KEY POINT

Observation status admissions may be to a specified observation area or to another hospital floor. The location of the bed is not as important as the patient's designated status of "observation" versus "inpatient."

"observation status," whether the patient was admitted to an observation unit or some other hospital unit for observation purposes.

- For reporting these services, unit/floor intraservice time includes both bedside services and those services rendered while on the hospital unit. Unit/floor time includes chart review, patient examination, record documentation, and communication with the patient's family and facility staff.

- In general, code 99218 is used when a patient is admitted for problems of low severity, code 99219 for problems of moderate severity and code 99220 for problems of high severity.

- It is important to remember that hospitals have their own guidelines regarding how long a patient can remain in observation status. Many hospitals do not allow a patient to remain in observation for longer than 23 hours, although Medicare guidelines under the outpatient prospective payment system (OPPS) allow for payment of up to 48 hours of observation, for certain conditions.

- For a patient admitted and discharged from observation status (or inpatient hospital status) on the same date, see codes 99234–99236. Observation care discharge, code 99217, is not reported in conjunction with a hospital admission immediately following discharge from observation status (i.e., subsequent to the patient being "changed" from observation status to hospital inpatient status. This change may or may not require the patient to be moved from a hospital observation unit to a hospital inpatient care unit).

APC Note: Under the OPPS, also known as ambulatory payment classifications (APCs), hospitals should not report as observation care, services that are part of another Part B service, such as postoperative monitoring during a standard recovery period. In the case of patients who undergo diagnostic testing in a hospital outpatient department, routine preparation services furnished prior to the testing and recovery afterwards are included in the payments for those diagnostic services. When the procedure(s) interrupt observation services, a hospital should determine the most appropriate way to account for this time. The hospital may record the beginning and ending time for each period of observation services during the encounter. The total length of time for the two periods of observation services would be the total number of units reported on the claim for the hourly observation services. A hospital may also deduct the average length of time of the interrupting procedure from the total duration of time that the patient receives observation services.

Facilities billing for observation services are required to report HCPCS Level II codes G0378 Hospital observation service, per hour, and G0379 Direct referral for hospital observation care.

Facilities should bill HCPCS code G0378 when observation services are provided to any patient admitted to observation status, whether an inpatient or outpatient. In addition to HCPCS code G0378, hospitals should bill code G0379 when observation services are the result of a direct referral to observation status without an associated emergency room visit, clinic visit, or critical care service on the day of or day before the observation services. These HCPCS codes will trigger OPPS Outpatient Code Editor (OCE) logic during the processing of the claim to determine whether the observation service is packaged with the other separately payable hospital

---

✓ **QUICK TIP**

Check with the hospitals where the provider has privileges to determine whether observation status must be limited to 23 hours or 48 hours.

---

services provided or whether a separate APC payment for observation services is appropriate.

Physicians should be diligent about documenting the admission of a patient from the observation unit to inpatient status. Under the Medicare APC system, if an "inpatient-only" procedure is performed on a patient still considered to be in observation, the procedure may not be paid under the APC system because the patient is still considered outpatient without an order to admit by the physician.

ISSUES IN THIS CODE RANGE

- Code 99218—Observation at the low level of decision making is a bit hard to explain. This code, and the code for the lowest level of hospital admission, indicates decision making of low complexity. It is highly unlikely that a patient will be placed in observation or admitted to the hospital unless they have either a new problem or a previous problem with at least mild exacerbation or progression. Unless there are limited diagnostics, or for some reason the history or physical is less than detailed—this code will not likely see much use. Both AMA tables place observation or admission at moderate level decision making at the least.

99217

QUICK TIP

Inpatient discharge codes have two levels based upon time, and observation discharge has a single code without time parameters.

DOCUMENTATION REQUIREMENTS

Parameters
- Includes final physical examination
- Includes discussion(s) regarding hospital stay and post-discharge patient care guidelines
- Includes preparation of discharge records
- Report this code only when the observation care discharge occurs on a date other than the initial date of observation status; for same-day observation care and discharge, see codes 99234–99236.

Duration of Time
- There are no time parameters set for reporting of this code.

Coding Exclusions
- Excludes *observation* encounters by other providers (i.e., other than the supervising physician); use codes 99202–99215 office or other outpatient service codes.
- Excludes services performed for patients admitted and discharged on the same date from an observation unit or observation care, and inpatient hospitalization (see codes 99234–99236 for further information).

99218

DOCUMENTATION REQUIREMENTS

Medical Decision Making: straightforward or low
- Minimal or limited number of diagnoses or management options considered
- Minimal or limited amount and complexity of data reviewed
- Minimal or low risk of complications or morbidity or mortality

Problem Severity: low
- Expectation of full recovery without functional impairment, or uncertain outcome or increased probability of prolonged functional impairment.
- Expectation of full recovery without functional impairment
- Low risk of morbidity without treatment

History: detailed
- Chief complaint
- Extended history of present illness (four or more HPI elements or the status of three chronic problems)
- Extended system review (two to nine systems)
- Pertinent past, family and/or social history (one of the history areas)

Examination: detailed
- 1995: two to seven organ systems or body areas with an extended exam of affected area(s)
- 1997: at least two bullet (•) elements from at least six organ systems or body areas, OR at least 12 bullet (•) elements from two or more organ systems or body areas. Eye and psychiatric single-system exams must include at least nine bullet (•) elements.

Code Indicators (from tables of risk—including some AMA indicators in italic)

Presenting Problem(s)
- One or more self-limited or minor problem, one stable chronic illness
- Acute uncomplicated illness or injury

Management Options
- Over the counter drugs, *medication management with minimal risk*
- Elastic bandages or superficial dressings
- Minor surgery, with no identified risk factors
- IV fluids, without additives

Counseling and/or Coordination of Care
- As appropriate for the problem

QUICK TIP

The history level is detailed, as there is not a complete ROS documented.

Sample Documentation—99218

Level I Initial Observation Care

S: A 52-year-old female was admitted to the hospital observation unit today after the sudden onset of left-sided renal colic this a.m. She is a known hypercalcemic stone former, from primary hyperparathyroidism, and has passed eight calculi in the past six years. She underwent a resection of her parathyroid adenoma four mos. ago, without complications. At that time, two nonobstructing calculi were seen in the left renal pelvis by x-ray. She has mild parathyroid bone disease without bone pain. Her pain is intermittent, severe and radiates to the vulva. She has vomited four times and is unable to keep down any liquids or oral pain meds. The pain is not relieved by any position, and she finds it difficult to lie still. Today's presentation is "exactly like my other episodes" of renal colic.

She has urinated several times today, small amounts, without dysuria or hematuria noted. No fever, sweats, chills, shakes. No diarrhea/constipation. No history of pyelonephritis. Pulmonary: no cough. Heart: no pain, palpitations or SOB. Current medications include Os-Cal and Rocaltrol, on taper.

PMH: No DM, HTN. Positive for appendectomy at age 21.

FH: Renal calculi in father; mother died of MI at age 70. NKA.

SH: Smokes one pack per day for 25 years; social drinker; lives with husband.

O: T: 97.4; R: 24; P: 104; BP: 138/84. General: well-developed, well-nourished slightly heavyset female in acute distress. Skin is dry without rashes; normal turgor. HEENT: unremarkable. Neck: parathyroidectomy scar midline below thyroid, healing well. No masses. Lungs: clear to percussion and auscultation. Heart: regular rate and rhythm. No gallops, murmurs, or rubs. Spine: nontender. Mild left flank tenderness. Abdomen: rounded, healed appendectomy scar RLQ, without tenderness; no hepatosplenomegaly. No mass. Rare bowel sounds. GU: deferred due to pain. Rectal: normal tone, nontender. Stool heme negative. Extremities: no clubbing, cyanosis, edema, tenderness. Pulses normal. Neuro: alert; oriented x 3. No gross focal deficits.

Labs: UA: pH 6; color clear yellow; Spec gravity 1.022; trace blood; 0-4 WBC/HPF; no bacteria; no casts. CBC w/ diff and chemistries pending.

A: 1. Recurrent renal colic; no signs infection.
2. S/P partial parathyroidectomy for adenoma.

P: 1. Admit to Observation. Patient is unable to maintain hydration or take oral pain medications secondary to vomiting.
2. IV hydration, parenteral analgesia.
3. Strain urine for stone passage. No need to send the calculus for analysis as we already know the composition of previous stones, the etiology, and she has received definitive treatment (partial parathyroidectomy).
4. Urine C&S.
5. Urology consultation requested.

(General multisystem)

99219

DOCUMENTATION REQUIREMENTS

Medical Decision Making: moderate
- Multiple number of diagnoses or management options considered
- Moderate amount or complexity of data reviewed
- Moderate risk of complications or morbidity or mortality

Problem Severity: moderate
- Moderate risk of morbidity without treatment
- Moderate risk of mortality without treatment
- Uncertain outcome or increased probability of prolonged functional impairment or increased probability of prolonged functional impairment

History: comprehensive
- Chief complaint
- Extended history of present illness (four or more HPI elements or the status of three chronic problems)
- Complete system review (10 systems)
- Complete past, family, social history (at least one element from all history areas)

Examination: comprehensive
- 1995: eight or more organ systems
- 1997: multisystem exam must include all bullet (•) elements from at least nine organ systems or body areas unless specific instructions limit content of the exam; at least two bullet elements from each area/system reviewed are expected to be documented.
  Single organ system/body area exam must include all bullet (•) elements in shaded boxes PLUS at least one element in each unshaded box.

Code Indicators (from tables of risk—including some AMA indicators in italic)

Presenting Problem(s)
- One or more chronic illness with mild exacerbation, progression, or side effects of treatment
- Two or more stable chronic illnesses
- Undiagnosed new *illness, injury,* or problem with uncertain prognosis
- Acute illness, with systemic symptoms (pyelonephritis, pleuritis, colitis)
- Acute complicated injury, e.g., head injury, with brief loss of consciousness

Management Options
- Prescription drug management
- Closed treatment of fracture or dislocation, without manipulation
- IV fluids with additives
- Minor surgery, with identified risk factors
- Elective major surgery (open, percutaneous, endoscopic), with no identified risk factors
- Therapeutic nuclear medicine

Counseling and/or Coordination of Care
- As appropriate for the problem

KEY POINT

Note that history is comprehensive due to addition of documentation "ROS otherwise negative."

✓ **QUICK TIP**

Comprehensive exam per 1995 guidelines are for eight or more organ systems.

Sample Documentation—99219

Level II Initial Observation Care

S: A 52-year-old female was admitted to the hospital observation unit today after the sudden onset of left-sided renal colic this a.m. She is a known hypercalcemic stone former, from primary hyperparathyroidism, and has passed eight calculi in the past six years. She underwent a resection of her parathyroid adenoma four mos. ago, without complications. At that time, two nonobstructing calculi were seen in the left renal pelvis by x-ray. She has mild parathyroid bone disease without bone pain. Her pain is intermittent, severe and radiates to the vulva. She has vomited four times and is unable to keep down any liquids or oral pain meds. The pain is not relieved by any position, and she finds it difficult to lie still. Today's presentation is "exactly like my other episodes" of renal colic.

She has urinated several times today, small amounts, without dysuria or hematuria noted. No fever, sweats, chills, shakes. No diarrhea/constipation. No history of pyelonephritis. Pulmonary: no cough. Heart: no pain, palpitations or SOB. Current medications include Os-Cal and Rocaltrol, on taper. *ROS otherwise negative.*

PMH: No DM, HTN. Positive for appendectomy at age 21.

FH: Renal calculi in father; mother died of MI at age 70. NKA.

SH: Smokes one pack per day for 25 years; social drinker; lives with husband.

O: T: 97.4; R: 24; P: 104; BP: 138/84. General: well-developed, well-nourished slightly heavyset female in acute distress. Skin is dry without rashes; normal turgor. HEENT: unremarkable. Neck: parathyroidectomy scar midline below thyroid, healing well. No masses. Lungs: clear to percussion and auscultation. Heart: regular rate and rhythm. No gallops, murmurs, or rubs. Spine: nontender. Mild left flank tenderness. Abdomen: rounded, healed appendectomy scar RLQ, without tenderness; no hepatosplenomegaly. No mass. Rare bowel sounds. GU: deferred due to pain. Rectal: normal tone, nontender. Stool heme negative. Extremities: no clubbing, cyanosis, edema, tenderness. Pulses normal. Neuro: alert; oriented x 3. No gross focal deficits.

Labs: UA: pH 6; color clear yellow; Spec gravity 1.022; trace blood; 0-4 WBC/HPF; no bacteria; no casts. Stat KUB: radiopaque calculus, 0.6 diameter, at the utero-vesicular junction. CBC w/ diff and chemistries pending.

A: 1. Recurrent renal colic; no signs infection.
    2. S/P partial parathyroidectomy for adenoma.

P: 1. Admit to Observation. Patient is unable to maintain hydration or take oral pain medications secondary to vomiting.
    2. IV hydration, parenteral analgesia.
    3. Strain urine for stone passage. No need to send the calculus for analysis as we already know the composition of previous stones, the etiology, and she has received definitive treatment (partial parathyroidectomy).
    4. Urine C&S.
    5. Urology consultation requested.

Note: This is the same example as the 99218 example with additions in italic. This should indicate the minor differences between these code levels and documentation requirements.

(General multisystem)

99220

DOCUMENTATION REQUIREMENTS

Medical Decision Making: high
- Extensive number of diagnoses or management options considered
- Extensive amount or complexity of data reviewed
- High risk of complications or morbidity or mortality

Problem Severity: high
- Moderate to extreme risk of morbidity without treatment
- Moderate to high risk of mortality without treatment
- Uncertain outcome or increased probability of prolonged functional impairment or high probability of severe prolonged functional impairment

History: comprehensive
- Chief complaint
- Extended history of present illness (four or more HPI elements or the status of three chronic problems)
- Complete system review (10 systems)
- Complete past, family, social history least one element from all history areas)

Examination: comprehensive
- 1995: eight or more organ systems
- 1997: multisystem exam must include all bullet (•) elements from at least nine organ systems or body areas unless specific instructions limit content of the exam; at least two bullet elements from each area/system reviewed are expected to be documented.
- 1997: single organ system/body area exam must include all bullet (•) elements in shaded boxes PLUS at least one element in each unshaded box.

Code Indicators (from tables of risk—including some AMA indicators in italic)

Presenting Problem(s)
- One or more chronic illness with severe exacerbation, progression, or side effects of treatment
- Acute or chronic illness or injury that poses a threat to life or bodily function, e.g., multiple traumas, acute MI, pulmonary embolism, severe respiratory distress, progressive severe rheumatoid arthritis, psychiatric illness, with potential threat to self or others, peritonitis, ARF
- An abrupt change in neurological status, e.g., seizure, TIA, weakness, sensory loss

Management Options
- Elective major surgery with identified risk factors or emergency major surgery (open, percutaneous, endoscopic)
- Decision not to resuscitate or to deescalate care because of poor prognosis

- Parenteral controlled substances
- Drug therapy requiring intensive monitoring for toxicity

Counseling and/or Coordination of Care
- As appropriate for the problem

Sample Documentation—99220

Level III Initial Observation Care

S: Today a 32-year-old mother presents with her six-year-old daughter in my office. History of present illness earlier today revealed the child, well-known to me and my staff, developed a temperature elevation after a several day bout with what was believed to be a URI. Pt. was treated by her mother with OTC medications, including ASA. The illness progressed to nausea and vomiting, severe headache, lethargy and bilateral earaches.

ROS: General: lethargy, as noted. HEENT: mild symptoms of coryza initially including sore throat, bil. otalgia, nasal congestion. Resp: cough. CV: no complaints. GI: N&V, as stated. No diarrhea reported. Decreased appetite. GU: Normal urine output though mother thinks urine may be slightly darker. Neuro: noncontributory data. Musculoskeletal: multi-arthralgias that mother thought were associated with URI. Psych: irritable and not feeling well. ROS otherwise negative.

PMH: Benign medical history. Surgery: bil. myringotomies with tubes. Up-to-date with immunizations.

SH: Unremarkable. Lives with mother, father and two siblings—one older, one younger.

FH: Unremarkable. Sibling History: Unremarkable.

O: T: 104.0. P: 112; R: 24; BP: 90/60. General: well-developed, well-nourished very ill-appearing and lethargic little girl. Alert. Oriented. Appears of above-average intelligence. Listens intently to questions; responds appropriately. HEENT: atraumatic; normocephalic. Eyes with injected, non-icteric sclerae. PERRLA. Ears: canals clean. Fluid levels visible in middle ear spaces. Myringotomy tubes not seen. Nose: congested with exudates. Throat: pharynx red and injected. Tonsils +2 enlarged without exudates. Red. Dentition consistent with that of her age, in good health. Neck: stiff; resistant to movement. Positive Kernig sign. No cervical lymphadenopathy. Resp: No wheezing or rales. Lung fields clear to P&A. Good inspiratory/expiratory movements. Abdomen: soft; nontender. No hepatomegaly or splenomegaly. BS normoactive to hyperactive. Skin: fine macular rash over fleshy parts of limbs. Pt. denies pruritus. No petechiae. GU: normal genitalia. Rectal deferred. Musculoskeletal: F/AROM all extremities. Neuro: no deficits. DTRs WNL. Equivocal Babinski.

Labs: STAT CBC w/diff; blood chemistries with SGOT/SGPT and prothrombin time. UA. Lumbar puncture.

A: Differential diagnoses (1) Meningitis; (2) Meningo-encephalitis; poss. Reye's syndrome; (3) viral exanthem; (4) Bilateral serous otitis media.

P: Admit to pediatric observation unit. Lumbar puncture STAT for opening pressures, gram stain, cell count, glucose, protein cultures. Antibiotic therapy; hold treatment pending CSF gram stain and cell count. IV hydration; limit fluids initially. Infectious disease consultation requested. Discussed all of the above with parent; consent forms signed.

(General multisystem)

Level III Initial Observation Care

S: This 83-year-old male, diet-controlled diabetic, well-known to me for many years, presented to the ED complaining of increased angina. He has a history of HTN for 50 years, angina for 30 years and a previous inferior MI. This angina is similar to his usual symptoms: substernal, dull, nonradiating chest pain, without shortness of breath or diaphoresis. However, in the past three days it has occurred eight times during previously well-tolerated activities (card playing, short walks, lifting groceries). He has not been lightheaded. Pain is not pleuritic. The angina was relieved within 2–3 minutes by sublingual nitroglycerin until today, when he developed angina three hours ago while walking the dog, and it is only partially alleviated after three sublingual nitroglycerin tablets. Patient takes Atenolol 100 mg q.d. and ASA on a daily basis.

(continued)

 KEY POINT

Note that the patient is admitted to observation status in the pediatric unit.

Sample Documentation—99220 (Continued)

ROS: HEENT: treated diabetic retinopathy. Wears glasses to watch TV. No recent URIs. Admits to sl. headache after the nitroglycerin ingestion earlier. Chest/Resp: No recent lower resp. tract infections. No cough. Cardio: See HPI. GI: no generalized dyspepsia. No NVD. No abdominal pain. GU: Stable nocturia due to BPH. Musculoskeletal: joint stiffness generalized. Worse in a.m. Neuro: no weakness. Endo: diabetes, as stated. Psych: Denies depression. ROS o/w neg.

PMH: Appendectomy 30 years ago; no recent surgeries or injuries except laser treatment for diabetic retinopathy.

FH: Positive for CAD in both mother and father. Only child; no siblings. One son, age 60 with hypertension.

SH: Smoked 2 PPD; ETOH—2–3 beers/day until 30 years ago. Quit both after initial MI. Wife deceased. Lives with grandson; leads fairly active life.

O: T: 98.4. P: 60. R: 24. BP: 138/88; Ht: 5'7"; Wt: 130 pounds. General: alert; oriented X 3. Normal affect. General: Slender gentleman appearing in relatively good health. HEENT: normocephalic; atraumatic. Ears, eyes, nose, throat all WNL. Dentition poor. PERRLA. Sclerae noninjected. Conjunctivae clear. EOMI. Fundi: evidence of laser treatment. Cardio: normal S1, S2. No rub, murmur. S4 gallop. RRR. Neck: jugulars nondistended; carotid bruits bilaterally. Thyroid: palpable, normal size. No nodules. Chest: normal but sl. shallow breath sounds. No rales/ rhonchi. No sternal tenderness. GI: abdomen scaphoid; nontender. No organomegaly. BS active. GU: deferred. Rectal deferred. Musculoskeletal: Gait WNL. FROM. Some joint tenderness over knees, hips. No lower extremity edema. Sl. dorsal kyphosis. Neuro: no deficits. DTRs +1, normal. Skin: pale. No cyanosis; no decrease in subcutaneous tissue or muscle mass.

EKG: similar to last EKG (six mos. ago). RRR 60. PR 0.2; QRS 0.10; axis +15. Old inferior Q-waves. No new T-wave inversion or ST-segment changes.

A: R/O MI; R/O unstable angina.

P: Admit to Observation Area.
1. Cardiac monitor.
2. Two liters O2.
3. Oximetry.
4. Serial EKGs and cardiac enzymes q 8 hrs.
5. Continue Atenolol, ASA.
6. Nitro drip titrates to relieve angina.
7. Morphine 1–2 mg IV PRN severe pain.
8. Cardiology consultation requested.
9. Tylenol for nitro H/A PRN.
10. If patient develops an MI, TPA is relatively contraindicated due to advanced age and diabetic retinopathy.

(General multisystem)

Subsequent Hospital Observation Services (99224–99226)

QUICK COMPARISON

Hospital Observation Services—Subsequent Care[1]

E/M Code [3]	Medical Decision Making[2]	History[2]	Exam[2]	Counseling and/or Coordination of Care	Time Spent Face to Face/Floor/Unit (avg.)
99224	Straightforward or low complexity	Problem focused interval	Problem focused	Consistent with problems and patient's or family's needs	15
99225	Moderate complexity	Expanded problem focused interval	Expanded problem focused	Consistent with problems and patient's or family's needs	25
99226	High complexity	Detailed interval	Detailed	Consistent with problems and patient's or family's needs	35

1   All subsequent levels of service include reviewing the medical record, diagnostic studies and changes in patient's status, such as history, physical condition and response to treatment since last assessment.

2   Key component. For subsequent hospital observation services, at least two of the three components (history, exam, and medical decision making) are needed to select the correct code.

3   These codes are resequenced and are included in the CPT book following code 99220.

GENERAL GUIDELINES

- Hospital observation services codes are used to report services provided to patients designated under "observation status" in a hospital.
- Three codes (99224, 99225, and 99226) describe "subsequent observation care, per day, with the evaluation and management of a patient." CPT code selection depends on the level of complexity of the service, as defined by the three key components—history, examination, and medical decision making.
- Codes 99224–99226 are appropriate for any subsequent visit to a patient that has been designated as observation status. The patient does not need to be physically located in an observation unit but does need to have a status of "observation" and not "inpatient."
- Use 99224–99226 for any observation service/visit provided to a patient on a calendar day that is different from the date that the patient was designated as "observation status," admission, or discharge.
- For reporting these services, unit/floor intraservice time includes both bedside services and those services rendered while on the hospital unit. Unit/floor time includes chart review, patient examination, record documentation, and communication with the patient's family and facility staff.
- It is important to remember that hospitals have their own guidelines regarding how long a patient can remain in observation status. Many hospitals do not allow a patient to remain in observation for longer than 23 hours, although Medicare guidelines under the outpatient prospective payment system (OPPS) allow for payment of up to 48 hours of observation, for certain conditions.

- When a patient receives observation services for a minimum of eight hours and is discharged from observation status (or inpatient hospital status) on the same date, see codes 99234–99236.

ISSUES IN THIS CODE RANGE

- Frequently history and decision making are the most contributory components in this code range. Given that a patient will have had a complete history and physical on admission to observation, the subsequent exam is often limited to the affected area

- These codes are also one of the few code sets where an interval history is described. The specific elements of these histories are not defined in CPT or federal guidelines, but the labels of each level are suggested. A problem-focused interval history would focus on HPI since the last visit. The expanded problem-focused version would include some ROS. The detailed version would simply have more of the above in each area, but again as limited by what has occurred since the last visit.

- Also remember that floor/unit time can be counted towards these codes when applicable. Extra time spent reviewing labs or looking at films (not for them) can count towards the level of service.

- According to the Medicare guidelines, outpatient observation services are classified as acute services and usually do not exceed one day (24 hours). Some patients may require a second day of outpatient observation (48 hours or two calendar days). And, in some rare and exceptional cases, an outpatient observation placement may span more than 48 hours. Providers billing 99224–99226 should pay close attention to the number of days a patient was held in observation. Unless the provider has requested an exception to the denial of services, Medicare will deny all observation services after the third day.

- When a patient's condition worsens after the initial day of observation and the provider feels that an inpatient admission is warranted, the provider must admit the patient to inpatient status. Extended days on an observation unit are not a substitute for a medically appropriate inpatient admission.

99224

DOCUMENTATION REQUIREMENTS

Medical Decision Making: straightforward or low
- Minimal or limited number of diagnoses or management options considered
- Minimal or limited amount and complexity of data reviewed
- Minimal or low risk of complications or morbidity or mortality

Problem Severity
- Stability, recovery, or improvement

History: problem focused *interval* **history**
- Brief history of present illness or problem (one to three HPI elements)

Examination: problem focused
- 1995: one organ system or body area
- 1997: one to five bullet (•) elements in one or more organ systems/body areas

Code Indicators (from tables of risk—including some AMA indicators in italic)

Presenting Problem(s)
- One or more self-limited or minor problem, one stable chronic illness
- Acute uncomplicated illness or injury

Management Options
- Over-the-counter drugs, *medication management with minimal risk*
- IV fluids without additives
- Elastic bandages or superficial dressings
- Minor surgery, with no identified risk factors

Counseling and /or Coordination of Care
- As appropriate for the problem

Time Spent Bedside and on Floor/Unit (average)
- 15 minutes

✓ QUICK TIP

The history and physical exam documented are interval and appropriate for subsequent observation care services.

Sample Documentation—99224

Level I Subsequent Observation Care

Patient with progressive urinary urgency and frequency. Condition now improved. The patient has received Terazosin to improve voiding and Finasteride to help reduce the size of the prostate.

General: Alert, feels well, except as noted above: Temp: 94.7, BP: 140/90, pulse 72. GU exam unchanged from yesterday. No new symptoms or complaints

PSA moderately elevated, > 3 ng/mL, transrectal ultrasound detects abnormally large prostate

A: BPH

P:
1. Continue drug therapy
2. Refer for TURP if unresponsive to drug therapy
3. Discharge from observation

(General multisystem)

99225

DOCUMENTATION REQUIREMENTS

Medical Decision Making: moderate
- Multiple number of diagnoses or management options considered
- Moderate amount or complexity of data reviewed
- Moderate risk of complications or morbidity or mortality

Problem Severity
- Inadequate response to treatment or development of a minor complication

History: expanded problem focused *interval* **history**
- Brief history of present illness (one to three HPI elements)
- Problem pertinent system review (one or two systems)

Examination: expanded problem focused
- 1995: two to seven organ systems or body areas
- 1997: at least six bullet (•) elements in one or more organ systems/body areas

Code Indicators (from tables of risk—including some AMA indicators in italic)

Presenting Problem(s)
- One or more chronic illness with mild exacerbation, progression, or side effects of treatment
- Two or more stable chronic illnesses
- Undiagnosed new *illness, injury,* or problem with uncertain prognosis
- Acute illness, with systemic symptoms (pyelonephritis, pleuritis, colitis)
- Acute complicated injury, e.g., head injury, with brief loss of consciousness

Management Options
- Prescription drug management
- IV fluids with additives
- Minor surgery, with identified risk factors
- Elective major surgery (open, percutaneous, endoscopic), with no identified risk factors
- Therapeutic nuclear medicine

Counseling and/or Coordination of Care
- As appropriate for the problem

Time Spent Bedside and on Floor/Unit (average)
- 25 minutes

Sample Documentation—99225

Level II Subsequent Observation Care

Elderly white male with a history of stroke, atrial fibrillation, on anticoagulants referred to observation status yesterday with slurred speech and expressive aphasia.

No new complaints on today. No rash, fevers, or night sweats. No double vision or blurry vision, no speech or swallow difficulties. No memory or concentration complaints. All other systems unrevealing.

General Exam:

BP 208/86 | Pulse 78 | Temp 98.1 °F (36.7 °C) | Resp 18 | Wt 115 lb (52.164 kg) | NAD, pleasant and cooperative. CV, RRR Lungs CTA, Ab- soft and nontender

Neurologic Exam:

MENTAL STATUS

He is awake, alert, and oriented to person and place incorrect day, date but normal year and month. He follows simple and only some 2-step commands, no complex commands. Language impaired in naming, poor repetition, intact fluency and only mild difficulties in comprehension. Speech intact. Normal attention. Intact simple calculations.

SENSATION

Intact sensation to pin and proprioception. Vibration decreased to the ankles. There is no extinction to double simultaneous stimulation.

COORDINATION

No tremor at rest, posture, or intention. Rapidly alternating movements mildly slow in the UEs. [upper extremities]

GAIT and STANCE

Not tested.

CT Head without contrast

Impression: Stable pattern of chronic infarcts. No acute intracranial hemorrhage. No CT evidence of new infarction.

PT   32.1

INR   3.6

Patient discussed with Dr. Stephens from neurology

P: 1.   Differential diagnosis includes CVA/TIA, migraine, and myasthenia gravis. The most likely diagnosis in this patient is a CVA/TIA, since he has an extensive history of CVAs and TIAs. While a migraine can cause focal neurological symptoms such as dysarthria, the patient has no history of migraines and denies any headaches.

2.   Pure hypercholesterolemia - Pt's triglyceride is 127, HDL is 65 and LDL is 114 -Order Cardiac risk panel

3.   Hold Coumadin

(General multisystem)

99226

DOCUMENTATION REQUIREMENTS

Medical Decision Making: high
- Extensive number of diagnoses or management options considered
- Extensive amount or complexity of data reviewed
- High risk of complications or morbidity or mortality

Problem Severity
- Lack of stability or development of a significant complication or new problem

History: detailed *interval* history
- Extended history of present illness (four or more HPI elements or the status of three chronic problems)
- Extended systems review (two to nine)

Examination: detailed
- 1995: two to seven organ systems or body areas with an extended exam of affected area(s)
- 1997: at least two bullet (•) elements from at least six organ systems or body areas, OR at least 12 bullet (•) elements from two or more organ systems or body areas. Eye and psychiatric single-system exams must include at least nine bullet (•) elements.

Code Indicators (from tables of risk—including some AMA indicators in italic)

Presenting Problem(s)
- One or more chronic illness with severe exacerbation, progression, or side effects of treatment
- Acute or chronic illness or injury that poses a threat to life or bodily function, e.g., multiple traumas, acute MI, pulmonary embolism, severe respiratory distress, progressive severe rheumatoid arthritis, psychiatric illness, with potential threat to self or others, peritonitis, ARF
- An abrupt change in neurological status, e.g., seizure, TIA, weakness, sensory loss

Management Options
- Elective major surgery with identified risk factors or emergency major surgery (open, percutaneous, endoscopic)
- Parenteral controlled substances
- Drug therapy requiring intensive monitoring for toxicity
- Decision not to resuscitate or to de-escalate care because of poor prognosis

Counseling and/or Coordination of Care
- As appropriate for the problem

Time Spent Bedside and on Floor/Unit (average)
- 35 minutes

Sample Documentation—99226

Level III Subsequent Observation Care

S: A 71-year-old female with history of hypertension, chronic lymphedema, OSA, hypothyroidism, Sjögren's who was referred to observation yesterday for an evaluation of severe chest pain and tightness. Pain was reported to be sharp and towards the left side.

Denied chest pain this am. Said she had 2-3 BMs since last night and thinks that's what has helped her chest pain symptoms. Noted drop in Hgb 8.9 -->7.9 w/o any obvious acute bleeding.

ROS:

Constitutional: neg.

Respiratory: negative

Cardiovascular: negative

Gastrointestinal: constipation (resolved)

O: BP 106/58 | Pulse 64 | Temp 97.8 °F (36.6 °C) | Resp 20 | Ht 5' 3" (1.6 m) | Wt 100.608 kg (221 lb 12.8 oz) |

Head: Atraumatic. No tenderness or masses noted.

Neck: Neck supple. No tenderness. No adenopathy. Thyroid symmetric, normal size. Carotids 2+/4 without bruits

Lungs: clear to auscultation

CV: Regular rate and rhythm, NL s1, s2 and no murmurs, gallops or rubs

Abdominal: non-tender and non-distended, chronic lower ecchymosis edema

Ext: L shoulder w/ mild edema/ (post-op)

Neuro: no focal deficits

Tests/ Labs:

GLU 100, NA 137, K 3.7, CL 99, CO2 2, BUN 20, CREAT 0.4

PT   18.9 10/12/2010

INR   2.0 10/12/2010

PTT   29 9/3/2010

Pulse Ox (%): 98 %

CXR:

Cardiomegaly is unchanged. There is no congestion, acute infiltrate, or effusion.

Current Meds:

ALBUTEROL-IPRATROPIUM (DUONEB) 0.5-2.5	2.5 mL inhale every 4 hours. (3) MG/3ML IN SOLN Indications: Spasm of Lung Air Passages
Norco 10, Hydrocodone/APAP 10/325mg, 10-325 MG PO TABS	Take 1-2 Tabs by mouth every 4 hours as needed.
Metoprolol SR (TOPROL XL) 25 MG PO TB24	Take 0.5 Tabs by mouth once per day.
Docusate (COLACE) 100 MG PO CAPS	Take 1 Cap by mouth two times per day.
Polyethylene Glycol (MIRALAX) PO PACK	Take 1 Each by mouth twice daily as needed.
Senna (SENOKOT) 8.6 MG PO TABS	Take 2 Tabs by mouth every night at bedtime.
Omeprazole 20 MG PO CPDR	Take 1 Cap by mouth once per day.
Potassium Chloride (K-LOR) 20 MEQ PO PACK	Take 20 mEq by mouth four times per day.
Levothyroxine 137 MCG PO TABS	Take 137 mcg by mouth once per day.
Sertraline (ZOLOFT) 50 MG PO TABS	Take 50 mg by mouth once per day.
Multiple Vitamins-Minerals (CENTRUM CARDIO PO)	Take 1 Tab by mouth two times per day.

(continued)

Sample Documentation—99226 (Continued)

Furosemide 20 MG PO TABS	Take 2 Tabs by mouth two times per day. Limit sodium intake
Enalapril (VASOTEC) 5 MG PO TABS	Take 1 Tab by mouth two times per day. Limit potassium salt intake
HYDROCHLOROTHIAZIDE 50 MG PO TABS	1 Tablet every morning
Warfarin 2 MG PO TABS	Take by mouth. Use as directed.
Simvastatin (ZOCOR) 20 MG PO TABS	Take 2 Tabs by mouth every night at bedtime.

A/P:

A 63 YO with history of hypertension, OSA, SLE, hypothyroidism, with known abnormal stress test taken in last 30 days presents with complaints of severe chest pain. Workup remarkable for hypokalemia 3.2, hgb 8.9,

Given evidence of CAD on previous stress test, I personally reviewed the EKG tracing. Findings: EKG: with nonspecific TW changes (slight flatter) in V3-6.

1. CV: Chest pain, h/o CAD
   - likely non-cardiac given presentation (relief w/ BM).
   - cont ASA 81 mg daily
   - cont Toprol 12.5 mg daily, Vasotec 5 mg daily- with holding parameters
   - Lasix 40 mg bid on admission due to appearance of dehydration.
   - Noted drop in hgb while on IVF (? dilutional). Will stop IVF now and resume diuretics in am.
   - compression hose on.
2. Pulm: OSA
   - no longer wears CPAP per patient
3. Heme: anemia- hgb 8.9 --> 7.9, worsened by IVF dilution (baseline 10-11's)
   - stopped IVF
   - cont Coumadin for recent shoulder surgery
   - INR therapeutic
   - follow CBC
4. Endo: hypothyroidism, last TSH 4.036
   - cont levothyroxine 137 mcg daily
5. GI: constipation
   - senna S QHS, MiraLAX BID
   - Dulcolax suppository
6. Rheum: history of Sjögren's syndrome
   - off Plaquenil
7. Psych: depression
   - cont Zoloft 50 mg daily

(General multisystem)

QUICK TIP

Although the patient's current symptoms have resolved on the subsequent day of observation, the extensive past medical history and the management of several chronic conditions have resulted in high complexity medical decision making and detailed exam.

Initial Hospital Care (99221–99223)

QUICK COMPARISON

Hospital Inpatient Services—Initial Care, New or Established Patient

E/M Code	Medical Decision Making[1]	History[1]	Exam[1]	Counseling and/or Coordination of Care	Time Spent Face to Face/ Floor/Unit (avg.)
99221	Straight-forward or low complexity	Detailed or comprehensive	Detailed or comprehensive	Consistent with problems and patient's or family's needs	30 min.
99222	Moderate complexity	Comprehensive	Comprehensive	Consistent with problems and patient's or family's needs	50 min.
99223	High complexity	Comprehensive	Comprehensive	Consistent with problems and patient's or family's needs	70 min.

1 Key component. For initial hospital care, all three components (history, exam, and medical decision making) must be adequately documented in the medical record to substantiate the level of service reported, and are crucial for selecting the correct code.

CODING AXIOM

Medicare does not accept consultation codes. Use initial hospital care codes to report the first inpatient encounter by a physician. The admitting physician should append modifier AI Principal physician of record, to the initial hospital care code.

GENERAL GUIDELINES

- CPT guidelines indicate these services are reported only by the admitting/supervising provider; all other providers should report 99231–99233 or 99251–99255. Medicare and some payers may allow providers of different specialties to report initial hospital services and require the admitting/supervising provider to append modifier AI.
- Combine all E/M services performed on the same date by the same physician that are related to the admission, no matter where they were provided (e.g., emergency department, observation status, office or nursing facility), and report the appropriate initial hospital care code.
- Consider assigning the appropriate consultation code instead of these codes when an opinion or advice was provided about a patient for a specific problem at the request of another physician or other appropriate source.
- Report the lowest level of initial hospital care to Medicare when the admitting physician performed a detailed or comprehensive history and physical several days prior to admission and a lesser history and physical on the day of admission.
- Assign the appropriate critical care code if the physician provided constant attention to a critically ill patient on the same day of admission.
- For reporting these services, unit/floor intraservice time includes both bedside services and those services rendered while on the hospital unit. Unit/floor time includes chart review, patient examination, record documentation, and communication with the patient's family and facility staff.
- Report prolonged services codes 99356–99359 for E/M services that run 30 minutes beyond the typical time specified in the code narrative. The time must be clearly documented in the medical record.

- Assign modifier 24 to indicate that an E/M service performed during the postoperative period was not related to the prior procedure. The claim should show a different diagnosis from that for the surgery.

- Append modifier 25 to report that a separately identifiable E/M service was performed by the same physician on the same day as a procedure or service. Only the work involved in the separate E/M service should be considered when determining the appropriate code for the E/M service.

- Append modifier 57 to indicate that the decision to perform surgery was made at this visit. For Medicare, the decision must be to perform major surgery.

> ✓ **QUICK TIP**
>
> Modifiers 24, 25, and 57 are to be appended to the E/M code and not to the codes for other procedures or services that may be performed.

ISSUES IN THIS CODE RANGE

- If a patient is admitted late in the evening on the first day and the provider does not see the patient until the next day, the Admission H&P is billed on the second day when a face-to-face service is performed.

- Code 99221—Admissions at the low level of decision making is a bit hard to explain. This code, and the code for the lowest level of hospital observation, indicates decision making of low complexity. It is highly unlikely that a patient will be admitted to the hospital or placed in observation unless they have either a new problem or a previous problem with at least mild exacerbation or progression. Unless there are limited diagnostics, or for some reason the history or physical is less than detailed—this code will not likely see much use. Both AMA tables place observation or admission at moderate level decision making at the least.

- Remember that both the higher levels of admission require a complete ROS. Currently this is ten systems, and lacking a notation indicating that those systems not remarked upon are negative, a notation referencing at least ten systems is expected. This area is the cause of many failed documentation audits.

- Notes provided by NPPs resulting from a visit prior to that of the admitting physician's do not count toward the physician's documentation of an admission unless the detail is specifically referenced, such as the history area.

- In this section we find one of only a few E/M codes where the level of medical decision making is expressed as a range. Normally these levels are clearly indicated though the nature of presenting problem may state "low-moderate severity." In this case we see the level of decision making expressed as straightforward or low for code 99221.

99221

DOCUMENTATION REQUIREMENTS

Medical Decision Making: straightforward or low
- Minimal or limited number of diagnoses or management options considered
- Minimal or limited amount and complexity of data reviewed
- Minimal or low risk of complications or morbidity or mortality

Problem Severity: low
- Expectation of full recovery without functional impairment
- Low risk of morbidity without treatment

History: detailed
- Chief complaint
- Extended history of present illness (four or more HPI elements or the status of three chronic problems)
- Extended system review (two to nine systems)
- Pertinent past, family, and/or social history (one of the history areas)

Examination: detailed
- 1995: two to seven organ systems or body areas with an extended exam of affected area(s)
- 1997: at least two bullet (•) elements from at least six organ systems or body areas, OR at least 12 bullet (•) elements from two or more organ systems or body areas. Eye and psychiatric single-system exams must include at least nine bullet (•) elements.

Code Indicators (from tables of risk—including some AMA indicators in italic)

Presenting Problem(s)
- One or more self-limited or minor problem, one stable chronic illness
- Acute uncomplicated illness or injury

Management Options
- Over the counter drugs, *medication management with minimal risk*
- Elastic bandages or superficial dressings
- Minor surgery, with no identified risk factors
- Physical therapy
- IV fluids, without additives

Counseling and/or Coordination of Care
- As appropriate for the problem

Time Spent Bedside and on Floor/Unit (average)
- 30 minutes

Sample Documentation—99221

Level I Initial Hospital Care

Three-year old female admitted from office after presenting with three day history of fever, cough and malaise. Fevers to 102, cough worse at night described as 'wet and loose sounding'. OTC meds for cough and sinus ineffectual. Some night sweats, no chills, N/V, or GU problems. No Hx of respiratory problems, no prior surgeries. NKDA. Child attends daycare.

Physical Exam: Vitals per written chart WNL T: 103. Well-developed, well-nourished female child resting quietly, alert and oriented but somewhat lethargic. Head normocephalic. PERRLA-Fundi disc edges sharp. Both TMs red and injected. ENT: nose slight erythema, OP w/o exudates, neck supple, no nodes. No meningeal signs. Chest: breathing unlabored. CV RRR. ABD soft non-tender, no CVAT, no HSM. Neuro WNL. Skin warm to touch. Post tibial pulses +1 bilaterally. Muscle strength +2, and DTR's +1. X-ray reveals clear lungs.

Impression: Dehydration

Plan: 1.   Admit for IV hydration, pulse oximetry monitoring.

(General multisystem)

99222

DOCUMENTATION REQUIREMENTS

Medical Decision Making: moderate
- Multiple number of diagnoses or management options considered
- Moderate amount or complexity of data reviewed
- Moderate risk of complications or morbidity or mortality

Problem Severity: moderate
- Moderate risk of morbidity without treatment
- Moderate risk of mortality without treatment
- Uncertain outcome or increased probability of prolonged functional impairment or increased probability of prolonged functional impairment

History: comprehensive
- Chief complaint
- Extended history of present illness (four or more HPI elements or the status of three chronic problems)
- Complete system review (10 systems)
- Complete past, family, social history (at least one element from all history areas)

Examination: comprehensive
- 1995: eight or more organ systems
- 1997: multisystem exam must include all bullet (•) elements from at least nine organ systems or body areas unless specific instructions limit content of the exam; at least two bullet elements from each area/system reviewed are expected to be documented.
- 1997: single organ system/body area exam must include all bullet (•) elements in shaded boxes PLUS at least one element in each unshaded box.

Code Indicators (from tables of risk—including some AMA indicators in italic)

Presenting Problem(s)
- One or more chronic illness with mild exacerbation, progression, or side effects of treatment
- Two or more stable chronic illnesses
- Undiagnosed new *illness, injury,* or problem with uncertain prognosis
- Acute illness, with systemic symptoms (pyelonephritis, pleuritis, colitis)
- Acute complicated injury, e.g., head injury, with brief loss of consciousness

Management Options
- Prescription drug management
- Closed treatment of fracture or dislocation, without manipulation
- IV fluids with additives
- Minor surgery, with identified risk factors

- Elective major surgery (open, percutaneous, endoscopic), with no identified risk factors
- Therapeutic nuclear medicine

Counseling and/or Coordination of Care
- As appropriate for the problem

Time Spent Bedside and on Floor/Unit (average)
- 50 minutes

Sample Documentation—99222

Level II Initial Hospital Care

History: This is the fifth hospital admission for this 18-year-old female with significant history of chronic asthma since age eight. All of her prior admissions were for asthma. The patient is compliant with medication which currently includes Slo-bid 300 mg TID, Intal inhaler QID and PRN Albuterol inhaler. She was seen in the office two days ago with a flare-up of her chronic asthma requiring increased use of Albuterol. Chest x-ray and CBC were within normal limits; theophylline level was 12.0. Exam at that time showed bilateral expiratory wheezing with good air movement and no acute distress. At that time she was started on oral corticosteroids in addition to her usual drugs. She returned to our office today with no improvement of symptoms, and in fact, increased respiratory distress and dyspnea. She is admitted to the hospital in status asthmaticus. Denies fever, increased sputum, URI, or other asthma triggers. She lives with her parents and two siblings, and is a high-school senior. No prior surgery. No significant family illnesses. No known drug allergies. No alcohol, tobacco or drug use. She denies sexual activity and contraceptive use. Menstrual periods are regular. Immunizations are up to date. Review of systems is otherwise within normal limits except as noted.

Exam: BP 110/60, pulse 60, respiration 28 and labored, afebrile. Well-developed, well-nourished, anxious female in mild respiratory distress with audible expiratory wheezing. HEENT: Normocephalic; PERRLA; EOM intact; nasal septum midline, passages clear; dentition WNL; oropharynx clear. Neck supple with no JVD, adenopathy, bruits or thyromegaly. Chest is symmetrical with minimal costal retractions; nontender to palpation and percussion, breath sounds revealed bilateral expiratory wheezing with diminished air movement without rales or rhonchi. Heart shows S1 and S2 within normal limits without gallop, murmur, click or irregularity. Abdomen soft, nontender, no organomegaly. No CVA tenderness. Extremities revealed distal pulses intact; no cyanosis, clubbing or edema; no muscle atrophy. Skin WNL.

Labs: Admission chest x-ray within normal limits but with some evidence of pulmonary hyperaeration. No infiltrates noted. CBC within normal limits. Theophylline level 13.4.

| Impression: | Status asthmaticus |
| | Chronic asthma |

Plan:	1.	Admit for intravenous corticosteroids, intravenous aminophylline
	2.	Hydration and continue Intal Inhaler
	3.	Supplemental oxygen
	4.	See admitting orders

(Single organ system—respiratory)

- **History: CC:** "fifth hospital admission for this 18-year-old female with chronic asthma. She is admitted to the hospital in status asthmaticus. **HPI:** Extended, reviewing current status and recent status with specific data given. **ROS:** Integrated throughout the history portion of the note. "Review of systems is otherwise within normal limits except as noted" is acceptable documentation of unaffected systems/body areas. **PFSH:** Complete. History documentation equates to "comprehensive."

(continued)

Sample Documentation—99222 (Continued)

- **Physical Examination** (Single System—Respiratory): There are two constitutional bullet elements documented: (1) vital signs and (2) general appearance of patient. HEENT: Three bullet elements. Neck: Three bullet elements. Respiratory: Five bullet elements. Cardiovascular: Two bullet elements. GI: Two bullet elements are noted. Other systems noted in the documentation: Lymphatic: One bullet element. Musculoskeletal: One bullet element. Extremities: One bullet element. Skin: One bullet element. Neuro/Psych: One bullet element. Total number of elements noted in documentation: each element identified in the shaded boxes of the Single System—Respiratory exam and at least one bullet element in the remaining unshaded boxes. Therefore, the physical examination documentation equates to "comprehensive."

- **Medical Decision Making:** Diagnoses made by the physician are Status asthmaticus and Chronic asthma. There are blood tests ordered as well as a CXR. The patient is admitted to the hospital, and IV medications are started. The patient's problem is a chronic illness with severe exacerbation (high risk). With multiple diagnoses, moderate amount of data reviewed and high risk, the overall medical decision making is of "moderate complexity."

- **Final E/M Level of Service:** CPT code 99222 is assigned. If the patient had additional diagnoses or comorbidities, and if the attending physician had ordered more tests and/ or reviewed more clinical data, the level of service would have been reported as 99223.

Level II Initial Hospital Care

History: A 72-year-old white male admitted after falling down the stairs at home earlier today. He was in obvious pain in ED and was given sedating analgesics. Some of the history was obtained from his wife. He noted immediate severe pain in his left hip area and pain in his left shoulder. Denies head trauma, no LOC, no visual disturbances, no bleeding, neck or back pain. Past history is generally otherwise noncontributory. Family history non-contributory. He had an MI seven years ago followed by two-vessel CABG; he had gallbladder surgery at age 38 and a fractured ankle at age 19. He reports occasional problems with arthritis in his knees and shoulders. No medications and no allergies. All systems reviewed and are otherwise within normal limits. No dizziness, palpitations, tremor or muscle weakness; no GI or GU complaints.

Physical Exam: BP I40/85, temperature 98.7, pulse 80, respirations 22. Well-developed, well-nourished male, resting quietly in bed, alert, oriented and appropriate but drowsy secondary to administered med. HEENT: Head atraumatic. Negative Battles Sign. PERRLA-Fundi flat. ENT: no hemotympanum. Lungs clear with unlabored breathing. Neck/spine nontender. There is bruising over the left shoulder but no obvious deformity. Range of motion and muscle strength normal as far as can be assessed. Right shoulder and right and left upper extremities otherwise normal There is obvious deformity of the left lower extremity in the upper femoral area with eversion and foreshortening of the limb with marked tenderness and bruising over the area; knee and lower leg are normal; right lower extremity is normal. Both feet are warm to touch. Post tibial pulses +1 bilaterally. Normal finger to nose. No nystagmus. Muscle strength +2, and DTR's +1, with stocking response to touch and pinprick.

X-ray of both shoulders and upper extremities shows no bony or soft tissue abnormality. There are mild degenerative changes in the shoulder and elbow and generalized demineralization. X-ray of the left hip shows a comminuted fracture with dislocation of the fragments and subluxation of the shaft of the femur. The right hip is normal. There are mild degenerative changes in the hip joints, with some bony demineralization.

Impression: Comminuted fracture, left femur, as described on x-ray
Contusion, left shoulder

Plan:
1. Admit for open reduction, internal fixation of the left femur fracture after cardiology evaluation for cardiac risk.
2. UA for blood.
3. See admitting orders.

(General Multisystem)

QUICK TIP

It would be appropriate to append modifier 57 to indicate that this encounter determined the need for major surgery during this admission.

99223

DOCUMENTATION REQUIREMENTS

Medical Decision Making: high
- Extensive number of diagnoses or management options considered
- Extensive amount or complexity of data reviewed
- High risk of complications or morbidity or mortality

Problem Severity: high
- Moderate to extreme risk of morbidity without treatment
- Moderate to high risk of mortality without treatment
- Uncertain outcome or increased probability of prolonged functional impairment or high probability of severe prolonged functional impairment

History: comprehensive
- Chief complaint
- Extended history of present illness (four or more HPI elements or the status of three chronic problems)
- Complete system review (10 systems)
- Complete past, family, social history (at least one element from all history areas)

Examination: comprehensive
- 1995: eight or more organ systems
- 1997: multisystem exam must include all bullet (•) elements from at least nine organ systems or body areas unless specific instructions limit content of the exam; at least two bullet elements from each area/system reviewed are expected to be documented.
- 1997: single organ system/body area exam must include all bullet (•) elements in shaded boxes PLUS at least one element in each unshaded box.

Code Indicators (from tables of risk—including some AMA indicators in italic)

Presenting Problem(s)
- One or more chronic illness with severe exacerbation, progression, or side effects of treatment
- Acute or chronic illness or injury that poses a threat to life or bodily function, e.g., multiple traumas, acute MI, pulmonary embolism, severe respiratory distress, progressive severe rheumatoid arthritis, psychiatric illness, with potential threat to self or others, peritonitis, ARF
- An abrupt change in neurological status, e.g., seizure, TIA, weakness, sensory loss

Management Options
- Elective major surgery with identified risk factors or emergency major surgery (open, percutaneous, endoscopic)
- Parenteral controlled substances

- Drug therapy requiring intensive monitoring for toxicity
- Decision not to resuscitate or to deescalate care because of poor prognosis

Counseling and/or Coordination of Care
- As appropriate for the problem

Time Spent Bedside and on Floor/Unit (average)
- 70 minutes

Sample Documentation—99223

Level III Initial Hospital Care

History: This is a 49-year-old male presented to the ER with a 15-year history of alcohol abuse with known liver decompensation and cirrhosis. He came to the emergency room because of hematemesis which began about six hours before admission when he vomited three times. The first time he brought up bright red blood, the second and third times he brought up coffee-ground emesis. In the ED he was noted to be confused as to time and place and was febrile.

Past history: Reveals that his general health has otherwise been good with no hypertension, heart disease, renal disease, diabetes or other significant medical problems. He has two prior hospitalizations, one for nonspecific gastroenteritis with diarrhea and dehydration, and another episode about three years ago for mild liver decompensation with jaundice, ascites and peripheral ankle edema which responded to bed rest, diet and salt restriction. Review of systems at this time is otherwise within normal limits.

Family history: Father died at age 57 with acute varicocele hemorrhage with advanced Laennec's cirrhosis. His mother is age 69, in good health. One brother died at age 11 from complications of acute glomerulonephritis. No family history of hypertension, diabetes, coronary artery disease, or other hereditary or familial disorders. History was obtained primarily from his mother who accompanied him to the emergency room.

Social history: He is single, lives alone, and has a ninth-grade education; he is a construction worker but has been unemployed for seven months. He smokes a pack and one-half of cigarettes daily and uses alcohol on a daily basis, usually vodka. No regular medications; he drinks five or six cups of coffee daily.

Physical Exam: Well-developed/well-nourished male appearing older than his stated age. Temperature 100.1, blood pressure 112/84, pulse 68 and regular, respiration 28. He is lying in bed with purposeless movements of extremities, responds to questions but answers inappropriately. Conjunctivae pale, scleral icterus, PERRLA, EOMI. TM's intact; oral mucosa pale, teeth in poor repair, oropharynx not injected. Neck veins flat, no thyromegaly. Trachea midline. Lungs clear to percussion and auscultation. Heart regular rate and rhythm; no murmurs or thrills. Abdomen protuberant with a fluid wave; liver edge is 3 fingers below the right costal margin; spleen tip felt on the left; no tenderness. No abnormal venous pattern on the abdominal wall. No submandibular, cervical or inguinal adenopathy. 2+ pitting edema of the lower extremities; pulses normal. Cranial nerves intact; deep tendon reflexes diminished; Babinski negative, + Asterixis.

Labs: Lab results in the ED showed H&H of 6 and 19, WBC 21,000, with a shift to the left; bilirubin 6.2, 4.2 direct and 2 indirect; alkaline phosphatase 165; SGOT 310, SGPT 140; serum ammonia 174 (11-55); BUN 46; creat. 1.2; albumin 2.4; K 3-6; PT/PTT-prolonged.

Impression:	Hepatic encephalopathy	Rule out peptic ulcer disease
	Laennec's cirrhosis	Rule out alcoholic gastritis
	Hepatic decompensation	Rule out esophageal varices
	Portal hypertension	Rule out spontaneous bacterial peritonitis
	Esophageal varices with hematemesis	

Plan: He will be admitted and subsequently scheduled for immediate upper GI endoscopy. He will have blood cultures, urine cultures, peritoneal fluid culture, and chest x-ray to rule out infectious process. He will be transfused with packed RBCs to a hematocrit of at least 30. Lactulose enemas. NPO, careful diuresis. Follow electrolytes.

(General multisystem)

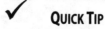

✓ QUICK TIP

The medical decision making is high with an extensive number of diagnoses and high risk with chronic illness with severe exacerbation and progression of disease.

Sample Documentation—99223 (Continued)

Level III Initial Hospital Care

This 42-year-old diabetic female Hispanic patient is admitted today with four-day history of fever, chills, harsh cough productive of moderate amounts of greenish and foul-smelling sputum, shortness of breath at rest and general malaise. Onset of symptoms occurred rather suddenly, though the patient admits to a mild dry cough for several weeks, changing to a productive cough over the last four days. Denies rhinorrhea or nasal congestion. Pt. fainted today after walking up a flight of steps; says she "could not find my breath and then got dizzy." Feeling weak and just "really sick." Temperature taken at home last night 102 degrees. Had TB as a child in her native country in South America. Was apparently treated successfully at that time without sequelae. No history of asthma.

ROS: Head: no complaints except for recent dizziness. Ears: no complaints. Eyes: wears glasses. Last exam five years ago in her native country. Nose: denies rhinitis, as above. Throat: extremely sore secondary to deep cough. Resp: Cough, SOB as above. Breasts: has never had mammograms; denies history of nodule/mass. Cardio: pt. is hypertensive, controlled with Monopril 20 mg/day. Takes her Bp every other day at local drug store. GI: no NVD. Appetite diminished. GU: no complaints. Last Pap some years ago—normal. Musculoskeletal: admits to general arthralgias with onset of fever. No history of arthritis. Neuro: Without complaint. Endo: pt. is diabetic; controlled on daily Glucophage 1500 mg/day. Last glucose level taken at home a few days ago by home glucometer—pt. doesn't remember the result. Admits to being less than compliant in taking the med and monitoring the blood glucose.

PMH: Hypertension and diabetes for years. No major surgeries. Usual childhood illnesses. Immunizations: unknown. Allergy: severely allergic to penicillins: hives, no anaphylaxis.

FH: Noncontributory. Mother was nonhypertensive; nondiabetic. Never knew her father and therefore history is unavailable. Three siblings, alive and well.

SH: No smoke/no ETOH. Doesn't exercise. Married, two children.

O: General: febrile-appearing female, short with barrel-shaped chest, lying supine in bed. T: 101.6; P: 72; R: 30, shallow, guarded. BP: 132/82. Head: normocephalic. No lesions, signs of trauma or fall. Eyes: PERRLA. Sclerae sl. yellow. Ears: Canals clear. TM's WNL. Nose: mucosa pale. No exudates. Turbinates sl. congested. Septum deviated to left. Throat: posterior pharyngeal wall erythematous. Tonsils small, red without exudates. Tongue geographic, thick. Dentition poor. Gold fillings throughout. Neck: +3 anterior cervical lymphadenopathy. Thyroid not palpable. Chest auscultation reveals LUL clear; LLL with high-pitched rales. RUL nonaudible; RML and RLL some wheezing. Chest percussion reveals dull sounds over RML/RLL but "tinny" sounds over RUL. Breasts: WNL. No mass or tenderness. Areolae WNL. No discharge. Cardio: Normal S1, S2. No murmur or rub. Abdomen: no hepato- or splenomegaly. Some tenderness over epigastrium. BS active. GU: deferred. Rectal: deferred. Skin: Dry; no petechiae or purpura. Extremities: Warm. No pedal edema. Pulses +2 in upper/lower extremities. No digital clubbing. No CVA tenderness. Neuro: no focal deficits. DTRs +2 upper extremities; +1 lower extremities.

STAT portable chest x-ray ordered. Laboratory tests ordered: SMA-12 including CBC w/diff. STAT ABG. Blood glucose; Hg A1c; UA; sputum culture/sensitivity, and gram stain, AFB x 3. Oximetry reported 90 percent.

A:
1. Community acquired pneumonia of LUL. Probably bacterial
2. R/O pneumothorax
3. R/O atypical pneumonitis
4. NIDDM
5. HTN

P: (1) Patient admitted today to Medical Service ward. (2) Await chest x-ray/labs. (3) Obtain pulmonary consult. (4) Begin IV antibiotics—erythromycin 500 mg q. 6 h. (5) Begin Tylenol for fever. (6) 1500 cal/day ADA diet. (7) Fingersticks before meals. (8) Lispro insulin before meals. (9) Hold Glucophage for now. (10) Resp. isolation. (11) Nasal oxygen 2 liters by nasal cannula.

Addendum: Patient now reports she thinks she has visited the ED about eight months ago for lower respiratory infection, at which time she underwent chest x-ray. Old films to be pulled for comparative review.

(General multisystem)

QUICK TIP

Addendum adds additional information that may be important to the treatment of the current illness.

CODING AXIOM

Codes 99224–99226 Subsequent hospital observation services, have been resequenced by the American Medical Association and can be found following codes 99217–99220.

Subsequent Hospital Care and Hospital Discharge Services (99231–99239)

QUICK COMPARISON

Hospital Inpatient Services—Subsequent Care[1]

E/M Code	Medical Decision Making[2]	History[2]	Exam[2]	Counseling and/or Coordination of Care	Time Spent Face to Face (avg.)
99231	Straightforward or low complexity	Problem focused interval	Problem focused	Consistent with problems and patient's or family's needs	15 min.
99232	Moderate complexity	Expanded problem focused interval	Expanded problem focused	Consistent with problems and patient's or family's needs	25 min.
99233	High complexity	Detailed interval	Detailed	Consistent with problems and patient's or family's needs	35 min.
99234	Straightforward or low complexity	Detailed or comprehensive	Detailed or comprehensive	Consistent with problems and patient's or family's needs	40 min.
99235	Moderate complexity	Comprehensive	Comprehensive	Consistent with problems and patient's or family's needs	50 min.
99236	High complexity	Comprehensive	Comprehensive	Consistent with problems and patient's or family's needs	55 min.
99238[3]	Hospital discharge day management				30 minutes or less [3]
99239[3]	Hospital discharge day management				more than 30 minutes [3]

1. All subsequent levels of service include reviewing the medical record, diagnostic studies and changes in patient's status, such as history, physical condition and response to treatment since last assessment.
2. Key component. For subsequent hospital care, at least two of the three components (history, exam, and medical decision making) are needed to select the correct code. Admission and discharge on the same date requires that all three key components (history, exam, and medical decision making) be adequately documented in the medical record to substantiate the level of service reported, as they are crucial for selecting the correct code.
3. These codes are not based on the three key elements of patient history, physical examination, and level of medical decision making. These codes are correctly assigned based on time, as the CPT code description indicates.

GENERAL GUIDELINES

- Use codes 99231–99233 for any inpatient evaluation and management (E/M) services provided after the first inpatient encounter, including reviewing diagnostic studies and noting changes in the patient's status. These codes also are used to report preoperative medical evaluation and/or postoperative care before discharge when these services were provided by a physician other than the surgeon.
- Use codes 99234–99236 for any E/M services provided by the admitting physician to an inpatient *or* an observation patient that is admitted and discharged on the same day.
- Consider assigning the appropriate consultation code instead of these codes when an opinion or advice was provided about a patient for a

specific problem at the request of another physician/qualified healthcare professional or other appropriate source.

- Consider assigning the appropriate critical care code instead of these codes if the physician/qualified healthcare professional provided constant attention to a critically ill patient.

- Codes 99238 and 99239 for hospital discharge services are appropriately assigned by the length of time devoted to performing the service (e.g., 99238 requires 30 minutes or less and 99239 requires more than 30 minutes). Use of these codes excludes services rendered on behalf of a patient who has been admitted and discharged from either observation status or inpatient status on the same day. See codes 99234–99236 for further instruction in these situations.

- For reporting these services, unit/floor intraservice time includes both bedside services and those services rendered while on the hospital unit. Unit/floor time includes chart review, patient examination, record documentation, and communication with the patient's family and facility staff.

- Report 99356–99359, as appropriate, for E/M services that run 30 minutes beyond the typical time specified in the code narrative. The time must be clearly documented in the medical record.

- Assign modifier 24 with this code for readmission during the postoperative period. The claim should show a different diagnosis from that for the surgery. For Medicare, subsequent hospital care reported with this modifier is reimbursed only if the service was for immunotherapy management by a transplant surgeon or critical care for a burn or trauma patient.

- Append modifier 25 to report that a separately identifiable E/M service was performed by the same physician on the same day as a procedure or service. Only the work associated with the separate E/M service should be considered when determining the correct E/M code to assign.

- Append modifier 57 to indicate that the decision to perform surgery was made at this visit. For Medicare, the decision must be to perform *major* surgery.

- For codes 99231–99233, append modifier 95 to indicate that the E/M service was rendered to a patient at a distant site via a real-time interactive audio and video telecommunications system. The communication between the physician or other qualified healthcare professional and the patient should be commensurate with the same key components or requirements of those that would be required if the service had been rendered in a face-to-face setting.

- If a patient is admitted as an inpatient with a discharge less than eight hours later on the same calendar date, codes 99221–99223 must be used for the admission, and no discharge service is billed.

Medicare requirements for observation codes: For a provider to use codes 99234–99236, the patient must be an inpatient or an observation care patient for a minimum of eight hours on the same calendar date. If the patient is admitted for less than eight hours, the appropriate codes are 99218—99220 and no discharge code.

The physician must satisfy the documentation requirements for both the admission to and discharge from inpatient or observation care to bill CPT

QUICK TIP

Modifiers 24, 25, and 57 are to be appended to the E/M code and not to the codes for other procedures or services that may be performed.

KEY POINT

For additional guidance regarding telehealth services during the public health emergency (PHE) due to COVID-19, refer to the Medicare FAQ, Section P, at https://www.cms.gov/files/document/03092020-covid-19-faqs-508.pdf.

codes 99234, 99235, or 99236. The length of time for observation care or treatment status must also be documented.

ISSUES IN THIS CODE RANGE

- Frequently history and decision making are the most contributory components in this code range. Given that a patient will have had a complete history and physical on admission, the exam is often quite limited to the affected area.

- These codes are also one of the few code sets where an interval history is described. The specific elements of these histories is not defined in CPT or federal guidelines, but the labels of each level are suggestive. A problem focused interval history would focus on HPI, since the last visit. The expanded problem focused version would include some ROS. The detailed version would simply have more of the above in each area, but again as limited by what has occurred since the last visit.

- These codes are best not assigned until the following day, particularly with patients whose condition is changing or in question. Remember that these are daily visit codes, a provider can't really know what the final level of service will be for that entire 24-hour period until after morning rounds.

- Also remember that floor-time can be counted towards these codes when applicable. Extra time spent reviewing labs, or looking at films (not for them), can count towards the level of service.

- Many providers have established conventions of coding inpatients by location in the hospital, for example, all patients in the ICU are critical care or 99233, while all patients on a general floor might be coded as 99231. Relative to coding, these types of conventions are a bad idea. The nature of the presenting problem for these codes is especially useful as they are typically one-line descriptors of the status of the patient, for example, "improving, inadequate response, serious complication," etc.

- In this section we find one of only a few E/M codes where the level of medical decision making is expressed as a range. Normally these levels are clearly indicated though the nature of presenting problem may state "low-moderate severity." In this case we see the level of decision making expressed as straightforward or low for codes 99231 and 99234.

- Swing beds billed by the hospital as inpatient services should be reported as inpatient services according to *Medicare Claims Processing Manual,* Pub. 100-04, chapter 12, section 30.6.9.D.

99231

DOCUMENTATION REQUIREMENTS

Medical Decision Making: straightforward or low
- Minimal or limited number of diagnoses or management options considered
- Minimal or limited amount and complexity of data reviewed
- Minimal or low risk of complications or morbidity or mortality

Problem Severity
- Stability, recovery, or improvement

History: problem focused *interval* history
- Brief history of present illness or problem (one to three HPI elements)

Examination: problem focused
- 1995: one organ system or body area
- 1997: one to five bullet (•) elements in one or more organ systems/body areas

Code Indicators (from tables of risk—including some AMA indicators in italic)

Presenting Problem(s)
- One or more self-limited or minor problem, one stable chronic illness
- Acute uncomplicated illness or injury

Management Options
- Over the counter drugs, *medication management with minimal risk*
- Elastic bandages or superficial dressings
- Minor surgery, with no identified risk factors
- Physical therapy
- IV fluids, without additives

Counseling and/or Coordination of Care
- As appropriate for the problem

Time Spent Bedside and on Floor/Unit (average)
- 15 minutes

Sample Documentation—99231

Level I Subsequent Hospital Visit

Gastric ulcer, now stable. Since admission, she has received three units of packed RBCs; hematocrit 29.9, hemoglobin 9.2. Tolerating clear liquids well. No GI complaints at this time. NG tube was removed. Stools remain somewhat melanotic and heme +.

Blood pressure, pulse, respirations are stable; temperature normal. Abdominal exam is basically unchanged from yesterday.

Endoscopy yesterday showed a large gastric ulcer at the lesser curvature of the angulus covered with a large clot; ulcer was benign in appearance, pathology report pending. She is now hungry and can be fed. I think that her acute bleed has stabilized, and she will be discharged in the next two to three days; there are no apparent cardiovascular or pulmonary complications.

(General multisystem)

 QUICK TIP

The history and physical exam documented are interval and appropriate for subsequent inpatient documentation.

99232

DOCUMENTATION REQUIREMENTS

Medical Decision Making: moderate
- Multiple number of diagnoses or management options considered
- Moderate amount or complexity of data reviewed
- Moderate risk of complications or morbidity or mortality

Problem Severity
- Inadequate response to treatment or development of a minor complication

History: expanded problem focused *interval* history
- Brief history of present illness (one to three HPI elements)
- Problem pertinent system review (one or two systems)

Examination: expanded problem focused
- 1995: two to seven organ systems or body areas
- 1997: at least six bullet (•) elements in one or more organ systems/body areas

Code Indicators (from tables of risk—including some AMA indicators in italic)

Presenting Problem(s)
- One or more chronic illness with mild exacerbation, progression, or side effects of treatment
- Two or more stable chronic illnesses
- Undiagnosed new *illness, injury,* or problem with uncertain prognosis
- Acute illness, with systemic symptoms (pyelonephritis, pleuritis, colitis)
- Acute complicated injury, e.g., head injury, with brief loss of consciousness

Management Options
- Prescription drug management
- Closed treatment of fracture or dislocation, without manipulation
- IV fluids with additives
- Minor surgery, with identified risk factors
- Elective major surgery (open, percutaneous, endoscopic), with no identified risk factors
- Therapeutic nuclear medicine

Counseling and/or Coordination of Care
- As appropriate for the problem

Time Spent Bedside and on Floor/Unit (average)
- 25 minutes

Sample Documentation—99232

Level II Subsequent Hospital Visit

S: Both the patient and the nursing staff note increasing redness around venous stasis ulcers. The patient is complaining of more pain in the area of the pretibial ulcer on the right lower extremity.

O: The patient is resting quietly in bed, but he is increasingly anxious about his condition. Blood pressure, respiration and pulse stable; temperature now elevated to 100.6. Lungs clear, CV RRR, + S4, No S3, no murmur. Large stasis ulcer in the pretibial area of the right lower extremity measuring 1 x 2.5 cm, unchanged from the last exam 24 hours ago. There is obvious erythema covering the ulcerated area about 3 cm. with a definite red streak extending proximally to just below the level of the knee. Skin is warm to touch, exquisitely tender adjacent to the ulcer and moderately tender over the red streak. The left leg shows two 2-cm ulcers, unchanged from the last exam with no surrounding erythema. The ulcer craters are filled with dry, intact eschar and there is 1+ edema of the left lower extremity.

A: Hospital-acquired secondary infection of the stasis ulcer with surrounding cellulitis and early ascending lymphangitis.
Edema due to local stasis.

P: 1. Debride eschar.
2. Swab ulcer crater for C&S of the purulent drainage, and stat gram stain.
3. Unasyn IV Q 6 hrs, pending results of gram stain and culture.
4. Elevate lower extremities on pillows to four inches above the level of the right atrium.
5. Start wet-to-dry dressings for large ulcer on the right lower extremity.

(Single organ system—skin)

QUICK TIP

Both history and physical exams are interval in nature. As the patient has had worsening of symptoms, the exam is expanded problem focused using 1995 guidelines and detailed using 1997 guidelines.

99233

DOCUMENTATION REQUIREMENTS

Medical Decision Making: high
- Extensive number of diagnoses or management options considered
- Extensive amount or complexity of data reviewed
- High risk of complications or morbidity or mortality

Problem Severity
- Lack of stability or development of a significant complication or new problem

History: detailed *interval* **history**
- Extended history of present illness (four or more HPI elements or the status of three chronic problems)
- Extended system review (two to nine)

Examination: detailed
- 1995: two to seven organ systems or body areas with an extended exam of affected area(s)
- 1997: at least two bullet (•) elements from at least six organ systems or body areas, OR at least 12 bullet (•) elements from two or more organ systems or body areas. Eye and psychiatric single-system exams must include at least nine bullet (•) elements.

Code Indicators (from tables of risk—including some AMA indicators in italic)

Presenting Problem(s)
- One or more chronic illness with severe exacerbation, progression, or side effects of treatment
- Acute or chronic illness or injury that poses a threat to life or bodily function, e.g., multiple traumas, acute MI, pulmonary embolism, severe respiratory distress, progressive severe rheumatoid arthritis, psychiatric illness, with potential threat to self or others, peritonitis, ARF
- An abrupt change in neurological status, e.g., seizure, TIA, weakness, sensory loss

Management Options
- Elective major surgery with identified risk factors or emergency major surgery (open, percutaneous, endoscopic)
- Parenteral controlled substances
- Drug therapy requiring intensive monitoring for toxicity
- Decision not to resuscitate or to deescalate care because of poor prognosis

Counseling and/or Coordination of Care
- As appropriate for the problem

Time Spent Bedside and on Floor/Unit (average)
- 35 minutes

Sample Documentation—99233

Level III Subsequent Hospital Visit

History: The patient reports 20 minutes of squeezing, substernal chest pain associated with shortness of breath, diaphoresis, and nausea. Pain was not relieved by two sublingual nitroglycerin, does not change with position. There has been no sharp chest pain. The pain began when she went to the bathroom. This was her first BM since admission and she had to "strain" a fair amount. Otherwise, system review is negative and unchanged since admission.

Exam: She appears to be in moderate discomfort. Temperature 98.6, pulse 80, respirations 22 and blood pressure 122/84. HEENT: EOMI, PERRLA, TM's normal, oropharynx clear. Neck: no jugular venous distention or abdominal jugular reflux. Chest: clear to auscultation and percussion; Heart: PMI midline. Regular rate and rhythm, no gallop or murmur or rubs. Pulses are full and equal in all extremities. Abdomen flat and soft, bowel sounds normoactive; no hepatosplenomegaly. Extremities: no edema, full range of motion without cyanosis, clubbing or edema. Skin is cool and clammy. EKG inverted T-waves laterally with acute I mm ST elevation and new reciprocal changes inferiorly.

Assessment: Four days status post subendocardial myocardial infarction with new onset of chest pain and EKG changes. Unstable angina, possibly extension of MI. Discussion with the patient and her family included discussion of diagnostic results, management options, potential medication side effects, and the need for consultation to evaluate patient for cardiovascular intervention.

Plan:
1. Nitroglycerin IV per protocol
2. Morphine IV per protocol
3. Stat cardiovascular surgery consultation
4. Begin heparin drip
5. Beta blocker, follow heart rate
6. Hold ace inhibitor

Note: This encounter could well require prolonged services or critical care by the time this day is over.

(Single organ system—cardiovascular)

Level III Subsequent Hospital Visit

S: Follow up note for 42-year-old female with pneumonia, HTN and DM. Patient feeling "a little better" today. Still feels SOB though this is improved. Appetite still diminished. Has tolerated small amounts of p.o. fluids. T-max 102 degrees/24 hours. No NVD. No polyuria/polydipsia.

ROS: No changes except as otherwise noted above.

PMH/FH/SH: Reviewed documented data with patient, now that she is feeling improved. No changes to note except that she does remember being ill at the time of her diagnosis of TB, though still cannot remember the details of medications, etc.

Admission CXR reveals diffuse infiltrates both lung fields, left greater than right. Apical scarring bilaterally. Small pneumothorax of LUL. No midline shift. No nodules. CBC/diff: WBCs 12,000. Diff—see lab report. Platelets 280,000. H/H 12/36. HgbA1c 9 (elevated). Fingerstick glucoses: 350, 220, 160 mg/dL. Admission ABG (room air): pH 7.29; PO2 64; PCO2 26; HCO3 18. A-a gradient 50. Oximetry 90-92 percent (2 liters O2). UA: WNL. AFB sputum #1 negative. Gram stain: gram + diplococci.

O: Vitals: Temp: 100.8. BP: 130/82. Resp: 26, shallow. Appearance: continues to appear ill though somewhat improved from admission. HEENT: no changes in eyes, ears. Throat: erythemic without lesion. No lesions over palate. Chest: auscultation reveals similar findings to that of yesterday. Neck: no change. Thyroid nonpalpable. Cardio: WNL. Abdomen: non-tender; no mass. Musculoskeletal/extremities: WNL. No joint tenderness. No peripheral clubbing or cyanosis. Neuro: no deficits. Remainder of PE within normal limits.

A:
1. Pneumonia, pneumococcal etiology
2. Pneumothorax, small, spontaneous, non tension
3. NIDDM
4. HTN

P:
1. Continue antibiotics as above, pending completion of Pulmonary consultation
2. Adjust IV fluids to 0.5 NSS at 40 cc/hour
3. I&Os
4. Continue sliding scale for NIDDM

(General multisystem)

QUICK TIP

The patient in this sample experienced an exacerbation or worsening of symptoms with resulting high medical decision making and detailed examination.

99234

DOCUMENTATION REQUIREMENTS

Observation or Inpatient Care Services (Including Admission and Discharge Services on the Same Day

Medical Decision Making: straightforward or low
- Minimal or limited number of diagnoses or management options considered
- Minimal or limited amount and complexity of data reviewed
- Minimal or low risk of complications or morbidity or mortality

Problem Severity: low
- Expectation of full recovery without functional impairment
- Low risk of morbidity without treatment

History: detailed
- Chief complaint
- Extended history of present illness (four or more HPI elements or the status of three chronic problems)
- Extended system review (two to nine)
- Pertinent past, family and/or social history (one of the history areas)

Examination: detailed
- 1995: two to seven organ systems or body areas with an extended exam of affected area(s)
- 1997: at least two bullet (•) elements from at least six organ systems or body areas, OR at least 12 bullet (•) elements from two or more organ systems or body areas. Eye and psychiatric single-system exams must include at least nine bullet (•) elements.

Code Indicators (from tables of risk—including some AMA indicators in italic)

Presenting Problem(s)
- One or more self-limited or minor problem, one stable chronic illness
- Acute uncomplicated illness or injury

Management Options
- Over the counter drugs, *medication management with minimal risk*
- Elastic bandages or superficial dressings
- Minor surgery, with no identified risk factors
- Physical therapy
- IV fluids, without additives

Counseling and/or Coordination of Care
- As appropriate for the problem

Time Spent Face to Face (average)
- 40 minutes

99235

DOCUMENTATION REQUIREMENTS

Medical Decision Making: moderate
- Multiple number of diagnoses or management options considered
- Moderate amount or complexity of data reviewed
- Moderate risk of complications or morbidity or mortality

Problem Severity: moderate
- Moderate risk of morbidity without treatment
- Moderate risk of mortality without treatment
- Uncertain outcome or increased probability of prolonged functional impairment or increased probability of prolonged functional impairment

History: comprehensive
- Chief complaint
- Extended history of present illness (four or more HPI elements or the status of three chronic problems)
- Complete system review (10 systems)
- Complete past, family, social history (at least one element from all history areas)

Examination: comprehensive
- 1995: eight or more organ systems
- 1997: multisystem exam must include all bullet (•) elements from at least nine organ systems or body areas unless specific instructions limit content of the exam; at least two bullet elements from each area/system reviewed are expected to be documented.
- 1997: single organ system/body area exam must include all bullet (•) elements in shaded boxes PLUS at least one element in each unshaded box.

Code Indicators (from tables of risk—including some AMA indicators in italic)

Presenting Problem(s)
- One or more chronic illness with mild exacerbation, progression, or side effects of treatment
- Two or more stable chronic illnesses
- Undiagnosed new *illness, injury*, or problem with uncertain prognosis
- Acute illness, with systemic symptoms (pyelonephritis, pleuritis, colitis)
- Acute complicated injury, e.g., head injury, with brief loss of consciousness

Management Options
- Prescription drug management
- Closed treatment of fracture or dislocation, without manipulation
- IV fluids with additives
- Minor surgery, with identified risk factors

QUICK TIP

Patients who are admitted and discharged on the same date should be seen by the provider at least twice, once for the decision to admit to observation or inpatient status, and once to determine that the patient is adequately improved for discharge.

- Elective major surgery (open, percutaneous, endoscopic), with no identified risk factors
- Therapeutic nuclear medicine

Counseling and/or Coordination of Care
- As appropriate for the problem

Time Spent Face to Face (average)
- 50 minutes

99236

DOCUMENTATION REQUIREMENTS

Medical Decision Making: high
- Extensive number of diagnoses or management options considered
- Extensive amount or complexity of data reviewed
- High risk of complications or morbidity or mortality

Problem Severity: high
- Moderate to extreme risk of morbidity without treatment
- Moderate to high risk of mortality without treatment
- Uncertain outcome or increased probability of prolonged functional impairment or high probability of severe prolonged functional impairment

History: comprehensive
- Chief complaint
- Extended history of present illness (four or more HPI elements or the status of three chronic problems)
- Complete system review (10 systems)
- Complete past, family, social history (at least one element from all history areas)

Examination: comprehensive
- 1995: eight or more organ systems
- 1997: multisystem exam must include all bullet (•) elements from at least nine organ systems or body areas unless specific instructions limit content of the exam; at least two bullet elements from each area/system reviewed are expected to be documented.
- 1997: single organ system/body area exam must include all bullet (•) elements in shaded boxes PLUS at least one element in each unshaded box.

Code Indicators (from tables of risk—including some AMA indicators in italic)

Presenting Problem(s)

- One or more chronic illness with severe exacerbation, progression, or side effects of treatment
- Acute or chronic illness or injury that poses a threat to life or bodily function, e.g., multiple traumas, acute MI, pulmonary embolism, severe respiratory distress, progressive severe rheumatoid arthritis, psychiatric illness, with potential threat to self or others, peritonitis, ARF
- An abrupt change in neurological status, e.g., seizure, TIA, weakness, sensory loss

Management Options

- Elective major surgery with identified risk factors or emergency major surgery (open, percutaneous, endoscopic)
- Decision not to resuscitate or to deescalate care because of poor prognosis
- Parenteral controlled substances
- Drug therapy requiring intensive monitoring for toxicity

Counseling and/or Coordination of Care

- As appropriate for the problem

Time Spent Face to Face (average)

- 55 minutes

99238

DOCUMENTATION REQUIREMENTS

Hospital Discharge Day Management

Duration of Time
- 30 minutes or less
- Constitutes the total duration of time spent performing the discharge service, even if the time spent on that date was not continuous

Parameters
- Includes final physical examination
- Includes discussion regarding hospital stay and post-discharge patient care guidelines
- Includes preparation of discharge records, prescriptions, and referral forms, among other documentation

Coding Exclusions
- Excludes services performed for patients admitted and discharged on the same date from an observation unit, observation care, or inpatient hospitalization (see codes 99234–99236 for further information)
- Excludes "discharge" of a patient from a specialist's care when the specialist is not the attending physician. These providers must report the subsequent hospital care codes to appropriately report these services (see codes 99231–99233 for more information).
- Excludes observation unit or care discharge; see code 99217 for patients classified as "observation status" when the discharge service is performed on a date other than the same date as observation status classification and/or admission
- Excludes nursing facility discharge (see codes 99315–99316 for further instruction)
- Excludes discharge services for newborns that are admitted and discharged on the same date (see code 99463 for more information)

Sample Documentation—99238

Hospital Discharge Day Management

S: This is the fourth hospital day for this 68-year-old white female admitted with congestive heart failure. She is totally symptom-free at this time. She has neither positional nor exertional dyspnea. She denies chest pain, she denies nausea. Her appetite has improved and is essentially back to normal.

O: This pleasant lady appears comfortable, she is neither dyspneic nor cyanotic. Inspection of the neck reveals no jugular venous distention. Auscultation of the heart is normal, sinus rhythm at 80 per minute without intermittencies or murmurs. Auscultation of the lungs: completely clear, no wheezes, rales or rhonchi. Examination of the lower extremities reveals no edema.

A: Congestive heart failure secondary to mild coronary artery disease, now compensated and stable.

P: Patient will be discharged home with the following discharge instructions:
1.   RX furosemide 20 mg p.o. q. a.m.
2.   RX Lanoxin 0.125 mg each a.m.
3.   RX isosorbide 10 mg p.o. TID
4.   Potassium chloride 6 mEq p.o. TID
5.   Arrangements for Meals on Wheels with no-salt-added diet
6.   Instruction sheet for no-salt-added diet given
7.   Arrange for visiting nurse home evaluation within 24 hours of discharge
8.   Arrange a follow-up visit at the office in one week, serum Lanoxin and potassium levels to be drawn at that time
9.   Family conference completed. Family members agreed to arrange for assistance for the patient with laundry services and housecleaning.

(Final hospital discharge, 30 minutes or less)

QUICK TIP

If the provider fails to indicate the time spent preparing the patient for discharge in the documentation, the time is presumed to be 30 minutes or less.

99239

DOCUMENTATION REQUIREMENTS

Hospital Discharge Day Management—Prolonged

Duration of Time
- Thirty-one minutes or more
- Constitutes the total duration of time spent performing the discharge service, even if the time spent on that date was not continuous

Parameters
- Includes final physical examination
- Includes discussion(s) regarding hospital stay and post-discharge patient care guidelines
- Includes preparation of discharge records, prescriptions, and referral forms, among other documentation.

Coding Exclusions
- Excludes services performed for patients admitted and discharged on the same date from an observation unit, observation care, or inpatient hospitalization (see codes 99234–99236 for further information)
- Excludes "discharge" of a patient from a specialist's care when the specialist is not the attending physician. These providers must report the subsequent hospital care codes to appropriately report these services (see codes 99231–99233 for more information).
- Excludes observation unit or care discharge; see code 99217 for patients classified as "observation status" when the discharge service is performed on a date other than the same date as observation status classification and/or admission
- Excludes nursing facility discharge (see codes 99315–99316 for further instruction).
- Excludes discharge services for newborns that are admitted and discharged on the same date. See code 99463 for more information.

☛ KEY POINT

The provider must document that the time spent was more than 30 minutes to report this code.

KNOWLEDGE ASSESSMENT CHAPTER 6

See chapter 19 for answers and rationale.

1. Based on the sample documentation for code 99219 on page 138, what is the chief complaint?
    a. Left-sided renal colic
    b. Hypercalcemic stone
    c. Hyperparathyroidism
    d. All of the above

2. Based on the sample documentation used for code 99219 on page 138, what level of MDM was documented?
    a. Minimal
    b. Low
    c. Moderate
    d. High

3. What elements pertaining to the MDM in the sample documentation starting on page 148 qualify the visit as a 99226 or high MDM?
   a. Numerous diagnoses
   b. Extensive amount of data reviewed
   c. New problem—chest pain
   d. All of the above

4. Documentation for a level 2 initial hospital visit (99222) requires a complete ROS. How many systems must be reviewed?
   a. Eight or more
   b. Ten or more
   c. Depends on what physician is documenting the visit
   d. Four or more

5. Based on the sample documentation for 99222 on page 155, what statement did the physician use to document that enough systems were reviewed to qualify as a complete ROS?

6. Codes 99234–99236 are used to report E/M services provided to an observation patient or inpatient admitted and discharged on the same day.
   a. True
   b. False

7. Based on the first documentation sample for 99233 on page 167 and using the Table of Risk provided with the 1995 and 1997 E/M documentation guidelines in appendix C or D, what elements were documented that qualify this visit as high complexity MDM? (Select all that apply.)
   a. Moderate discomfort
   b. Pain does not change with position
   c. New onset of chest pain with associated symptoms
   d. Starting a heparin drip

Chapter 7: Consultations (99241–99255)

Office or Other Outpatient Consultations (99241–99245)

QUICK COMPARISON

Consultations—Office or Other Outpatient, New or Established Patient

E/M Code	Medical Decision Making[1]	History[1]	Exam[1]	Counseling and/or Coordination of Care	Time Spent Face to Face (avg.)
99241	Straightforward	Problem focused	Problem focused	Consistent with problems and patient's or family's needs	15 min.
99242	Straightforward	Expanded problem focused	Expanded problem focused	Consistent with problems and patient's or family's needs	30 min.
99243	Low complexity	Detailed	Detailed	Consistent with problems and patient's or family's needs	40 min.
99244	Moderate complexity	Comprehensive	Comprehensive	Consistent with problems and patient's or family's needs	60 min.
99245	High complexity	Comprehensive	Comprehensive	Consistent with problems and patient's or family's needs	80 min.

1   Key component. For office or other outpatient consultations, all three components (history, exam, and medical decision making) must be adequately documented in the medical record to substantiate the level of service reported and are crucial for selecting the correct code.

GENERAL GUIDELINES

- Use these CPT® codes if the physician/qualified healthcare professional provided an opinion or gave advice regarding evaluation or management of a specific problem at the request of another physician/qualified healthcare professional or appropriate source. A consultation may also be necessary to determine whether the consultant is willing to accept transfer and ongoing management of the patient's entire care or for management of a specific problem. The consultant may initiate diagnostic or therapeutic services.

- Consultation codes are appropriate in many settings such as the physician's office, or outpatient or other ambulatory facility, hospital observation unit, patient's home, domiciliary/rest home, custodial care facility or emergency department.

- A written report must be sent to the requesting provider or source to be placed in the patient's permanent medical record. Required documentation includes the request for consultation, the need or reason for the consultation, consultant's opinion and any services that were ordered or performed.

 KEY POINT

Medicare and some commercial carriers do not accept CPT consultation codes.

- When a common chart is used, a separate report to the requesting provider does not need to be sent. Examples of a common chart include large multispecialty clinics with electronic medical records.
- Use the appropriate office consultation code if the consultant was asked again for an opinion or advice regarding the same problem or a new problem.
- Assign the appropriate critical care code instead of these codes if the physician provided constant attention to a critically ill patient.
- Assign the appropriate office visit code if the patient or family member and not another physician (or appropriate source) requested the consultation.
- Do not consider the time spent by other staff (e.g., nurse) as part of the face-to-face time.
- Report 99354–99359 for E/M services that run 30 minutes beyond the typical time specified in the code narrative. The time must be clearly documented in the medical record.
- Append modifier 25 to report that a separately identifiable E/M service was performed by the same physician/qualified healthcare professional on the same day as a procedure or service. Only the work involved in the separate E/M service should be considered when determining the correct level of service.
- Use modifier 32 when the services were mandated, such as by a third-party payer, or as a result of a governmental, legislative or regulatory requirement.
- Append modifier 57 to indicate that the decision to perform major surgery has been made.
- Append modifier 95 to indicate that the E/M service was rendered to a patient at a distant site via a real-time interactive audio and video telecommunications system. The communication between the physician or other qualified healthcare professional and the patient should be commensurate with the same key components or requirements of those that would be required if the service had been rendered in a face-to-face setting.
- Report separately the codes for the diagnostic tests or studies performed.
- Codes for high-level E/M services have been targeted in the CERT program as being overutilized. Medical necessity and the level of medical decision making should be verified for all high-level E/M services.
- Follow-up visits initiated by the physician consultant or patient are reported with the appropriate site-of-service codes (e.g., office visits) for established patients. However, if an additional request is documented in the record for an additional opinion or advice for the same or separate problem, the consultation codes may be reported again.
- Transfer-of-care services (for either specific condition or the patient's entire care) are reported with the appropriate new or established patient codes for the site of service.
- Medicare eliminated the use of all consultation codes with the exception of telehealth inpatient consultation G codes. See chapter 17 for more information on G codes. Report outpatient consultations with the appropriate E/M service code for the site of service and new or established patient.

✓ **QUICK TIP**

Modifiers 25, 32, and 57 are to be appended to the E/M code and not to the codes for the other procedures or services that may be performed.

99241

DOCUMENTATION REQUIREMENTS

Medical Decision Making: straightforward
- Minimal number of diagnoses or management options considered
- No or minimal amount and complexity of data reviewed
- Minimal risk of complications or morbidity or mortality

Problem Severity: minor or self-limited
- Little, if any, risk of morbidity without treatment
- Little, if any, risk of mortality without treatment
- Transient problem, low probability of permanently altered status
- Good prognosis

History: problem focused
- Chief complaint
- Brief history of present illness or problem (one to three HPI elements)

Examination: problem focused
- 1995: one organ system or body area
- 1997: one to five bullet (•) elements in one or more organ systems/body areas

Code Indicators (from tables of risk—including some AMA indicators in italic)

Presenting Problem(s)
- One self-limited or minor problem

Management Options
- Rest, gargles, elastic bandages, superficial dressings

Counseling and/or Coordination of Care
- As appropriate for the problem

Time Spent Face to Face (average)
- 15 minutes

Sample Documentation—99241

Level I Office/Outpatient Consultation

TO: Dr. Attending Physician

FROM: Dr. Consultant

This 26-year-old female is seen at the request of Dr. Attending Physician to evaluate a lump the patient found in her right breast. She states that she found the mass three days ago during a regular, monthly self-examination. She states that the mass is "a little sore." She has had no such masses before; no history of injury to the area. No other significant past history. No family history of breast cancer.

Menses are regular, and the patient is "within a couple of days" of beginning her menses.

The patient is not on oral contraceptives or other medications.

Px: BP 120/80, respirations 18, temperature 98.7, pulse 65. Neck shows no masses or palpable nodes. Breasts are small, symmetrical and generally nontender. There is a small, 1.5-cm nodule palpable in the right inner quadrant; it is easily movable, well circumscribed and feels cystic. There are no other masses. No nipple discharge or other abnormalities. No axillae lymphadenopathy.

Assessment: Cyst of breast, right

Recommendation: Patient was reassured that this mass is probably a cyst and not likely to be malignant, and this seemed to relieve her anxiety. We discussed the possibility of fine-needle aspiration of the cyst. The patient, however, indicates that she is "very afraid" of needles and prefers not to have this procedure done today. Because of the patient's concern over aspiration, I recommend ultrasound to distinguish simple vs. complex cyst. She agrees to the ultrasound, which our office will schedule.

Thank you for asking me to see your patient. I recommend that we proceed with the needle aspiration in the near future if the ultrasound shows the cyst to be suspicious.

(Single organ system—GYN)

✓ **QUICK TIP**

The consulting provider initiated a diagnostic procedure and made follow-up recommendations based upon the outcome of the testing.

99242

DOCUMENTATION REQUIREMENTS

Medical Decision Making: straightforward
- Minimal number of diagnoses or management options considered
- No or minimal amount and complexity of data reviewed
- Minimal risk of complications or morbidity or mortality

Problem Severity: low
- Expectation of full recovery without functional impairment, or uncertain outcome or increased probability of prolonged functional impairment
- Expectation of full recovery without functional impairment
- Low risk of morbidity without treatment

History: expanded problem focused
- Chief complaint
- Brief history of present illness (one to three HPI elements)
- Problem pertinent system review (one or two systems)

Examination: expanded problem focused
- 1995: two to seven organ systems or body areas
- 1997: at least six bullet (•) elements in one or more organ systems/body areas

Code Indicators (from tables of risk—including some AMA indicators in italic)

Presenting Problem(s)
- One self-limited or minor problem

Management Options
- Rest, gargles, elastic bandages, superficial dressings

Counseling and/or Coordination of Care
- As appropriate for the problem

Time Spent Face to Face (average)
- 30 minutes

(See "General Guidelines" for additional documentation considerations.)

Sample Documentation—99242

Level II Office/Outpatient Consultation

TO: Dr. Attending Psychiatrist
FROM: Dr. Consultant
RE: Admitting evaluation

Chief complaint: "They brought me for a checkup."

History: This 24-year-old white male is seen for the first time for medical evaluation at the request of Dr. Attending Psychiatrist at the County Mental Health Facility where he was sent from County Correctional Facility after being charged with assault. He was admitted to CMHF for treatment. He is seen today for an admitting H&P.

(continued)

Sample Documentation—99242 (Continued)

Past history: He states that he has had no serious medical problems. His only past illness was chickenpox and occasional upper respiratory infections. He smokes about a pack of cigarettes a day and drinks "some," but would not elaborate further.

Allergies: He states that he was given Haldol while in a reformatory eight years ago which caused him to choke and stutter. No other allergies.

Illicit drug use: He reports using cocaine and smoking marijuana in the past but "none in the past few months." Admitting drug screens at CCF were normal.

Family history: Father is 43, mother 41, both living and well. He has an older sister age 25, and a brother age 21, both living and well. He has an aunt who is alcoholic and an uncle who died at age 28 of testicular cancer. His maternal grandmother died of myocardial infarction. Other grandparents are living and well.

Review of systems: No specific complaints on general review but admits to feeling anxious and depressed. Cardiorespiratory: No chest pain, shortness of breath, palpitations or hemoptysis. GI: No nausea, vomiting, diarrhea, constipation. GU: No dysuria, urgency, frequency. Neuromuscular: no myalgia, arthralgia.

Physical exam: This is a well-developed, well nourished, moderately obese white male in no acute distress. Height 5'6", weight 185, temperature 98.3, pulse 72, respirations 20, blood pressure l35/88.

HEENT: Some male pattern alopecia starting; he has a large sebaceous cyst on the scalp, midline, measuring about 2 cm in diameter. He states that this is getting larger and would like it removed because it is sometimes tender. Eyes: EOM intact. PERRLA, Snellen Chart tests reveal vision 20/ 25 on right and 20/20 on the left, uncorrected. Ears: TM's intact; hearing is grossly normal. Nose, mouth and throat: nose patent, tongue midline; pharynx not injected.

Neck: Supple; no bruits; no lymphadenopathy; thyroid normal.

Chest: Symmetrical expansion; lungs clear to auscultation and percussion.

Heart: regular sinus rhythm; no murmurs or gallops. S1, S2 normal.

Abdomen: Moderately obese; no organomegaly, masses, tenderness or hernia. Bowel sounds normal and active in all quadrants.

Rectal/genital: Circumcised, no lesions of penis; both testes descended; no inguinal hernia; rectal negative to inspection; sphincter tone normal; prostate normal; stool guaiac negative.

Neurological: Sensation to touch and pain normal. Cranial nerves II-XII intact; No pathological reflexes. Babinski negative. Deep tendon reflexes +2 and symmetrical.

Extremities: No varicosities or edema. Full range of motion in all extremities. Muscle strength normal.

Skin: Normal except for sebaceous cyst of scalp.

Impression:
1. Sebaceous cyst of scalp
2. Probable non-allergic intolerance to Haldol
3. R/O situational depression

Medical Management Recommendations:
1. Avoid Haldol.
2. Consider excision of scalp cyst in near future.
3. No other medical problems at this time.
4. Psychiatric consultation to follow.

Thank you for allowing me to see your patient.

(General multisystem)

✓ **QUICK TIP**

Note that this is a medical consultation for a psychiatric patient. Although the psychiatrist is a licensed physician, most defer treatment of medical conditions to the care of other healthcare providers. Psychologists may not treat medical conditions and should refer out care for all nonpsychiatric conditions.

99243

DOCUMENTATION REQUIREMENTS

Medical Decision Making: low
- Limited number of diagnoses or management options considered
- Limited amount and complexity of data reviewed
- Low risk of complications or morbidity or mortality

Problem Severity: moderate
- Moderate risk of morbidity without treatment
- Moderate risk of mortality without treatment
- Uncertain outcome or increased probability of prolonged functional impairment or increased probability of prolonged functional impairment

History: detailed
- Chief complaint
- Extended history of present illness (four or more HPI elements or the status of three chronic problems)
- Extended system review (two to nine systems)
- Pertinent past, family, and/or social history (one of the history areas)

Examination: detailed
- 1995: two to seven organ systems or body areas with an extended exam of affected area(s)
- 1997: at least two bullet (•) elements from at least six organ systems or body areas, OR at least 12 bullet (•) elements from two or more organ systems or body areas. Eye and psychiatric single-system exams must include at least nine bullet (•) elements

Code Indicators (from tables of risk—including some AMA indicators in italic)

Presenting problem(s)
- Two or more self-limited or minor problem(s)
- One stable chronic illness (e.g., well controlled hypertension or non-insulin-dependent diabetes, cataract, BPH)
- Acute uncomplicated illness or injury (e.g., cystitis, allergic rhinitis, simple sprain)

Management options
- Physical therapy, *rest or exercise, diet, stress management*
- Over the counter drugs, *medication management with minimal risk*
- Minor surgery, with no identified risk factors
- Occupational therapy
- IV fluids, without additives

Counseling and/or Coordination of Care
- As appropriate for the problem

Time Spent Face to Face (average)
- 40 minutes

QUICK TIP

Note that specialists perform most consultations, as is the case with this ophthalmology consultation.

Sample Documentation—99243

Level III Office/Outpatient Consultation

TO: Dr. Attending Physician
FROM: Dr. Consultant
RE: Evaluation of retinopathy

This is a 32-year-old insulin-dependent diabetic being seen at the request of her family physician for evaluation of diabetic retinopathy. Her diabetes was diagnosed at age 12, and she has been controlled with insulin since that time. Her diabetes is basically stable and controlled by diet and medication. She is periodically evaluated for retinopathy. With the last examination about one year ago, reportedly she had very minimal nonproliferative retinopathy. The patient is not hypertensive. She has had no visual changes or problems, no blurring of vision, vision loss, scotoma, floaters, pain or photophobia. No dizziness, unsteadiness, lightheadedness or impairment of night vision. Review of systems otherwise within normal limits; she has no other health problems. She checks her blood sugar daily and adheres to her diabetic regimen. She takes no medications except her sliding scale insulin.

Exam: Visual acuity good with current corrective lenses; conjunctivae are clear. No icterus. Gross visual fields intact. Extraocular movements intact; no nystagmus. Pupils equal, round react normally to light and accommodation. Pupils were dilated. Slit lamp examination showed no corneal abnormalities. Anterior chambers normal. Lenses clear. Intraocular pressures normal. Minimal nonproliferative retinopathy with a few very small areas of pinpoint exudate. Optic discs are flat and normal; posterior segments otherwise normal.

Assessment: Minimal nonproliferative retinopathy
                   Insulin dependent diabetes mellitus

Discussion & Recommendations: In comparing her current findings to my charts and mapping from her examination a year ago, I believe there has been no progression of her retinopathy in the past year. No intervention needs to be undertaken at this time. The patient should be cautioned to be particularly watchful for any change in visual symptomatology, to report any changes promptly, and to continue her efforts to follow her diabetic treatment plan faithfully. She should, of course, continue to receive yearly ophthalmologic evaluations.

Thank you for allowing me to participate in the care of your patient. I will be happy to see her again if any problems should arise.

(Single organ system—eye)

99244

DOCUMENTATION REQUIREMENTS

Medical Decision Making: moderate
- Multiple number of diagnoses or management options considered
- Moderate amount or complexity of data reviewed
- Moderate risk of complications or morbidity or mortality

Problem Severity: moderate to high
- Moderate to high risk of morbidity without treatment
- Moderate to high risk of mortality without treatment
- Uncertain outcome or increased probability of prolonged functional impairment or high probability of severe prolonged functional impairment

History: comprehensive
- Chief complaint
- Extended history of present illness (four or more HPI elements or the status of three chronic problems)
- Complete system review (10 systems)
- Complete past, family, social history (at least one element from all history areas)

Examination: comprehensive
- 1995: eight or more organ systems
- 1997: multisystem exam must include all bullet (•) elements from at least nine organ systems or body areas unless specific instructions limit content of the exam; at least two bullet elements from each area/system reviewed are expected to be documented.
- 1997: single organ system/body area exam must include all bullet (•) elements in shaded boxes PLUS at least one element in each unshaded box.

Code Indicators (from tables of risk—including some AMA indicators in italic)

Presenting Problem(s)
- One or more chronic illness with mild exacerbation, progression, or side effects of treatment
- Two or more stable chronic illnesses
- Undiagnosed new *illness, injury,* or problem with uncertain prognosis
- Acute illness, with systemic symptoms (pyelonephritis, pleuritis, colitis)
- Acute complicated injury, e.g., head injury, with brief loss of consciousness

Management Options
- Prescription drug management
- Closed treatment of fracture or dislocation, without manipulation
- IV fluids with additives
- Minor surgery, with identified risk factors

- Elective major surgery (open, percutaneous, endoscopic), with no identified risk factors
- Therapeutic nuclear medicine

Counseling and/or Coordination of Care
- As appropriate for the problem

Time Spent Face to Face (average)
- 60 minutes

Sample Documentation—99244

Level IV Office/Outpatient Consultation

Dr. Internal Medicare Consult
1234 Anyway Place
Scottsville, Ohio 45111
January 6, 20XX

Dear Dr. Orthopaedic Surgeon:

Thank you for your request for an Internal Medicine consultation on this 49-year-old male, who presents for pre-operative physical examination and clearance, scheduled for a right hip replacement in two weeks. The patient is hypertensive, has multifocal osteoarthritis with femoral head and acetabular degeneration of the right hip, and status-post polypectomy of the large intestine one year ago. The patient presents today with no new complaints though does need refills on antihypertensive med. Currently takes Ziac 5mg/6.25 mg daily. Takes Motrin PRN, Voltaren 100 mg/day for arthritic exacerbation and pain. The OA of the right hip has grossly interfered with the patient's ADLs, and subjects him to constant pain and impaired gait.

PMH: Usual childhood diseases. T&A age 14; fracture right wrist at age eight. Degenerative arthritis for "years." Fell and injured the right hip some years ago, without apparent sequelae until recently.

SH: Married; wife alive and well. Children: three, all well.

FH: As above. Siblings: two older brothers, both alive and well but history of DM and cataracts; one with history of colon CA. Mother and father died of "old age." History of HTN in brother and mother. No endocrine diseases, no thyroid problems, CA as noted.

ROS: HEENT: no complaints. Throat: T&A as noted. Ears: hears well without tinnitus. Cardio: HTN as noted, controlled on combination beta blocker/diuretic medication with good results. Denies other problems (angina, SOB). Resp/chest: no complaints. GI: occasional dyspepsia. Occasional diarrhea. Previous surgery as noted; no CA sequelae. Submits to annual colonoscopies by GI specialist. GU: urine dribbling; no other complaints. Skin: no complaints. Heme: no history excess bleeding. Musculoskeletal: Old fx as noted. OA as described, followed by orthopaedic surgeon. Takes meds as noted with some relief. Endo: no complaints. Neuro: no complaints. Psych: leads active life, OA-permitting. Occasional frustrations secondary to OA pain/debility.

O: Ht. 5'11"; Wt. 195 lbs. T: 98.6; P: 68; BP: 136/88. General: well-developed, well-nourished adult male in no acute distress, who walks with guarded gait with slight limp, favoring to the left. Alert, oriented X 3. Head: WNL. No suspicious lesions. Ears, nose, throat: All WNL. Nasal mucosa pale; no exudates. Pharynx WNL. Ear canals hairy with minimal cerumen present. TM's clear. Eyes: PERRLA. EOMI. Sclerae and conjunctivae clear. Fundi: discs flat with narrowed arterioles. Neck: no cervical lymphadenopathy. No tenderness. FROM. No JVD or bruits. CV: normal heart sounds; S1, S2. Has S4 gallop. No murmur or rub noted. Resp: good breath sounds, clear to P&A. Abd: no mass, tenderness, organomegaly (spleen/liver). BS sl. hyperactive. Genitals: WNL. Testicles nontender and without mass. Some varicosities noted. Penis uncircumcised; several small papillomas in fold of prepuce noted but otherwise WNL. Rectal: no masses or hemorrhoids. Prostate nontender, +2 firm, not boggy. Skin: normal in color, turgor and without lesion.

(continued)

Sample Documentation—99244 (Continued)

Extremities/Joints: FROM though with obvious discomfort when performing SLR on the right. Hip ROM limited by pain. No arthritic changes noted over hands. There is minimal muscle atrophy noted at the right thigh, though not marked. Neuro: alert and oriented x 3. DTRs +2 in upper extremities and lower extremities.

The patient is accompanied by x-rays of the right and left hips, with a full report by Radiology. On re-view of the films, there is severe degenerative joint disease of the right hip with mild changes on the left. Report states "severe osteoarthritis of the right hip involving the femoral head and acetabular rim."

EKG: NSR at 70; PR 0.12; QRS 0.08. Normal axis; no ischemic changes. UA: neg for glucosuria; WBCs neg; RBCs neg; ketones neg; protein neg; neg for bacteria; color: light yellow, clear; specific gravity: 1.018; pH 7.5.

A: Cleared for surgery pending labs. Bilateral OA, worse in right hip vs. left. Mild HTN, med-controlled. S/P polypectomy.

P: OK for surgery. Follow HTN. Refill Ziac. Anesthesia will manage HTN perioperatively. Handicapped parking sticker application completed and provided to patient.

This comprises the consultation note for this patient. I have suggested to the patient, who recently moved to this area and does not have a preferred Internist, that I can follow him for the above IM findings. The patient's blood was drawn and sent to the health plan's lab for CBC w/diff, platelets, SMA-20, clotting studies. A pre-op CXR has been ordered. Results of these tests will be provided to the pre-op center upon their arrival. Thank you for your kind request of this most pleasant patient. If I can be of further service to you, please let me know.

Internal Medicine Physician

(General multisystem)

Level IV Office/Outpatient Consultation

TO: Dr. Surgeon

FROM: Dr. Consultant

RE: Preoperative evaluation

This 45-year-old diabetic female is seen at the request of Dr. Surgeon for a preoperative evaluation of her condition. She is scheduled for laparoscopic TAH-BSO on Monday at Local Hospital due to uterine fibroids. The fibroids were discovered about three years ago, when she complained of increasing pelvic pain and fullness, and menses becoming longer in duration and heavier in flow. Currently, the patient reports over the past four months, her menses last from 10 days to two weeks, are very heavy, sometimes going through a box of pads in a day, and with increasing cramping and abdominal pain.

Her Type II diabetes, diagnosed five years ago, is well controlled by diet and Glucotrol; the patient checks her blood sugar at home every other day which is generally about 120 postprandial. She was also diagnosed with hypertension about two years ago. She has been on Captopril with blood pressures of about 130–140/80. Her past history is otherwise unremarkable. She is G2, P2, uneventful pregnancies and deliveries, 26 and 28 years ago. No surgical history. The patient has seasonal allergies and at times develops asthmatic bronchitis and uses inhalers to relieve shortness of breath. She says that stress sometimes brings on asthmatic symptoms. She is not currently having any asthma problems. No history of significant trauma; no other hospitalizations and no other significant past medical history.

Family history and social history are otherwise noncontributory. Both children are living and well; patient manages a convenience store and lives with her husband. No tobacco use, minimal alcohol; no illicit drugs usage reported. See the self-history form completed by the patient. No family history of cancer; mother is hypertensive; father is type II diabetic. One sister, age 42, living and well.

Review of systems: The patient reports increasing fatigue, irritability and depression as her gynecologic symptoms have increased. Otherwise, she describes herself as generally happy and easy-going. She has lost about six pounds over the past six months, which she attributes to being "too tired to eat" and to getting less exercise than she is used to getting. Otherwise, review of systems was within normal limits; see form completed by the patient.

PX: BP 130/80, pulse 70, respirations 20, temperature 98.5; patient is 5'7" and weighs 142 pounds. Well-developed, well-nourished female in no acute distress but appearing tired and pale.

(continued)

QUICK TIP

Preoperative clearance consultations may have additional requirements according to the payer. Check your local carrier LCD or payer guidelines for additional information.

QUICK TIP

Preoperative clearance of a patient with a known medical condition is often requested by surgical specialties.

Sample Documentation—99244 (Continued)

HEENT: Normocephalic. Eyes, PERRLA; EOMI; conjunctivae clear; retinae no exudates or hemorrhages. **ENT:** TM's normal; nose and throat normal. Neck: no masses or bruits. Trachea midline. Thyroid normal. Chest clear to auscultation and percussion; no rales or wheezes. Heart: regular rate and rhythm. No murmurs. Breasts normal; no masses or tenderness. Abdomen, soft, no tenderness; no organomegaly, no masses. BS wnl. Pelvic exam deferred. Rectal exam deferred. Extremities full range of motion. Pulses normal. Neurological: DTR's +2 symmetrical.

Labs: Blood sugar was 115 mg/dL; patient had eaten normally and taken her medications this morning. Pre-op hemoglobin and hematocrit, and chest x-ray pending.

Assessment:
1. Patient with known uterine fibroids scheduled for surgery in five days.
2. Type II diabetic well-controlled on current regimen of Glucotrol and diet.
3. Hypertension, well-controlled on captopril.
4. History of asthmatic bronchitis, controlled with PRN inhalers.

Recommendation: Cleared for surgery. Hold all meds. Cover blood sugars with insulin on sliding scale. Oximetry.

Thank you for allowing me to see your patient. I will be happy to follow her along with you if you wish.

(General multisystem)

99245

DOCUMENTATION REQUIREMENTS

Medical Decision Making: high
- Extensive number of diagnoses or management options considered
- Extensive amount or complexity of data reviewed
- High risk of complications or morbidity or mortality

Problem Severity: moderate to high
- Moderate to extreme risk of morbidity without treatment
- Moderate to high risk of mortality without treatment
- Uncertain outcome or increased probability of prolonged functional impairment or high probability of severe prolonged functional impairment

History: comprehensive
- Chief complaint
- Extended history of present illness (four or more HPI elements or the status of three chronic problems)
- Complete system review (10 systems)
- Complete past, family, social history (at least one element from all history areas)

Examination: comprehensive
- 1995: eight or more organ systems
- 1997: multisystem exam must include all bullet (•) elements from at least nine organ systems or body areas unless specific instructions limit content of the exam; at least two bullet elements from each area/system reviewed are expected to be documented.
- 1997: single organ system/body area exam must include all bullet (•) elements in shaded boxes PLUS at least one element in each unshaded box.

Code Indicators (from tables of risk—including some AMA indicators in italic)

Presenting Problem(s)
- One or more chronic illness with severe exacerbation, progression, or side effects of treatment
- Acute or chronic illness or injury that poses a threat to life or bodily function, e.g., multiple traumas, acute MI, pulmonary embolism, severe respiratory distress, progressive severe rheumatoid arthritis, psychiatric illness, with potential threat to self or others, peritonitis, ARF
- An abrupt change in neurological status, e.g., seizure, TIA, weakness, sensory loss

Management Options
- Elective major surgery with identified risk factors or emergency major surgery (open, percutaneous, endoscopic)
- Parenteral controlled substances

- Drug therapy requiring intensive monitoring for toxicity
- Decision not to resuscitate or to deescalate care because of poor prognosis

Counseling and/or Coordination of Care
- As appropriate for the problem

Time Spent Face to Face (average)
- 80 minutes

Sample Documentation—99245

Level V Office/Outpatient Consultation

TO: Dr. Attending Physician
FROM: Dr. Consultant
RE: Evaluation of chest pain

History: This 63-year-old female is seen at the request of Dr. Attending Physician for evaluation of exertional chest pain. The patient reports upper chest pain radiating to the throat for the last 10 days with one episode a day; each episode lasts 10 to 15 minutes occurring with normal physical activity such as housework. Another episode occurred at rest in the early AM hours, awakening the patient from sleep, associated with shortness of breath and fatigue. Also complains of an episode of syncope lasting about three minutes, 48 hours ago while standing at the sink. Her husband says the patient suddenly fell to the floor, bruising herself, but she exhibits no seizure-like activity.

Past history: No allergies. Hysterectomy/oophorectomy age 56; usual childhood diseases; peptic ulcer age 52. She smokes a pack a day of cigarettes, and has borderline hypertension. No diabetes, hyperlipidemia or obesity. No other surgery or significant illnesses. She drinks three to four cups of coffee a day; ETOH socially. Three grown children, all healthy. No family history of MI. Mother died of early renal failure at age 46; father died of liver cancer at age 73. Two sisters, both well. See self-history forms completed by the patient.

Review of systems: She says a murmur was noted once on an insurance physical. She has aching in her legs below the calf, left more than right, on exertion such as walking up steps gradually increasing over the past three years, but the aching goes away with rest. No palpitations, shortness of breath, tremors, edema, dizziness, rheumatic fever, current GI or GU complaints, although she was treated for an ulcer in the past. She had migraines in the past. No problems with easy bruisability or unsteadiness or musculoskeletal problems. GYN: no problems since hysterectomy. Review of systems otherwise within normal limits.

Physical Exam:
General: BP 140/90, no orthostatic changes, pulse 72, respirations 14, afebrile. Well developed, slender white female in no acute distress, well oriented, communicative, and verbalizing some apprehension about her health.
Neck: Jugular venous pressure normal. Carotid pulses full with bruit or transmitted murmur.
Lungs: Clear to percussion and auscultation. No intercostal retractions.
Cardiovascular: PMI normal, S1 and S2 and S4, present; no S3 or gallop or rub. Grade III/VI systolic murmur, radiates to carotids and a grade 1/6 diastolic blowing murmur radiating to the carotids. No abdominal bruits. No carotid bruits.
Abdomen shows no masses, tenderness, organomegaly.
Extremities: Bilateral soft femoral bruits. Pulses are diminished in DP/PT arteries bilaterally. No pedal edema or varicosities.
Skin: Normal in color, without lesions
EKG: Sinus rhythm at 72. PR 0.16, Axis +30, no old MI or ischemic changes. QRS 0.08.

(continued)

Sample Documentation—99245 (Continued)

Impression:
1. Crescendo Angina
   A. R/O CAD
   B. R/O Aortic Stenosis
2. Syncope
   A. due to cardiac arrhythmia secondary to ischemia
   B. R/O aortic stenosis
3. Aortic stenosis
   A. no history of rheumatic fever
   B. consider congenital bicuspid aortic valve type
4. Claudication
   A. consistent with peripheral atherosclerosis
   B. level below knee L>R

Recommendations:
1. Stat admission to CCU
2. R/O MI protocol
3. Check lipids, thyroid function, CBC
4. Stat echocardiogram
5. Possible cardiac catheterization
6. Smoking cessation emphasized

I discussed the above recommendations and risks with the patient and her husband, who both understand and agree with the need for emergency admission. As you recall, I telephoned your office and as per our discussion arranged for the emergency admission.

We also discussed various medications that may be used for angina with aortic stenosis and claudication before it is begun.

Thank you for allowing me to participate in the care of your patient.

(Single organ system—cardiovascular)

 QUICK TIP

At the request of the consultant, the primary care physician arranged for admission and was the admitting physician; therefore, the consultation was a separate service.

Inpatient Consultations (99251–99255)

QUICK COMPARISON

Consultations—Inpatient[1], New or Established Patient

E/M Code[1]	Medical Decision Making[2]	History[2]	Exam[2]	Counseling and/or Coordination of Care	Time[3] (avg.)
99251	Straightforward	Problem focused	Problem focused	Consistent with problems and patient's or family's needs	20 min.
99252	Straightforward	Expanded problem focused	Expanded problem focused	Consistent with problems and patient's or family's needs	40 min.
99253	Low complexity	Detailed	Detailed	Consistent with problems and patient's or family's needs	55 min.
99254	Moderate complexity	Comprehensive	Comprehensive	Consistent with problems and patient's or family's needs	80 min.
99255	High complexity	Comprehensive	Comprehensive	Consistent with problems and patient's or family's needs	110 min.

1   These codes are used for hospital inpatients, residents of nursing facilities or patients in a partial hospital setting.
2   Key component. For initial inpatient consultations, all three components (history, exam, and medical decision making) must be adequately documented in the medical record to substantiate the level of service reported and are crucial for selecting the correct code.
3   For reporting these services, unit/floor intraservice time includes both bedside services and those services rendered while on the hospital unit. Unit/floor time includes chart review, patient examination, record documentation, and communication with the patient's family and facility staff.

CODING AXIOM

Medicare does not accept consultation codes. Use initial hospital care codes to report the first inpatient encounter by a physician. The admitting physician should append modifier AI Principal physician of record, to the initial hospital care code.

GENERAL GUIDELINES

- Use these codes if the physician/qualified healthcare professional provided an opinion or gave advice regarding evaluation and/or management of a specific problem at the request of another physician/qualified healthcare professional or appropriate source. A consultation may also be necessary to determine whether the consultant is willing to accept transfer and ongoing management of the patient's entire care or for management of a specific problem. The consultant may initiate diagnostic or therapeutic services.

- Consultation codes are appropriate only if the service was provided in the hospital, nursing facility or partial hospital setting. A written report must be sent to the requesting provider or source to be placed in the permanent medical record for that patient. Required documentation includes the request for consultation, need for the consultation, consultant's opinion and any services that were ordered or performed.

- When a common chart is used, a separate report to the requesting provider does not need to be sent.

- Consider assigning the appropriate critical care code instead of these codes if the physician provided constant attention to a critically ill patient.

- Do not consider the time spent by other staff (e.g., nurse) as part of face-to-face time.

- For reporting these services, unit/floor intraservice time includes both bedside services and those services rendered while on the hospital unit. Unit/floor time includes chart review, patient examination, record documentation, and communication with the patient's family and facility staff.

- Report 99356–99359 for E/M services that exceed 30 minutes beyond the typical time specified in the code narrative. The time must be clearly documented in the medical record.

- Append modifier 25 to report that a separately identifiable E/M service was performed by the same physician/qualified healthcare professional on the same day as a procedure or service. Only the work associated with the separate E/M service should be considered when assigning the correct E/M code.

- Use modifier 32 when the services were mandated, such as by a third-party payer, or as a result of a governmental, legislative, or regulatory requirement.

- Append modifier 57 to indicate that the decision to perform surgery was made at this visit. For Medicare, the decision must be to perform major surgery.

- Append modifier 95 to indicate that the E/M service was rendered to a patient at a distant site via a real-time interactive audio and video telecommunications system. The communication between the physician or other qualified healthcare professional and the patient should be commensurate with the same key components or requirements of those that would be required if the service had been rendered in a face-to-face setting.

- A consultant may report only one inpatient consultation per admission. Any subsequent services (e.g., completion of initial consult, monitoring of progress, revision of recommendations, addressing new problems) during the admission are reported using the appropriate subsequent inpatient care codes.

- Do not report an inpatient and outpatient consultation on the same day for services related to an inpatient stay. All evaluation and management services provided by consultant related to a hospital admission are reported with the appropriate inpatient consultation service codes.

- However, if a consultant sees a patient in outpatient consultation prior to admission, the consultant may report the appropriate outpatient consultation code. However, if the patient is seen by the consultant on the inpatient unit on the date of admission, all related services are reported with either the initial inpatient consultation or initial inpatient admission service codes, as appropriate.

- Transfer-of-care services (i.e., for either specific condition or the patient's entire care) are reported with the appropriate new or established patient codes for the site of service.

- As stated earlier, the Medicare program eliminated the use of all consultation codes except for telehealth inpatient consultation G codes; these codes are discussed in greater detail in chapter 17.

Special Instructions for Consultations Performed in the Hospital or Nursing Facility

Medicare requires that the initial hospital care code (99221–99223) be reported for each physician's first visit with a patient during a specific hospitalization. As only one physician can be the admitting physician, CMS created HCPCS Level II modifier AI that is to be appended to the initial

QUICK TIP

Modifiers 25, 32, and 57 are to be appended to the E/M code and not to the codes for the other procedures or services that may be performed.

hospital care code by the attending physician. All other physicians and consultants report the initial hospital care code without appending a modifier. Subsequent inpatient encounters by any physician are reported using codes 99231–99233.

- For Medicare beneficiaries, append modifier AI to the initial hospital care code (99221–99223) or initial nursing facility care code (99304–99306) reported by the attending physician
- Only the admitting physician of record who oversees the patient's care reports modifier AI
- It is inappropriate for consulting physicians to report modifier AI with their initial hospital care code

Do not append modifier AI to subsequent hospital care codes (99231–99233) or inpatient consultation codes (99251–99255).

Admitting Provider vs. Consultant

Medicare allows only one physician to be the admitting physician of record for hospital inpatient and nursing facility admissions. To identify the admitting physician of record who oversees the patient's care, CMS requires the use of HCPCS Level II modifier AI Principal physician of record, be reported by the admitting physician on the initial hospital care or initial nursing facility care code. Note that private payers may choose whether to follow the CMS policy regarding modifier AI; therefore, providers should verify consultation code policies with individual payers before using AI.

99251

DOCUMENTATION REQUIREMENTS

Medical Decision Making: straightforward
- Minimal number of diagnoses or management options considered
- No or minimal amount and complexity of data reviewed
- Minimal risk of complications or morbidity or mortality

Problem Severity: minor or self-limited
- Little, if any, risk of morbidity without treatment
- Little, if any, risk of mortality without treatment
- Transient problem, low probability of permanently altered status
- Good prognosis

History: problem focused
- Chief complaint
- Brief history of present illness or problem (one to three HPI elements)

Examination: problem focused
- 1995: one organ system or body area
- 1997: one to five bullet (•) elements in one or more organ systems/body areas

Code Indicators (from tables of risk—including some AMA indicators in italic)

Presenting Problem(s)
- One self-limited or minor problem

Management Options
- Rest, gargles, elastic bandages, superficial dressings

Counseling and/or Coordination of Care
- As appropriate for the problem

Time Spent Bedside and on Floor/Unit (average)
- 20 minutes

QUICK TIP

Consultations do not differentiate between new and established patients. A provider may be asked by a physician of another specialty to consult on a known patient.

Sample Documentation—99251

Level I Inpatient Consultation

TO: Dr. Attending Physician
FROM: Dr. Consultant
RE: Management of pernicious anemia

This 68-year-old male was admitted to the hospital last night following a fall down an escalator with resultant exacerbation of his chronic back problems. The patient has known pernicious anemia, diagnosed about three years ago and receives monthly B12 shots which have controlled the anemia well. The patient had his last B12 shot one week ago. No other pertinent history or complaints.

Exam: Vitals were reviewed and are stable. There is some bruising over the back area, including lower lumbar and buttocks, and upper thigh, and there are a few areas of ecchymosis over the left arm and shoulder. No other ecchymosis or bruising observed. HEENT within normal limits. No pallor or glossitis. Heart and lungs clear to auscultation and percussion; regular rate and rhythm. No abdominal tenderness or masses. No peripheral edema. Neuro—alert and oriented x3. No ataxia.

Admitting laboratory blood work all within acceptable limits. HGB 12g, HCT 35%, MCV 95.

Impression: Known pernicious anemia currently well controlled in a trauma patient.

Recommendations: Observe, but anticipate no problems with anemia at this time. Continue current B12 regimen.

Thank you for asking me to see this patient; I will be happy to see him again if any problems arise.

(Single organ system—hematology/immunology/lymphatics)

99252

DOCUMENTATION REQUIREMENTS

Medical Decision Making: straightforward
- Minimal number of diagnoses or management options considered
- No or minimal amount and complexity of data reviewed
- Minimal risk of complications or morbidity or mortality

Problem Severity: low
- Expectation of full recovery without functional impairment, or uncertain outcome or increased probability of prolonged functional impairment
- Expectation of full recovery without functional impairment
- Low risk of morbidity without treatment

History: expanded problem focused
- Chief complaint
- Brief history of present illness (one to three HPI elements)
- Problem pertinent system review (one or two systems)

Examination: expanded problem focused
- 1995: two to seven organ systems or body areas
- 1997: at least six bullet (•) elements in one or more organ systems/body areas

Code Indicators (from tables of risk—including some AMA indicators in italic)

Presenting Problem(s)
- One self-limited or minor problem

Management Options
- Rest, gargles, elastic bandages, superficial dressings

Counseling and/or Coordination of Care
- As appropriate for the problem

Time Spent Bedside and on Floor/Unit (average)
- 40 minutes

Sample Documentation—99252

Level II Inpatient Consultation

TO: Dr. Attending Physician
FROM: Dr. Consultant
RE: Evaluation of hearing loss

I was called in consultation to evaluate this 45-year-old male for progressive hearing loss. The patient was admitted four days ago for bleeding ulcers, and upon history and physical examination was noted to have decreased hearing. The patient denies any history of chronic middle ear disease as a child. He does report minimal tinnitus when he is sitting in a quiet room, but denies any dizziness. His wife has complained that she has to repeat things and wondered if he needed a hearing aid. He has a past history of noise exposure while hunting and while working in a manufacturing plant in his early 20s. He has worn ear protection while using firearms or around machinery for the past l2 years.

Physical exam: External auditory canals are clear; TM's are intact with no scarring or bulging. normal mobility. Rinne and Weber tests are normal. Exam of the nose and sinuses shows no obstructions, discharge, tenderness or other abnormalities. Oral cavity is clear; teeth are in good repair. Oropharynx and posterior pharynx all within normal limits.

Audiometry shows bilateral sloping, moderate high frequency sensorineural hearing loss from 2 kHz without an air-bone gap. Impedance studies were normal.

Impression:
    Bilateral moderate high frequency sensorineural hearing loss

Recommendations:
    Hearing aid evaluation and fitting
    Hearing conservation program to reduce and protect him from noise trauma

Thank you for allowing me to see your patient.

(Single organ system—ENT)

QUICK TIP

Append modifier 25 to the consultation code if reporting the audiology testing performed by the provider and not by the facility or facility staff.

99253

DOCUMENTATION REQUIREMENTS

Medical Decision Making: low
- Limited number of diagnoses or management options considered
- Limited amount and complexity of data reviewed
- Low risk of complications or morbidity or mortality

Problem Severity: moderate
- Moderate risk of morbidity without treatment
- Moderate risk of mortality without treatment
- Uncertain outcome or increased probability of prolonged functional impairment or increased probability of prolonged functional impairment

History: detailed
- Chief complaint
- Extended history of present illness (four or more HPI elements or the status of three chronic problems)
- Extended system review (two to nine systems)
- Pertinent past, family, and/or social history (one of the history areas)

Examination: detailed
- 1995: two to seven organ systems or body areas with an extended exam of affected area(s)
- 1997: at least two bullet (•) elements from at least six organ systems or body areas, OR at least 12 bullet (•) elements from two or more organ systems or body areas. Eye and psychiatric single-system exams must include at least nine bullet (•) elements.

Code Indicators (from tables of risk—including some AMA indicators in italic)

Presenting Problem(s)
- Two or more self-limited or minor problem(s)
- One stable chronic illness (e.g., well controlled hypertension or non-insulin-dependent diabetes, cataract, BPH)
- Acute uncomplicated illness or injury (e.g., cystitis, allergic rhinitis, simple sprain)

Management Options
- Physical therapy, *rest or exercise, diet, stress management*
- Over the counter drugs, *medication management with minimal risk*
- Minor surgery, with no identified risk factors
- Occupational therapy
- IV fluids, without additives

Counseling and/or Coordination of Care
- As appropriate for the problem

Time Spent Bedside and on Floor/Unit (average)
- 55 minutes

Sample Documentation—99253

Level III Inpatient Consultation

TO: Dr. Attending Physician
FROM: Dr. Consultant
RE: Evaluation of cataracts

History: This 79-year-old white female with multiple problems was transferred from her nursing home two days ago for chest pain, nausea and vomiting which are being treated by her attending physician. He has requested that I evaluate the patient for possible cataract surgery. The patient is somewhat difficult to communicate with, and history is taken from the hospital record and from her daughter. The daughter states that her mother was diagnosed with cataracts some time ago and had declined surgery although she was warned about the possibility of losing her sight if the cataracts progressed. The daughter states that her mother's vision has gradually gotten worse over the past few years, and her mother has recently indicated that she can no longer read, see the television, or distinguish among utensils at the table. The patient has stated that she would be willing to have the procedure done.

The patient has a past history of arthritis, mild hypertension, diverticulosis with occasional diverticulitis, status post hysterectomy; has one child, age 55, living and well; and was widowed in her 50s when her husband died in an accident. Review of systems is generally as recorded in the admitting note except that her gastrointestinal symptoms and mentation are markedly improved with treatment and hydration. No known allergies; no other significant history or complaints.

Physical examination: Elderly, thin, well-developed white female, oriented to time and place, BP 148/86. The patient is pleasant but clearly prefers that her daughter speak for her. She responds appropriately to direct questions. The patient hears well.

Examination of the eyes shows limited visual acuity due to mature cataracts in both eyes. Extraocular movements intact. Conjunctivae pink. Pupils' equal, reactive to light and accommodation. Slit lamp exam shows normal anterior chambers, mature posterior subcapsular cataracts. Discs and posterior segments normal as far as can be determined at this time but examination is obscured by the cataract. Intraocular pressures normal.

Impression: Bilateral mature posterior subcapsular cataracts

Recommendations: The patient will clearly benefit from removal of the cataracts and replacement with intraocular lens. After discussion with the patient and her daughter, we decided to schedule the first cataract procedure as soon as possible, with the second to follow at a suitable interval. Intraocular lens will be placed at the time of surgery with anticipated visual correction to 20/25. The daughter asked whether or not the first procedure could be done before her mother was discharged. I advised her that surgery would not be done until her GI symptoms are completely resolved, and therefore she would be discharged prior to the procedure.

Thank you for allowing me to see this patient.

(Single organ system—eye)

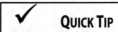

QUICK TIP

Only nine elements or bullets are required for the detailed eye exam using the 1997 guidelines.

99254

DOCUMENTATION REQUIREMENTS

Medical Decision Making: moderate
- Multiple number of diagnoses or management options considered
- Moderate amount or complexity of data reviewed
- Moderate risk of complications or morbidity or mortality

Problem Severity: moderate to high
- Moderate to high risk of morbidity without treatment
- Moderate to high risk of mortality without treatment
- Uncertain outcome or increased probability of prolonged functional impairment or high probability of severe prolonged functional impairment

History: comprehensive
- Chief complaint
- Extended history of present illness (four or more HPI elements or the status of three chronic problems)
- Complete system review (10 systems)
- Complete past, family, social history (at least one element from all history areas)

Examination: comprehensive
- 1995: eight or more organ systems
- 1997: multisystem exam must include all bullet (•) elements from at least nine organ systems or body areas unless specific instructions limit content of the exam; at least two bullet elements from each area/system reviewed are expected to be documented.
- 1997: single organ system/body area exam must include all bullet (•) elements in shaded boxes PLUS at least one element in each unshaded box.

Code Indicators (from tables of risk—including some AMA indicators in italic)

Presenting Problem(s)
- One or more chronic illness with mild exacerbation, progression, or side effects of treatment
- Two or more stable chronic illnesses
- Undiagnosed new *illness, injury,* or problem with uncertain prognosis
- Acute illness, with systemic symptoms (pyelonephritis, pleuritis, colitis)
- Acute complicated injury, e.g., head injury, with brief loss of consciousness

Management Options
- Prescription drug management
- Closed treatment of fracture or dislocation, without manipulation
- IV fluids with additives
- Minor surgery, with identified risk factors

- Elective major surgery (open, percutaneous, endoscopic), with no identified risk factors
- Therapeutic nuclear medicine

Counseling and/or Coordination of Care
- As appropriate for the problem

Time Spent Bedside and on Floor/Unit (average)
- 80 minutes

(See "General Guidelines" for additional documentation considerations.)

Sample Documentation—99254

Level IV Inpatient Consultation

TO: Dr. Attending Physician
FROM: Dr. Consultant:
RE: New onset—seizure activity

History: This 7-year-old male was admitted because he experienced three episodes of seizure activity in the week prior to admission. All three episodes occurred early in the morning, shortly after awakening, and all were observed by family members. The episodes reportedly lasted from two to three minutes on each occasion and involved generalized tonic-clonic movements and loss of consciousness; with loss of bladder control. The patient experienced a definite postictal state, sleeping for three hours and complaining of muscle aches and pains upon awakening with no memory of the seizure activity. The family states that they believe that each episode seems progressively longer. The patient has had no seizures observed in the hospital. The only aura-type prodrome that may be present is tingling in the left leg the night before each event. No fevers in association with the seizures.

Past History: Product of a normal pregnancy, labor and delivery. Normal developmental milestones. Detailed history from both parents elicited no etiology for seizure onset. The patient's immunizations are up to date. He has no past history of chronic conditions including infections, asthma or any other conditions. He sprained an ankle last fall. He is active, participating in sports activities, has a normal diet, and has no past or recent history of other trauma, especially head trauma. He has had no illnesses within the past several weeks, no colds, fevers, flu, GI or GU disturbances and no neurological symptoms. He lives with his family, is a second grader and does well in school, and has no learning difficulties. No one in the family has been ill with the past several weeks. No alcohol, tobacco or drug use. Past, family, social history and review of systems is otherwise within normal limits. No known exposure to toxic substances.

Physical examination: Vitals including blood pressure, pulse, temperature, respirations, height and weight all within normal limits for age. Well developed, well-nourished child. Alert and oriented, lying quietly in bed, somewhat mischievous, but cooperative and relaxed.

HEENT: Eyes show flat discs, EOMI, PERRLA, no abnormalities. ENT clear. Neck supple, no masses or tenderness. Lungs clear. Heart regular rhythm, no murmur.

Neurological: Gait and station are normal. Muscle strength and tone equal and age-appropriate in all extremities. Recent and distant memory appropriate. Attention span excellent for his age. Language and fund of knowledge appropriate for his age group. Cranial nerves II through XII all completely normal. Sensation normal to touch and pinprick. Deep tendon reflexes +2 in all four extremities. Cerebellar finger to nose, upper and lower rapid alternating movements, heel to shin all normal for age. Fine motor coordination appropriate for his age.

Lab: EEG done as an outpatient prior to last seizure showed spike discharges from left temporal lobe.

Impression: Tonic-clonic seizure. Possibly following a partial seizure with secondary generalization.

Discussion: Workup will include fasting glucose, calcium, magnesium and electrolyte. Further investigation with neuro-imaging in a child with a normal history and neuro exam is not indicated at this time. Will begin phenobarbital 4mgm/KG/Day.

I have discussed these recommendations with his parents, and they agree to proceed with the workup and treatment plan if you agree. Thank you for allowing me to participate in the care of your patient.

(Single organ system—neurology)

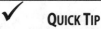

QUICK TIP

The consultant documented the counseling/coordination of care for this patient although time was not the key component in determining the level of code to report.

99255

DOCUMENTATION REQUIREMENTS

Medical Decision Making: high
- Extensive number of diagnoses or management options considered
- Extensive amount or complexity of data reviewed
- High risk of complications or morbidity or mortality

Problem Severity: moderate to high
- Moderate to extreme risk of morbidity without treatment
- Moderate to high risk of mortality without treatment
- Uncertain outcome or increased probability of prolonged functional impairment or high probability of severe prolonged functional impairment

History: comprehensive
- Chief complaint
- Extended history of present illness (four or more HPI elements or the status of three chronic problems)
- Complete system review (10 systems)
- Complete past, family, social history (at least one element from all history areas)

Examination: comprehensive
- 1995: eight or more organ systems
- 1997: multisystem exam must include all bullet (•) elements from at least nine organ systems or body areas unless specific instructions limit content of the exam; at least two bullet elements from each area/system reviewed are expected to be documented.
- 1997: single organ system/body area exam must include all bullet (•) elements in shaded boxes PLUS at least one element in each unshaded box.

Code Indicators (from tables of risk—including some AMA indicators in italic)

Presenting Problem(s)
- One or more chronic illness with severe exacerbation, progression, or side effects of treatment
- Acute or chronic illness or injury that poses a threat to life or bodily function, e.g., multiple traumas, acute MI, pulmonary embolism, severe respiratory distress, progressive severe rheumatoid arthritis, psychiatric illness, with potential threat to self or others, peritonitis, ARF
- An abrupt change in neurological status, e.g., seizure, TIA, weakness, sensory loss

Management Options
- Elective major surgery with identified risk factors or emergency major surgery (open, percutaneous, endoscopic)
- Parenteral controlled substances

- Drug therapy requiring intensive monitoring for toxicity
- Decision not to resuscitate or to deescalate care because of poor prognosis

Counseling and/or Coordination of Care
- As appropriate for the problem

Time Spent Bedside and on Floor/Unit (average)
- 110 minutes

Sample Documentation—99255

Level V Inpatient Consultation

TO: Dr. Attending Physician
FROM: Dr. Consulting Gastroenterologist
RE: Evaluation for GI bleed

History: This is the first Community Hospital admission for this 76-year-old female who noted the onset of black, tarry stools and lightheadedness some three days prior to admission. She has a known history of recurrent peptic ulcer disease over the past 10 years for which she has been treated with the usual dietary restrictions, H2 blockers and antacids. She also is a long-standing hypertensive, without complications, for which she is presently on Vasotec 10 mg a day and HCTZ 25 mg a day. There is no past history of renal involvement or cardiac involvement. The day prior to admission, her lightheadedness increased with dizziness on mild exertion. Her black stools became more frequent. She had the onset of the sensation of substernal chest pressure, which on the morning of admission progressed to anterior chest pain with some radiation into the neck and toward the left shoulder.

On admission to the hospital in the ER, she was noted to have hematocrit and hemoglobin of 22 and 7. Her EKG revealed ST depression and T-wave inversion in the lateral precordial leads, consistent with subendocardial ischemia. Her blood pressure was 98/64. She responded to the use of sublingual nitrates and the addition of parenteral calcium channel blocker to her regimen. She also received three units of packed RBC's with her hematocrit now 30 and hemoglobin of 10, with resolution of her angina.

Past History: Previous hospitalization was for hysterectomy at age 42, for menometrorrhagia. No other surgery. Only other hospitalization was for childbirth, gravida 2, para 1, AB 1. No other significant medical problems or chronic illness. All systems reviewed and are otherwise within normal limits.

Family History: Father died at age 81, acute myocardial infarction; he was hypertensive with NIDDM controlled by diet. Mother died at age 59 of ovarian cancer. Three brothers, all deceased, one of complications of alcohol abuse, one of coronary heart disease and one of complications of diabetes. Her sister, age 69, is living with mild hypertension, controlled with medications. No other relevant family history. She is married; her husband is 77 and in good health except for diffuse degenerative joint disease. She has one living daughter, age 50, mild hypertensive. She is a high-school graduate, retired clerk. Uses alcohol sparingly; uses caffeine moderately. Regular medications include H2 blockers, Vasotec and HCTZ as noted above. She occasionally uses enteric-coated aspirin to relieve aches and pains.

Physical Exam: Respirations 22 and somewhat labored, temperature 99.3, pulse 96, BP 112/78. The patient is pale and somewhat dyspneic, otherwise in no acute distress. **HEENT:** Eyes: PERRLA; EOMI; Ears, nose, mouth and throat all clear with no signs of infection. Neck supple, trachea midline; no thyromegaly; no cervical or submandibular nodes. Neck vein distension to 14cm. Normal carotids. Breasts are negative with no masses, no nipple discharge. Lungs reveal occasional fine rales at both bases, otherwise clear to auscultation and percussion; no use of accessory muscles of respiration. Heart: PMI, normal sinus rhythm, soft third heart sound, no murmurs. Abdomen soft, nontender, without palpable masses or organomegaly. Bowel sounds are normal. Extremities are negative with good pulses, no edema. cyanosis or clubbing. Neurological exam is grossly normal; cranial nerves intact. DTR's equal. Pelvic exam deferred. Rectal exam revealed soft, mushy black stool strongly heme positive.

(continued)

 QUICK TIP

The documentation supports a consultation noting who requested the consult and the purpose of the consult; this report is part of the patient's permanent hospital record. The consultant has made recommendations and will initiate treatment when the patient is stable.

> **Sample Documentation—99255 (Continued)**
>
> **Impression:**
> 1. Massive upper GI hemorrhage, probable secondary to reactivation of known peptic ulcer disease
> 2. Hypotension, resolved with transfusions
> 3. Angina pectoris, secondary to acute anemia and hypotension
> 4. Mild CHF secondary to blood transfusion fluid overload
>
> **Recommendations:**
> 1. Admit to ICU R/O MI protocol
> 2. Transfuse with RBC's to maintain hematocrit of 30 or above
> 3. Once the patient is stabilized, therapeutic endoscopy for management of GI bleed
> 4. Hold antihypertensives until needed
> 5. Bumetanide for fluid overload/CHF
> 6. Biopsy for H. Pylori during endoscopy
>
> Thank you for asking me to see your patient.
>
> **(General multisystem)**

KNOWLEDGE ASSESSMENT CHAPTER 7

See chapter 19 for answers and rationale.

1. Which of the following are appropriate places of service for use of office or other outpatient consultation codes (99241–99245)?
   a. Physician office
   b. Patient's home
   c. Hospital inpatient
   d. Emergency department

2. Codes 99241–99255 may be used to report consults initiated by a physician or the patient themselves.
   a. True
   b. False

3. Medicare no longer recognizes consultation codes but they are still used and reimbursable by some carriers.
   a. True
   b. False

4. Based on the documentation for code 99243 on page 184, which data element qualifies the PFSH as pertinent?
   a. Periodically evaluated for retinopathy
   b. Diabetes was diagnosed at age 12
   c. The patient is not hypertensive
   d. She has had no vision changes or problems

5. Select the HPI elements documented in the coding sample on page 196.
   a. Duration
   b. Severity
   c. Modifying factors
   d. Context

Chapter 8: Other Hospital-Based Services (99281–99292)

Emergency Department Services, New or Established Patient (99281–99288)

QUICK COMPARISON

Emergency Department Services, New or Established Patient

E/M Code	Medical Decision Making[1]	Problem[3] Severity	History[1]	Exam[1]	Counseling and/or Coordination of Care	Time Spent Face to Face (avg.)[2]
99281	Straight-forward	Minor or self-limited	Problem focused	Problem focused	Consistent with problems and patient's or family's needs	N/A
99282	Low complexity	Low to moderate	Expanded problem focused	Expanded problem focused	Consistent with problems and patient's or family's needs	N/A
99283	Moderate complexity	Moderate	Expanded problem focused	Expanded problem focused	Consistent with problems and patient's or family's needs	N/A
99284	Moderate complexity	High; requires urgent evaluation	Detailed	Detailed	Consistent with problems and patient's or family's needs	N/A
99285	High complexity	High; poses immediate/ significant threat to life or physiologic function	Comprehensive	Comprehensive	Consistent with problems and patient's or family's needs	N/A
99288[4]	Physician direction of EMS					N/A

1   Key component. For emergency department services, all three components (history, exam, and medical decision making) are crucial for selecting the correct code and must be adequately documented in the medical record to substantiate the level of service reported.

2   Typical times have not been established for this category of services.

3   NOTE: The severity of the patient's problem, while taken into consideration when evaluating and treating the patient, does not automatically determine the level of E/M service unless the medical record documentation reflects the severity of the patient's illness, injury, or condition in the details of the history, physical examination, and medical decision making process. Federal auditors will "downcode" the level of E/M service despite the nature of the patient's problem when the documentation does not support the E/M code reported.

4   Code 99288 is used to report two-way communication with emergency medical services personnel in the field.

GENERAL GUIDELINES

- Use these CPT® codes when an unscheduled, episodic evaluation and management (E/M) service was rendered to a patient who needed immediate medical attention. The services must have been provided in a hospital-based facility open 24 hours a day. These codes apply to new and established patients.

- Consider assigning the appropriate consultation code instead of these codes when an opinion or advice was provided about a patient for a specific problem at the request of another physician or other appropriate source.

- Report only the appropriate initial hospital care, initial hospital observation care or comprehensive nursing facility assessment code if the patient was admitted to the hospital or a nursing facility on the same day as the emergency department visit.

- Consider assigning the appropriate critical care codes (99291, 99292) instead of these codes if the physician provided constant attention to a critically ill patient.

- Append modifier 25 to report that a separately identifiable E/M service was performed by the same physician/qualified healthcare professional on the same day as a procedure or service. Only the content of the work associated with the separate E/M service should be considered when assigning the correct E/M level.

- Append modifier 57 to indicate that the decision to perform surgery was made at the visit. For Medicare, the decision must be to perform major surgery.

APC Note: Also, it is important to note that the use of the CPT E/M codes in provider-based clinics and emergency departments for APC billing is not determined or reported the same as for a facility. Unlike physician E/M codes, facility E/M codes are assigned according to internal coding guidelines. There are currently no national guidelines for distinguishing between the five levels of service. Some professional organizations have made recommendations for determining each level of service; however, at this time it is still each facility's responsibility to set internal standards. Many facilities require nursing staff to determine the level of service according to the types of diagnosis and treatment, while others may use a point system.

Under OPPS, CMS defines a type A emergency department as one that is licensed and advertised to be available to provide emergent care 24 hours a day, seven days a week. A type B emergency department is licensed and advertised to provide emergent care less than 24 hours a day, seven days a week. The type B emergency department may be the only emergent care portion of a hospital or it may be a separately carved out portion of the type A emergency department. Facilities should verify with their contractor to determine the types of emergency department they operate. Type A services are reported with codes 99281–99285, while type B services are reported with codes G0380–G0384. CMS notes that the designation of type A or B is based upon hours of operation of the hospital area and not the methodology to triage patients.

Under the Medicare ambulatory payment classification (APC) system, the type B emergency department services are classified into five APC groups:

- Code G0380 groups to level 1 type B emergency visit APC category 5031.
- Code G0381 groups to level 2 type B emergency visit APC category 5032.
- Code G0382 groups to level 3 type B emergency visit APC category 5033.
- Code G0383 groups to level 4 type B emergency visit APC category 5034.
- Code G0384 groups to level 5 type B emergency visit APC category 5035.

Each facility should develop a system for mapping the provided services or combination of services furnished to the different levels of effort represented by the codes. Each facility will be accountable for following its own system for assigning the different levels of HCPCS codes. As long as the services furnished are documented and medically necessary and the facility is following its own system, which reasonably relates the intensity of hospital resources to the different levels of HCPCS codes, CMS assumes compliance with these reporting mechanisms. They do not expect to see a high correlation between the code reported by the physician and the code reported by the facility. When a patient presents to the ER for a screening, and no other services are provided, it is reasonable to bill a low-level emergency department code. The screening services must be documented in the medical record, and the patient's leaving against medical advice—or whatever other facts are pertinent to the case—needs to be documented in the record.

ISSUES IN THIS CODE RANGE

- Emergency department professional coding and documentation has some different issues than many of the other code types and ranges. Practitioners in this area have long been taught to treat all presentations as new with uncertain outcomes, and perform fairly comprehensive histories and exams. The tendency is to have the history and physical exams better documented than decision making. Decision making is often undervalued by these providers because of the often critical conditions encountered. In other words, ER providers have a tendency to undervalue their decision making. In terms of the various decision making tables, these providers often score quite high on diagnostic tests performed and ordered because of the ready availability of these facilities.
- Greater use of the critical care codes would be expected as these providers routinely deal with unstable patients. When the level of patient care supports the use of critical care services it is imperative that the documentation supports the service and that time spent providing critical care services is documented in the record. When using these codes, coders must be cognizant of all the codes that are bundled in to these services to avoid unbundling. Critical care codes have a greater RVU value and are reported in lieu of emergency department codes. For detailed information on critical care codes and services included

 QUICK TIP

Services by nonemergency department providers are usually reported with other category E/M services. Some payers restrict the use of codes 99281–99285 to ED-based physicians only.

with these services, refer to the critical care services section later in this chapter.

- At the higher code ranges ROS and FH are usually the history components overlooked or under-documented. Use of the phrase "ROS o/w neg." goes a long way to help here if it is in fact taken. HPIs in this setting are usually quite complete.

- The 99285 code is the only code in the CPT book that has a caveat relative to the extent of history and exam recorded or taken. This states that all components, but most likely the history and exam, are required "within the constraints imposed by the urgency of the patient's clinical condition and/or mental status." Not enough providers reference this caveat in their notes although many patients present either unconscious, intubated, or confused.

- There is also an interesting shift on coding and documentation indicators in these codes. Both levels 99282 and 99283 have identical history and exam requirements with the only difference being the level of decision making. At the 99284 and 99285 levels we also see language used nowhere else in the nature of the presenting problem. The level IV code definition is stated as "urgent evaluation is required" while the level V code describes problems (or differentials) that "pose an immediate significant threat to life and physiologic function."

- The differences above are important to note as often the histories and exams are rather complete. With both level 99283 and 99284 assigned moderate level decision making—the real difference lies in the urgency of the problem.

- The single-system specialty exam for Heme/Lymph seems to most closely resemble the typical ER higher-end exams. The 1995 organ system level general system exam is by far the easiest to document in this setting.

- Codes for high-level E/M services have been targeted in the CERT program as being overutilized. Medical necessity and the level of medical decision making should be verified for all high-level E/M services.

99281

DOCUMENTATION REQUIREMENTS

Medical Decision Making: straightforward
- Minimal number of diagnoses or management options considered
- No or minimal amount and complexity of data reviewed
- Minimal risk of complications or morbidity or mortality

Problem Severity: minor or self-limited
- Little, if any, risk of morbidity without treatment
- Little, if any, risk of mortality without treatment
- Transient problem, low probability of permanently altered status
- Good prognosis

History: problem focused
- Chief complaint
- Brief history of present illness or problem (one to three HPI elements)

Examination: problem focused
- 1995: one organ system or body area
- 1997: one to five bullet (•) elements in one or more organ systems/body areas

Code Indicators (from tables of risk—including some AMA indicators in italic)

Presenting Problem(s)
- One self-limited or minor problem

Management Options
- Rest, gargles, elastic bandages, superficial dressings

Counseling and/or Coordination of Care
- As appropriate for the problem—no times are assigned these codes

Sample Documentation—99281

Level I Emergency Department Visit

A 7-year-old black male presents to the emergency department with his mother for a burn recheck. He was seen in this department two days ago after picking up an expended sparkler and sustaining a minor burn to the right palm which was cleaned and dressed.

He is a well-developed, well-nourished black child in no acute distress. He has had no fever and examination of the palmate surface shows a healing 5 centimeter linear area of burn. Neurovascularly intact, good range of motion all digits.

Apply clean dressing. Burn care sheet provided.

(General multisystem)

 QUICK TIP

Code 99281 is more appropriate than 16020 Dressing change, small outpatient burn. Code 16020 usually applies to burns greater than first degree or minor burns as described in the documentation.

99282

DOCUMENTATION REQUIREMENTS

Medical Decision Making: low
- Limited number of diagnoses or management options considered
- Limited amount and complexity of data reviewed
- Low risk of complications or morbidity or mortality

Problem Severity: low to moderate
- Expectation of full recovery without functional impairment, or uncertain outcome or increased probability of prolonged functional impairment
- Low to moderate risk of morbidity, if any, without treatment

History: expanded problem focused
- Chief complaint
- Brief history of present illness (one to three HPI elements)
- Problem pertinent system review (one or two systems)

Examination: expanded problem focused
- 1995: two to seven organ systems or body areas
- 1997: at least six bullet (•) elements in one or more organ systems/body areas

Code Indicators (from tables of risk—including some AMA indicators in italic)

Presenting Problem(s)
- Two or more two self-limited or minor problem(s)
- One stable chronic illness (e.g., well controlled hypertension or non-insulin-dependent diabetes, cataract, BPH)
- Acute uncomplicated illness or injury (e.g., cystitis, allergic rhinitis, simple sprain)

Management Options
- Physical therapy, *rest or exercise, diet, stress management*
- Over the counter drugs, *medication management with minimal risk*
- Minor surgery, with no identified risk factors
- Occupational therapy

Counseling and/or Coordination of Care
- As appropriate for the problem—no times are assigned these codes

Sample Documentation—99282

Level II Emergency Department Visit

A 22-year-old female presents to the ED with nonmenstrual vaginal hemorrhage. Bleeding is described as mild, beginning at about 5:00 p.m. last evening, occurring only periodically between now and the time it began last night. Denies clots or other debris. Denies pregnancy; is sexually active. Intermittent use of condoms. No other contraception. LMP six weeks ago. No other symptoms. Denies breast/nipple changes. Last GYN exam one year ago. Gravida 0; para 0. Positive history of dysmenorrhea in mother and maternal grandmother.

(continued)

Sample Documentation—99282 (Continued)

O: General: well-developed, well-nourished thin female in no acute distress. Vitals: T: 98.4; R: 18; P: 88; BP: 116/68. HEENT deferred. Abdomen: soft, flat, no organomegaly. No mass. External genitalia essentially WNL. Vagina: no sign of blood in vault. No signs of trauma. Urethra WNL. Bimanual exam of uterus: 12 cm nontender uterus. No adnexal mass/tenderness.

Labs: b-HCG reported negative.

A: R/O development of dysmenorrhea.

P: Office appointment made with patient's OB/GYN for tomorrow in a.m. Strict bedrest. If hemorrhage should become heavy in the interim, she should return to the ED.

(General multisystem)

How This Level of E/M Service Was Assigned

- **History:** CC: A 22-year-old female presents to the ED for evaluation of minimal nonmenstrual vaginal hemorrhage. HPI: extended. ROS: problem pertinent. PFSH: The past, family, and social history data qualify as complete. The history, considering its elements of CC, HPI, ROS, and PFSH, ranges from expanded problem focused to comprehensive. All elements must meet or exceed the specific requirements for a level of service; therefore, the final assessment of the history is a level of "expanded problem focused."

- **Physical Examination (multisystem):** Constitutional: Two bullet elements: (1) vital signs and (2) general appearance. GI: Two bullet elements are noted. GU: Four bullet elements noted. Total number of elements noted in documentation equals eight; therefore, physical examination documentation minimally exceeds the level requirements for "expanded problem focused." Three organ systems are assessed qualifying for expanded problem focused under 1995 guidelines as well.

- **Medical Decision Making:** Diagnosis made by the physician is R/O dysmenorrhea. One laboratory test is performed and assessed. The patient is instructed to observe the flow of hemorrhage (if any) and is referred to a specialist. The elements in the medical decision making, at this point in the patient's presentation for this condition, range from minimal to low. The number of diagnoses/management options is low, with a new problem to both the patient and examiner; the amount/complexity of data reviewed is minimal; the risk is minimal to low. Therefore, the final medical decision making level is assessed as being "low."

- **Final E/M Level of Service:** CPT code 99282 is assigned. ED services must have the three key components (history, exam, and medical decision making) documented in the chart and all of the key components must meet or exceed a specific level of service to be appropriately assigned. In this particular case, the history and exam both qualify as expanded problem focused (code 99282) as does the medical decision making. Therefore, code 99282 is the final assignment.

Level II Emergency Department Visit

This 33-year-old male presents today in the ED for evaluation and treatment of NVD, fever, and chills of over four-hour duration. Patient noticed symptoms began about six hours after ingesting a buffet "all you can eat" meal at a local restaurant. Had various dishes at that time including chicken, chicken casseroles, spaghetti and meatballs, and fresh salad. Tried an OTC antiemetic to no avail.

ROS: Negative for other GI or CV indications. Past Medical Hx: no history gastritis; appendicitis. Usual childhood illnesses. Adenoidectomy age 5. Tonsils intact. Social Hx reveals NKA. Nonsmoker; occasional ETOH at parties

O: T: 99.4; R: 24; P: 60; BP: 124/76. General: adult male in obvious distress; worried. Mouth: pharynx WNL. Heart: RSR, no murmurs. Chest: clear. Abd: muscular with sl. epigastric tenderness. BS hyperactive..

Laboratory Findings: Blood profile: normal chemistries. WBCs 7,500 with no shift. UA: specific gravity 1.030.

A: Probable staphylococci gastroenteritis.

P: Compazine 25 mg IM. Encourage p.o. fluids. Prescription for Lomotil sig: 2 tabs q.i.d. #32. Follow up with Primary Care Physician if no improvement. If worsening occurs return to ED.

(General multisystem)

 KEY POINT

This service is reported with 99282 as the medical decision making is documented at the low level. Higher levels of E/M require a higher level of medical decision making.

99283

DOCUMENTATION REQUIREMENTS

Medical Decision Making: moderate
- Multiple number of diagnoses or management options considered
- Moderate amount or complexity of data reviewed
- Moderate risk of complications or morbidity or mortality

Problem Severity: moderate
- Moderate risk of morbidity without treatment
- Moderate risk of mortality without treatment
- Uncertain outcome or increased probability of prolonged functional impairment or increased probability of prolonged functional impairment

History: expanded problem focused
- Chief complaint
- Brief history of present illness (one to three HPI elements)
- Problem pertinent system review (one or two systems)

Examination: expanded problem focused
- 1995: two to seven organ systems or body areas
- 1997: at least six bullet (•) elements in one or more organ systems/body areas

Code Indicators (from tables of risk—including some AMA indicators in italic)

Presenting Problem(s)
- One or more chronic illness with mild exacerbation, progression, or side effects of treatment
- Two or more stable chronic illnesses
- Undiagnosed new *illness, injury,* or problem with uncertain prognosis
- Acute illness, with systemic symptoms (pyelonephritis, pleuritis, colitis)
- Acute complicated injury, e.g., head injury, with brief loss of consciousness

Management Options
- Prescription drug management
- Closed treatment of fracture or dislocation, without manipulation
- IV fluids with additives
- Minor surgery, with identified risk factors
- Elective major surgery (open, percutaneous, endoscopic), with no identified risk factors
- Therapeutic nuclear medicine

Counseling and/or Coordination of Care
- As appropriate for the problem—no times are assigned these codes

Sample Documentation—99283

Note: This encounter is almost the same as the second example for 99282. The only differences in these levels occur in decision making and severity of the presenting problem. You will see that a few diagnostic services and further treatment make the difference between low and moderate. Additions in italic.

Level III Emergency Department Visit

This 33-year-old male presents today in the ED for evaluation and treatment of NVD, fever, and chills of over four-hour duration. Patient noticed symptoms began about six hours after ingesting a buffet "all you can eat" meal at a local restaurant. Had various dishes at that time including chicken, chicken casseroles, spaghetti and meatballs, and fresh salad. Tried an OTC anti-emetic to no avail.

ROS negative for other GI or CV indications. Past Medical Hx: no history gastritis; appendicitis. Usual childhood illnesses. Adenoidectomy age 5. Tonsils intact. Social Hx reveals NKA. Nonsmoker; occasional ETOH at parties

O: T: 99.4; R: 24; P: 60; BP: 124/76. General: adult male in obvious distress; worried. Mouth: pharynx WNL. Heart: RSR, no murmurs. Chest: clear. Abd: muscular with sl. epigastric tenderness. BS hyperactive. *Psoas-negative.*

Laboratory Findings: Blood profile: normal chemistries. WBCs 7,500 with no shift. UA: specific gravity 1.030. *KUB within normal limits as read by me.*

A: Probable staphylococci gastroenteritis; *dehydration.*

P: *IV hydration.* Compazine 25 mg IM. Encourage p.o. fluids. Prescription for Lomotil sig: 2 tabs q.i.d. #32. Follow up with Primary Care Physician. If worsening occurs return to ED.

(General multisystem)

 KEY POINT

The level of decision making is appropriate based upon the nature of the presenting problem.

99284

DOCUMENTATION REQUIREMENTS

Medical Decision Making: moderate
- Multiple number of diagnoses or management options considered
- Moderate amount or complexity of data reviewed
- Moderate risk of complications or morbidity or mortality

Problem Severity: high
- High to extreme risk of morbidity without treatment
- Moderate to high risk of mortality without treatment
- No immediate significant threat to life or physiological function, but urgent physician care required

History: detailed
- Chief complaint
- Extended history of present illness (four or more HPI elements or the status of three chronic problems)
- Extended system review (two to nine systems)
- Pertinent past, family, and/or social history (one of the history areas)

Examination: detailed
- 1995: two to seven organ systems or body areas with an extended exam of affected area(s)
- 1997: at least two bullet (•) elements from at least six organ systems or body areas, OR at least 12 bullet (•) elements from two or more organ systems or body areas. Eye and psychiatric single-system exams must include at least nine bullet (•) elements.

Code Indicators (from tables of risk—including some AMA indicators in italic)

Presenting Problem(s)
- One or more chronic illness with mild exacerbation, progression, or side effects of treatment
- Two or more stable chronic illnesses
- Undiagnosed new *illness, injury,* or problem with uncertain prognosis
- Acute illness, with systemic symptoms (pyelonephritis, pleuritis, colitis)
- Acute complicated injury, e.g., head injury, with brief loss of consciousness

Management Options
- Prescription drug management
- Closed treatment of fracture or dislocation, without manipulation
- IV fluids with additives
- Minor surgery, with identified risk factors
- Elective major surgery (open, percutaneous, endoscopic), with no identified risk factors
- Therapeutic nuclear medicine

Counseling and/or Coordination of Care

- As appropriate for the presenting problem—no times are assigned these codes

Sample Documentation—99284

Level IV Emergency Department Visit

This is a 23-year-old female, on active duty in the military but home at this time on military leave, with a three-day history of lower right back pain secondary to muscle strain she thinks she had sustained at that time. Several hours prior to her presentation here, she developed rapid onset of fever, severe shaking chills and nausea and vomiting. No diarrhea. She also c/o headaches at this time. Denies dysuria, polyuria, and change in urine color or stool color/consistency. Denies any real injury to her back, just thought she might have strained something carrying her suitcase. Positive history of frequent UTIs. Has not self-treated. No increase in fluid intake.

ROS: Feels well in general except for this episode. CV: history of heart murmur present since a child. She has been told by her military doctors that this murmur presents no problems for her. No resp. problems. Neg. GI or GU symptomatology, but frequent UTIs as noted. Psych: likes the military, relatively happy as she is stationed close to home. Skin: No complaints. Tends to scar easily. Has developed keloids about the earlobes, removed twice now but she no longer wears pierced earrings. Musculoskeletal: no arthritis. Neuro: without complaint. Allergic: severely allergic to bee stings and is "deathly" afraid to have these insects around her.

PMH: gravida 1, para 1 vaginal delivery three years ago.

SH: Taking BCPs now. Smokes 1/2 pack cigarettes/day. Drinks occasionally. Unmarried. Child lives with the patient's mother.

FH: positive for CA of lungs, HTN in paternal grandfather, CAD in maternal grandmother, and DM in mother.

O: Vitals: T; 104.4; BP: 124/82; R: 22. General: well-developed, well-nourished female appearing her stated age. HEENT: unremarkable. Nasopharynx normal. Eyes WNL. Ears WNL. Throat WNL. Chest: clear to P&A. Heart auscultation reveals grade II/VI holosystolic murmur along the left sternal border; otherwise WNL. GI: Sl. tenderness over epigastrium referred to the right flank region. No guarding or rebound. Negative psoas sign. No organomegaly. No mass. Right CVA tenderness. Unable to touch her chin to her chest. Negative Kernig's sign. Neuro: unremarkable. Normal DTRs. Musculoskeletal exam: entirely WNL. No muscle spasm. Lymph: Axillary/cervical/inguinal nodes negative. GU: deferred.

Labs: CBC, UA with culture and sensitivity, and blood chemistries ordered. KUB ordered. (all STAT labs)

A: Right acute pyelonephritis.

P: Patient is well hydrated and tolerating oral agents well; therefore, begin Cipro 500 mg q.12h. for two weeks. Re-check in three to four days. PRN sooner. Tylenol for temperature elevations. Encourage fluids.

(General multisystem)

Level IV Emergency Department Visit

This 19-year-old male presents in the ER after office hours with complaints of abdominal pain of a two-day duration, beginning as an epigastric discomfort and culminating in today's presentation of sharp RLQ and diffuse LLQ pain. The pain has been gradually increasing. Has not been exercising the past few days secondary to abdominal pain. Does admit to N&V for past 24 hours. Fever spiked to 102 today. Loss of appetite and fatigue. No history of appendectomy. Pt. is accompanied to the ER by his mother.

PMH: Negative abdominal history. No childhood surgeries. Usual illnesses including chickenpox. Typically gets seasonal coryza every few years. Otherwise, negative. No known drug allergies. Immunizations up-to-date.

SH: Lives at home with parents; in community college taking general studies curriculum. Does not smoke or drink. Exercises daily using free weights and nautilus-type machines.

FH: Noncontributory.

(continued)

✓ **QUICK TIP**

Note that the medical decision making is of moderate level.

Sample Documentation—99284 (Continued)

ROS: General: as above. GI: see HPI. GU: no dysuria. No polyuria. No flank pain. Musculoskeletal: no complaints. Denies recent or probable abdominal strain secondary to weightlifting.

O: General appearance: young man appearing moderately ill and uncomfortable. T: 102.8. BP: 122/78. Ht: 6'1". Wt: 200 lbs. HEENT: sclerae/conjunctivae clear. Oral mucosa slightly dry. Remainder negative. Resp: lung fields clear. No rales, rhonchi, wheezing. Clear to P. CV: RSR. Normal S1, S2. No rub, murmur or gallop. Abd: right lower quadrant tenderness with rebound tenderness at McBurney's point. BS normal to hypoactive. No organomegaly. No mass. Positive psoas sign. Rectal: tender rectal vault. Lymph: no cervical or axillary lymphadenopathy. Inguinal nodes nontender. Neuro: no focal deficits. DTRs normal. Skin warm to touch.

Laboratory Findings reveal WBC of 15,800 with a shift to the left. Normal HCT, SMA-24, UA and CXR. KUB revealed evidence of mass in RLQ.

A: Probable appendicitis.

P: Admit to General Medical service. Hydrate. Begin on IV Cleocin and Garamycin. Emergency call to Dr. General Surgeon for exploratory lap ASAP.

(General multisystem)

How This Level of E/M Service Was Assigned

- **History:** CC: A 19-year-old male presents in the ER with complaints of abdominal pain, HPI: Extended. ROS: Three distinct systems are mentioned in the note—all problem pertinent—including the ROS data integrated into the HPI, qualifying this element of the history as detailed. PFSH: the past, family, and social history data qualify as complete. The history, considering its elements of CC, HPI, ROS, and PFSH, ranges from detailed to comprehensive. All elements must meet or exceed the specific requirements for a level of service; therefore, the final assessment of the history is a level of detailed.

- **Physical Examination (Multisystem):** Constitutional: Two bullet elements: (1) vital signs and (2) general appearance. HEENT (includes multisystem exam requirements for eyes, ears, nose, mouth, and throat): Three bullet elements are noted. Respiratory: Two bullet points. Cardiovascular: One bullet point. GI: Three bullet elements are noted. Lymphatic: Three bullet elements. Neuro: Two bullet points. Skin: one bullet point. Total number of elements noted in documentation equals 17; therefore, physical examination documentation exceeds the level requirements for detailed but does not meet the requirements for comprehensive per the 1997 guidelines. By 1995 or 2000 guidelines the exam qualified for comprehensive. The final exam level of service assessment equates to "detailed" or "comprehensive."

- **Medical Decision Making:** Diagnosis made by the physician is Probable appendicitis; R/O surgical abdomen. Several laboratory tests are performed and assessed; an x-ray is also ordered and reviewed. The patient is admitted to the inpatient service. IV antibiotics are begun, and a call is placed to a general surgeon for exploratory surgery. The number of diagnoses/management options is extensive; the amount/complexity of data reviewed is extensive; the risk is high considering the pending surgery. The final medical decision making level is assessed as being high.

- **Final E/M Level of Service:** CPT code 99284 is assigned. ED services must have the three key components (history, exam, and medical decision making) documented in the chart and all of the key components must meet or exceed a specific level of service to be appropriately assigned. In this particular case, the patient history qualifies as detailed(code 99284), the physical examination meets the requirements for a detailed level (99284) under 1997 guidelines or comprehensive (99285) under 1995, and the medical decision making qualifies as high (99285). As only one of the three key elements qualifies for reporting code 99285, the final code assignment is 99284. As appropriate, if the caveat had been referenced relative to history and exam this could have qualified for 99285. The addition or mention of a complete ROS was the difference here.

99285

DOCUMENTATION REQUIREMENTS

Medical Decision Making: high
- Extensive number of diagnoses or management options considered
- Extensive amount or complexity of data reviewed
- High risk of complications or morbidity or mortality

Problem Severity: high
- High to extreme risk of morbidity without treatment
- Moderate to high risk of mortality without treatment
- Immediate significant threat to life or physiological function

History: comprehensive
- Chief complaint
- Extended history of present illness (four or more HPI elements or the status of three chronic problems)
- Complete system review (10 systems)
- Complete past, family, social history (at least one element from all history areas)

Examination: comprehensive
- 1995: eight or more organ systems
- 1997: multisystem exam must include all bullet (•) elements from at least nine organ systems or body areas unless specific instructions limit content of the exam; at least two bullet elements from each area/system reviewed are expected to be documented.
- 1997: single organ system/body area exam must include all bullet (•) elements in shaded boxes PLUS at least one element in each unshaded box.

Code Indicators (from tables of risk—including some AMA indicators in italic)

Presenting Problem(s)
- One or more chronic illness with severe exacerbation, progression, or side effects of treatment
- Acute or chronic illness or injury that poses a threat to life or bodily function, e.g., multiple traumas, acute MI, pulmonary embolism, severe respiratory distress, progressive severe rheumatoid arthritis, psychiatric illness, with potential threat to self or others, peritonitis, ARF
- An abrupt change in neurological status, e.g., seizure, TIA, weakness, sensory loss

Management Options
- Elective major surgery with identified risk factors or emergency major surgery (open, percutaneous, endoscopic)
- Parenteral controlled substances
- Drug therapy requiring intensive monitoring for toxicity

- IV fluids, without additives
- Decision not to resuscitate or to deescalate care because of poor prognosis

Counseling and/or Coordination of Care
- As appropriate for the problem—no times are assigned these codes

---

Sample Documentation—99285

Level V Emergency Department Visit

A 73-year-old male presents this morning in the Emergency Department for evaluation and treatment of fever, chills and headache of one week duration. Patient had a home temperature of 103 degrees last evening. Also c/o productive cough, general malaise and muscle/joint aching. Occasional sputum, which is yellow-green in color, without blood and thick in consistency. The patient has had nocturnal diaphoresis and a several pound weight loss over the previous week. No history of previous pneumonitis or TB. The patient also c/o of concomitant symptoms of sore throat, mild earaches and decreased appetite. Other than this episode, he feels he has been in general good health and has a good sense of well-being.

PMH: Appendectomy at age 22; T&A at age 12. Laceration of hand many years ago while working on telephone lines, repaired with sutures.

FH: Unremarkable. No thyroid disease, no CA, no CVD, no DM no HTN. Only remarkable for "crazies" as he says, explaining that his mother and grandmother were manic-depressives. Denies any similar symptoms himself.

SH: Married, wife alive and well at age 70. No children. Mother, maternal grandmother as above. Father deceased of probable "old age."

ROS: Resp: does admit to SOB when coughing and with physical exertion over the last few days. Blames sore throat on cough. Heart: c/o some chest pain with deep inspiration over the last several days. Denies paroxysmal nocturnal dyspnea, orthopnea or dyspnea on exertion. No history MI or angina. GI: No NVD. No dark or clay-colored stools. GU: decreased urination this past week. Reports his urine seems darker during past week. No neuro complaints. Musculoskeletal: only "old age" complaints. O/w neg.

PE: General: well-developed male who appears ill and extremely fatigued. Answers all questions promptly; no signs disorientation. Alert. T: 103. Pulse 100. Resp: 20. Blood pressure 138/72. Skin is hot to touch without lesions or petechiae. Head normocephalic. Pupils are equal, round and reactive to light and accommodation. EOMs intact. Fundi: disc edges sharp. Ears: right TM red and injected; left TM WNL. Nose: mucosa slightly erythemic. Pharynx: erythematous without exudates. Neck supple without mass. Nontender, small cervical lymph nodes. No meningeal signs. Lungs: rhonchi audible bilaterally, lower lobes. Heart: regular rate and rhythm. There is a grade I/VI ejection murmur noted at the 5th left intercostal space without radiation. Abd: scaphoid, soft. Tenderness to percussion in RUQ. No mass. No rebound. Rectal within normal limits. Stool guaiac negative. Neuro: cranial nerves intact. Motor/sensory intact.

Laboratory tests ordered are blood chemistries, H&H and STAT CXR. UA also ordered as well as sputum culture and sensitivity, gram stain. ABGs: pH 7.0; PO2 65; PCO2 36.

STAT CXR reveals patchy infiltrate in the right and left lower lobes; remainder of lung fields is otherwise clear.

Admission Impression: 73-y/o male with probable community acquired pneumonia. Diff. dxs' include mycoplasma, Legionella, pneumococcus and gram negative infections.

P: (1) Admit due to age, temperature greater 101 degrees, and multi-lobe involvement. (2) Begin Erythromycin 500 mg q.i.d. (3) Patient unable to produce sputum—induce sputum for gram stain, C&S. (4) IV hydration. (5) Oxygen two liters by nasal cannula. Monitor with oximetry.

(General multisystem)

QUICK TIP

Although the patient will be admitted, the emergency department physician is not the admitting physician and it is appropriate to report code 99285.

99288

DOCUMENTATION REQUIREMENTS

Physician direction of emergency medical systems (EMS) emergency care, advanced life support

Parameters:

- Two-way voice communication by a physician or other qualified healthcare professional in a hospital emergency or critical care department with ambulance or rescue personnel outside the hospital
- Physician directs performance of necessary medical procedures taking place in the field
- Includes telemetry, cardiopulmonary resuscitation, intubation, administration of intravenous fluids and/or administration of intramuscular, intratracheal, or subcutaneous drugs, and/or defibrillation/electrical conversion of arrhythmia

Documentation:

- Typically, these communications are recorded, as well as entered into a written log.

Coding Issues:

- Medicare, as well as most other third-party payers, considers this service bundled into the evaluation and management (E/M) code billed by the emergency department physician at the time the patient arrives at the facility. Therefore, it would not typically be coded separately.

Special Instructions for E/M Coding of Trauma Care

The American College of Surgeons (ACS) published a bulletin titled "Effectively Using E/M Codes for Trauma Care." The bulletin provides coding guidance for surgeons on how to appropriately report E/M codes related to care rendered to injured or critically ill patients in the emergency department or inpatient setting including critical care services.

Highlights from the article are bulleted below:

- The ACS recommends the creation of a standardized evaluation form for the history and physical for both admissions and consultations. The Advanced Trauma Life Support (ATLS) initial assessment and management tool may be incorporated into the creation of the surgeon's initial assessment and management document to ensure capture of all necessary elements to code at the highest levels of E/M codes.
- Trauma admission forms usually cover a multisystem exam as the majority of trauma patients would receive a comprehensive evaluation.
- Complete, accurate, and detailed documentation is essential and should include times for time-based codes such as critical care services as well as the history, exam, and medical decision making for non-time-based codes.
- Because trauma care typically involves an evaluation in the ED and/or admission to the hospital, or transfer to another facility of observation, it is vitally important to ensure proper reporting of the patient's status

and the corresponding E/M code as well as the appropriate place of service code.

- In some circumstances, critical care services may be provided and reported in conjunction with other E/M codes for the same patient on the same date of service; for example, a patient may be admitted to the hospital (99223) and later in the day the patient's condition deteriorates to a degree where the physician must provide critical care to stabilize the patient. The total duration of time spent providing the critical care may also be reported.

Critical Care Services (99291–99292)

QUICK COMPARISON

Critical Care Services

E/M Code	Patient Status	Physician Attendance	Time
99291[1]	Critically ill or critically injured	Constant	First 30–74 min.
99292[2]	Critically ill or critically injured	Constant	Each additional 30 minutes beyond the first 74 minutes
1	Under outpatient prospective payment rules, only 99291 is submitted for critical care services in a hospital setting.		
2	Under outpatient prospective payment rules, 99292 is not an appropriate code for hospital outpatient use.		

Note: For critical care services provided in a facility to patients less than 71 months of age, see codes 99471–99476.

GENERAL GUIDELINES

- A minimum of 30 minutes must be rendered and appropriately documented in order to report the first hour of critical care. If total time documented is less than 30 minutes, report the appropriate level of E/M code. Critical care of less than 15 minutes duration is not reported separately.

- Record in the patient's record the time spent with the patient and the service provided.

- Append modifier 24 to code 99291 or 99292 to report postoperative critical care services that were unrelated to the surgery performed.

- Assign modifier 25 to code 99291 or 99292 to report preoperative critical care services that were unrelated to surgery but provided by the same physician on the same day as the surgery.

- A critical illness or injury acutely impairs one or more vital organ systems such that there is a high probability of imminent or life threatening deterioration in the patient's condition.

- Critical care involves high-complexity decision making to assess, manipulate, and support vital system functions to treat single or multiple vital organ system failure and/or to prevent further life threatening deterioration of the patient's condition.

- Examples of vital organ system failure include but are not limited to central nervous system failure, circulatory failure, shock, and renal, hepatic, metabolic, and/or respiratory failure. Although critical care typically requires interpretation of multiple physiologic parameters and/or application of advanced technologies, critical care may be provided in life threatening situations when these elements are not present.

- Providing medical care to a critically ill, injured, or postoperative patient qualifies as a critical care service only if both the illness and injury and the treatment being provided meet the above requirements.

- Critical care is usually, but not always, given in a critical care area, such as the coronary care unit, intensive care unit, pediatric intensive care unit, respiratory care unit, or the emergency care facility.

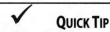

QUICK TIP

Inpatient critical care for 29 days to 24 months is reported with codes 99471 and 99472.

- Outpatient critical services for pediatric patients through 71 months old are reported with codes 99291 and 99292. See codes 99468–99476 for inpatient neonatal and pediatric critical services.
- Codes 99291 and 99292 should be used for physician attendance during a transport of a critically ill patient older than 24 months.
- Critical care and other E/M services may be provided to the same patient on the same date by the same physician based on CPT guidelines. However, there are NCCI edits in place bundling emergency room services and critical care services together. With appropriate modifiers and supporting documentation, they can be reported together on the same day, assuming they were provided at separate times and are separately identifiable services.
- Critical care services codes are time-based codes; thus, they are used to report the total amount of time spent by the physician providing critical care services to the patient.
- Critical care time does not have to be continuous and may encompass several critical care encounters per day.
- Time spent, per day, is added together for a total amount that aids in appropriate code selection. Note that a physician does not need to be in constant attendance at the patient's bedside, but does have to be directly involved in work related to the patient's care. The first hour of critical care can only be reported once per day. Assign the correct code for critical care provided to a hospital inpatient according to the following guidelines:

— less than 30 minutes	Appropriate E/M code
— 30–74 minutes	99291 x 1
— 75–104 minutes	99291 x 1 and 99292 x 1
— 105–134 minutes	99291 x 1 and 99292 x 2
— 135–164 minutes	99291 x 1 and 99292 x 3
— 165–194 minutes	99291 x 1 and 99292 x 4

Special Instructions for Reporting Critical Care Services

There are no absolute limits on the amount of critical care time that can be billed per day or hospital stay as long as the medical records can support the need for all critical care services provided. However, time spent performing procedures or services that can be reported separately should not be included in the time reported as critical care time.

- If, outside of the critical care period, the physician performs and adequately documents a complete E/M service, assignment of an additional E/M code reflecting this service is appropriate. Append modifier 25 to the additional E/M code to indicate that this was a separately identifiable service.
- Time spent providing services that do not directly relate and contribute to the care and treatment of the critical patient is not reported as critical care. This may include time spent outside of the unit, phone calls with other providers or patients, and remote supervision of a patient.
- For Medicare, however, only one physician may bill for a given hour of critical care even if more than one physician provided care to a critically ill or injured patient.

- According to *CPT 2021*, the following CPT codes are included in critical care codes and may not be billed on dates when critical care is billed:

36000	Introduction of needle or intracath, vein
36410	Venipuncture, over age 3, requiring physician's skill
36415	Venipuncture
36591	Collection of blood specimen from a completely implantable venous access device
36600	Arterial puncture
43752	Naso- or oro-gastric tube placement, necessitating physician's skill
43753	Therapeutic gastric intubation and aspiration(s), necessitating physician's skill
71045	Radiologic examination, chest; single view
71046	Radiologic examination, chest; 2 views
92953	Temporary transcutaneous pacing
93561	Indicator dilution studies with cardiac output measurements
93562	Indicator dilution studies, subsequent measurements
94002	Ventilation assist and management, initiation of pressure or volume preset ventilators for assisted or controlled breathing; hospital inpatient/observation, initial day
94003	Ventilation assist and management, initiation of pressure or volume preset ventilators for assisted or controlled breathing; hospital inpatient/observation, each subsequent day
94004	Ventilation assist and management, initiation of pressure or volume preset ventilators for assisted or controlled breathing; nursing facility, per day
94660	Continuous positive airway pressure ventilation (CPAP) initiation and management
94662	Continuous negative pressure ventilation initiation and management
94760	Noninvasive ear or pulse oximetry for oxygen saturation; single determination
94761	Noninvasive ear or pulse oximetry for oxygen saturation; multiple determinations (e.g., during exercise)
94762	Noninvasive ear or pulse oximetry for oxygen saturation; by continuous overnight monitoring (separate procedure)

- When additional procedures are reported on the same date as critical care services, the time involved in the procedures may not be included in total critical care time. For Medicare beneficiaries, the list of inclusive CPT codes when critical care is rendered may vary slightly from that published in *CPT 2021*. Check with your Medicare carrier for a correct listing of inclusive services when critical care is provided.

- CMS and other commercial carriers have been quite explicit in stating that physicians must be clear and thorough in noting the amount of time actually spent providing critical care services to a patient. Failure to accurately and appropriately document critical care times can result in a carrier downcoding the service or outright denying the claim.

Remember, the physician must devote his/her complete and full attention to the patient during the time specified as providing critical care.

- There are a number of templates and forms that can be used to capture all of the relevant information necessary to properly and correctly report critical care services. These forms and templates can be customized to the specific needs of a practice. A sample template is shown below.

Sample Documentation of Critical Care Time

Patient's Name:_____.
Patient's Medical Record Number:_____.
The services I provided to this patient were provided to treat_____
_____
(State the condition the patient was treated for)
The services I provided required the highest level of my skills with direct and personal management of the patient's treatment. These services included:

- Medical record documentation
- Vital sign assessments
- Medication orders and management
- Reviewing all notes and previous visits
- Collaborating with other physicians on treatment options
- Care, transfer of care, and discharge plans
- Interpreting/reviewing all tests and studies
- Discussions with family or surrogate decision makers
- Other
- _____

The total critical care time was_____hours _____minutes. The total time does not include treating other patients, performing separately reportable procedures, or activities that were not directly related to the care of the patient.
Physician's signature:_____Date:_____.

99291

DOCUMENTATION REQUIREMENTS

Patient Status:
- Lack of stability
- Conditions pose significant threat to life or risk of prolonged impairment

Physician Attendance
- Constant/intermittent
- Full attention devoted to the unstable critically ill or unstable critically injured patient

Time Spent Face to Face (average)
- First 30–74 minutes

Special Coding and Documentation Considerations
- Use this code to report critical care services rendered for a total of 30–74 minutes on a given day, even if the time spent by the physician is not continuous.
- Critical care performed on neonatal or pediatric patients less than 71 months of age may be reported with codes 99291 and 99292 when performed in an outpatient setting.

 KEY POINT

Time spent rendering critical care must be documented in the medical record. Documentation should support the need for constant attendance by the provider.

99292

DOCUMENTATION REQUIREMENTS

Patient Status
- Lack of stability
- Conditions pose significant threat to life or risk of prolonged impairment

Physician Attendance
- Constant/intermittent
- Full attention devoted to the unstable critically ill or unstable critically injured patient

Time Spent Face to Face (average)
- Each additional 30 minutes beyond the first 74 minutes

Special Coding and Documentation Considerations
- Never assign 99292 alone—it should be reported only with 99291
- Critical care performed on neonatal or pediatric patients less than 71 months of age may be reported with codes 99291 and 99292 when performed in an outpatient setting.

KNOWLEDGE ASSESSMENT CHAPTER 8

See chapter 19 for answers and rationale.

1. To qualify as an emergency department service, the encounter must be performed in a hospital-based facility that is open 24 hours a day.
   a. True
   b. False

2. Both 99283 and 99284 require moderate MDM. From an MDM standpoint, what distinguishes these two codes from one another?
   a. Amount of history reviewed
   b. Number of diagnoses
   c. How long the person has had the problem
   d. Problem severity or urgency

3. What code would be reported when a physician or other qualified health professional at the hospital is in two-way communication with rescue workers on site at a major traffic accident?
   a. This is not a billable service
   b. 99288
   c. 99285
   d. 99291

4. The physician documented that 75 minutes was spent monitoring a critical patient who was given fluids and pressors after becoming hypoxic and hypotensive. What critical-care code(s) would be reported?
   a. 99291 and 99292

   b. 99291

   c. 99292

   d. 99291, 99292 x 2

5. When additional procedures are performed by the same physician on the same date as critical care services, the time spent performing the additional procedures is counted toward the total critical-care time.
   a. True

   b. False

6. What code is assigned for 25 minutes of total critical-care time?
   a. 99291

   b. 99292

   c. Not reportable

   d. Another appropriate level of E/M but not a critical-care code

Chapter 9: Residential Care Services (99304–99340)

Nursing Facility Services (99304–99318)
Initial Nursing Facility Care (99304–99306)

QUICK COMPARISON

Nursing Facility Services—Comprehensive Nursing Facility Assessments

E/M Code	Medical Decision Making[1]	Problem Severity	History[1]	Exam[1]	Counseling and/or Coordination of Care	Time Spent[2] Face to Face (avg.)
99304	Straightforward or of low complexity	Low severity	Detailed or comprehensive	Detailed or comprehensive	Consistent with problems and patient's or family's needs	25 min.
99305	Moderate complexity	Moderate severity	Comprehensive	Comprehensive	Consistent with problems and patient's or family's needs	35 min.
99306	High complexity	High severity	Comprehensive	Comprehensive	Consistent with problems and patient's or family's needs	45 min.

1   Key component. For new patients, all three components (history, exam, and medical decision making) must be adequately documented in the medical record to substantiate the level of service reported and are crucial for selecting the correct code.

2   Time is not considered a key element; this information is provided here only as a guideline for assigning the appropriate level of service. Scenarios during which time becomes the critical factor in deciding the appropriate level of service include encounters for counseling and/or coordinating of care when these services constitute more than 50 percent of the time spent with the patient and/or family. This includes time spent with patient family members or others who will assume responsibility for the care of the patient or decision making whether or not they are family members (e.g., foster parents, person acting in locum parentis, legal guardian).

GENERAL GUIDELINES

- Use these CPT® codes to report initial nursing facility care provided in a hospital observation unit, office, nursing facility, domiciliary/non-nursing facility or the patient's home.
- Use these codes to report initial E/M services provided in a psychiatric residential treatment center.
- Per CPT guidelines, initial nursing facility assessments must be performed by a physician.
- Consider assigning the appropriate consultation code instead of these codes when an opinion or advice was provided about a patient for a specific problem at the request of another physician/qualified healthcare professional or other appropriate source.

- Assign these codes with a hospital discharge management code when a patient was discharged from the hospital and admitted to a nursing facility on the same day.
- For reporting these services, unit/floor intraservice time includes both bedside services and those services rendered while on the hospital unit. Unit/floor time includes chart review, patient examination, record documentation, and communication with the patient's family and facility staff.
- Use a domiciliary, rest home, or home care plan oversight services (99339–99340) code when coordination of care involved other providers or agencies but did not involve a patient encounter on that day.
- Append modifier 25 to report that a separately identifiable E/M service was performed by the same physician/qualified healthcare professional on the same day as a procedure or service. Only the content of work associated with the separate E/M service should be considered when assigning the correct level E/M code.
- Use modifier 32 when the services were mandated, such as by a third-party payer, or as a result of a governmental, legislative, or regulatory requirement.
- Report separately the codes for the diagnostic tests or studies performed.
- These codes include the services formerly known as residential care, skilled nursing facility (SNF), intermediate care facility (ICF) or long-term care facility (LTCF) services.

ISSUES IN THIS CODE RANGE

- In this section we find one of only a few E/M codes where the level of medical decision making is expressed as a range. Normally these levels are clearly indicated though the nature of presenting problem may state "low-moderate severity." In these cases, we see the levels of decision making expressed as straightforward or low, or moderate to high.
- Swing beds billed by the hospital as nursing facility care should be reported using nursing facility codes according to the *Medicare Claims Processing Manual*, Pub. 100-04, chapter 12, section 30.6.9.D.

99304

DOCUMENTATION REQUIREMENTS

Note: This code is to be used for an initial nursing facility assessment. Three of three components required.

Medical Decision Making: straightforward to low

- Minimal number of diagnoses or management options considered
- No or minimal amount or complexity of data reviewed
- Minimal risk of complications or morbidity or mortality

OR

- Limited number of diagnoses or management options considered
- Limited amount and complexity of data reviewed
- Low risk of complications or morbidity or mortality

Problem Severity: low

- Stability, recovery or improvement

History: detailed or comprehensive

- Chief complaint
- Extended history of present illness (four or more HPI elements or the status of three chronic problems)
- Extended system review (two to nine systems)
- Pertinent past, family, and/or social history (one of the history areas)

OR

- Chief complaint
- Extended history of present illness (four or more HPI elements or the status of three chronic problems)
- Complete system review (10 systems)
- Complete past, family, social history (at least one element from all history areas)

Examination: detailed or comprehensive

- 1995: two to seven organ systems or body areas with an extended exam of affected area(s)
- 1997: at least two bullet (•) elements from at least six organ systems or body areas, OR at least 12 bullet (•) elements from two or more organ systems or body areas. Eye and psychiatric singe-system exams must include at least nine bullet (•) elements OR
- 1995: eight or more organ systems
- 1997: multisystem exam must include all bullet (•) elements from at least nine organ systems or body areas unless specific instructions limit content of the exam; at least two bullet elements from each area/system reviewed are expected to be documented
- 1997: single organ system/body area exam must include all bulleted (•) elements in shaded boxes PLUS at least one element in each unshaded box

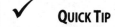

QUICK TIP

The purpose of this encounter should be the assessment or reassessment of a nursing facility patient. The same codes are used for new or established patients.

Code Indicators (from tables of risk—including some AMA indicators in italic)

Presenting Problem(s)

- Two or more self-limited or minor problem(s)
- One stable chronic illness (e.g., well controlled hypertension or non-insulin-dependent diabetes, cataract, BPH)
- Acute uncomplicated illness or injury (e.g., cystitis, allergic rhinitis, simple sprain)

Management Options

- Physical therapy, *rest or exercise, diet, stress management*
- Over the counter drugs, *medication management with minimal risk*
- Minor surgery, with no identified risk factors
- Occupational therapy
- IV fluids, without additives

Counseling and/or Coordination of Care

- As appropriate for the problem

Time Spent Bedside and on Floor/Unit (average)

- 25 minutes

Sample Documentation—99304

Level I Initial Nursing Facility

S: The patient is a 78-year-old female who has been cared for at home by an extended family member. The patient fell out of her chair today and injured her left arm. The patient has been uncooperative of late, not taking her medications for hypothyroid, arthritis, constipation, and hypertension. The family is concerned and determined it was appropriate to arrange for admission to the nursing facility as her needs have progressed.

The patient is calm and responds appropriately to questions. She states that she has been taking her medications although the care taker has found them throughout the house. The family is unsure how long she has been noncompliant with her medications. She states her arm is feeling better after taking Tylenol. Patient states she is sluggish throughout the day and has general joint aches and is otherwise doing okay.

ROS: General: no other complaints, HEENT: without complaints. CV: no complaints, GI: c/o constipation, MS: as above, Psych: is slightly depressed and upset that some family members have not been to visit.

PMH/SH/FH: As above, widowed for 5 years, quit smoking 20+ years ago.

O: General: alert; feels well, except as above. T: 97.4. P: 78; R: 18; BP: 144/88. HEENT: head normocephalic. Atraumatic. Eyes: PERRLA. EOMI. Conjunctivae clear. Bilateral cataracts. Fundi flat. Ears: WNL. Nose/Throat/Mouth: Oral cavity is dry. Throat WNL. No exudates. Resp: lung fields clear to P&A. Heart: normal S1, S2. NSR. No murmurs. S4 gallop present. GI: Soft, nontender. No organomegaly. BS hypoactive. GU: deferred. Rectal: vault full of hard feces. No hemorrhoids or blood. Musculoskeletal: left upper extremity ecchymotic just above the elbow, outer aspect. Some tenderness with palpation. No gross deformity. FROM. Remainder WNL except for global general discomfort with decreased ROM in all joints. Skin: pale, cool and dry. Neuro: alert and oriented x 2. DTRs +1 lower extremities and upper extremities. Delayed relaxation. Babinski equivocal. Motor/ sensory diffuse weakness 1/4.

A: (1) Noncompliant patient with contusion LUE. (2) hypothyroidism; (3) dementia; (4) bowel impaction, poss. secondary to hypothyroidism; (5) HTN

P: (1) Orders for T4, TSH; (2) ice to arm; acetaminophen for pain; (3) manual disimpaction followed by tap water enemas; (4) when patient is euthyroid, reevaluate for dementia work up; (5) admit to NF

(General multisystem)

99305

DOCUMENTATION REQUIREMENTS

Note: This code is to be used for an initial nursing facility assessment. Three of three components required.

Medical Decision Making: moderate
- Multiple number of diagnoses or management options considered
- Moderate amount or complexity of data reviewed
- Moderate risk of complications or morbidity or mortality

Problem Severity: moderate
- Moderate to high risk of morbidity without treatment
- Moderate to high risk of mortality without treatment
- Uncertain outcome or increased probability of prolonged functional impairment or high probability of severe prolonged functional impairment

History: comprehensive
- Chief complaint
- Extended history of present illness (four or more HPI elements or the status of three chronic problems)
- Complete system review (10 systems)
- Complete past, family, social history (at least one element from all history areas)

Examination: comprehensive
- 1995: eight or more organ systems
- 1997: multisystem exam must include all bullet (•) elements from at least nine organ systems or body areas unless specific instructions limit content of the exam; at least two bullet elements from each area/system reviewed are expected to be documented.
- 1997: single organ system/body area exam must include all bullet (•) elements in shaded boxes PLUS at least one element in each unshaded box.

Code Indicators (from tables of risk—including some AMA indicators in italic)

Presenting Problem(s)
- One or more chronic illness with mild exacerbation, progression, or side effects of treatment
- Two or more stable chronic illnesses
- Undiagnosed new *illness, injury*, or problem with uncertain prognosis
- Acute illness, with systemic symptoms (pyelonephritis, pleuritis, colitis)
- Acute complicated injury, e.g., head injury, with brief loss of consciousness

Management Options
- Prescription drug management
- Closed treatment of fracture or dislocation, without manipulation
- IV fluids with additives

- Minor surgery, with identified risk factors
- Elective major surgery (open, percutaneous, endoscopic), with no identified risk factors
- Therapeutic nuclear medicine

Counseling and/or Coordination of Care
- As appropriate for the problem

Time Spent Bedside and on Floor/Unit (average)
- 35 minutes

Sample Documentation—99305

Level II Initial Nursing Facility

This is a 73-year-old female who has been under my care for the last three years. She has severe hypertension, mixed arthritis secondary to rheumatoid and degenerative changes, and psoriasis. The staff telephoned my office this morning to report the patient has had nausea, vomiting and diarrhea during the night. Cannot correlate these symptoms with food ingestion. Patient began feeling nauseated an hour before bedtime, felt feverish and then awakened with the urge to vomit. Brown diarrhea culminated with fresh blood on the toilet paper. A few hours ago the patient reports cramping across the lower quadrants of the abdomen, relieved only with defecation and occurring every 45 minutes to an hour. Has vomited several times throughout the night without hematemesis; last episode of emesis about three hours ago. Now also c/o dizziness and slight disorientation. Has been unable to take anything p.o., including meds and liquids. Missed one dose HCTZ last evening.

ROS: General: On Cognex for dementia but seems unhappy with its effects; c/o "losing my memory." HEENT: without complaint with the exception of psoriatic lesions over forehead, with pruritus and some flaking of skin. Using Elocon cream with good response. Occasional dry mouth. Neck: no complaints except for stiffness. Chest/Resp: no cough. No real complaints. Heart: HTN, as above. On HCTZ 25 mg q.i.d. and Cardizem 240 mg q.d. without consistent control. Abdomen: as above. Reports early satiety at times. GU: without complaint. Skin: psoriasis, as stated. Psoriatic lesions also over elbows; these sometimes get tender as she leans on her elbows while doing some ADLs. Musculoskeletal: arthritis as described. Has been on various NSAIDS; now has good relief of symptoms by Daypro. Neuro: occasional peripheral paresthesias but no complaints at this time.

PMH: Partial salpingo-oophorectomy, right, 30 years ago. T&A in childhood. Last year was hospitalized secondary to malignant hypertension with CHF, peripheral edema and SOB.

SH: Married for over 50 years; husband deceased. Four children, none in immediate area.

FH: Mother had a history of hypertension and diabetes. Father killed in accident.

O: T: 100.8. BP: 148/98. R: 24. P: 96. General: feverish-appearing female in slight distress, not vomiting at this time. Head: no signs of active psoriasis. Normocephalic. A few benign-appearing senile keratotic lesions over forehead at margins of eyebrows, bilaterally. Eyes: clear. Fundi WNL. Some crusting over lower palpebral border, OD. Conjunctiva sl. erythematous, OD. Patient does admit to itching and watery eye. OS within normal limits. Nasal mucosa dry. No exudates. Pharynx: sl. irritation apparent at posterior pharyngeal wall with adherent mucus, probably due to vomiting. Yellowed dentition. Lips: sl. dry, especially at corners. No lesions. Neck: no lymphadenopathy. Thyroid without nodule. Chest: clear to A&P. No signs aspirate. Abdomen: flat, without rebound. Some discomfort RLQ/LLQ. Minimal distention. No signs obstruction/peritonitis. BS normal tones. No organomegaly. Skin: warm, dry. Flaking at elbows where active psoriasis is apparent. Musculoskeletal: Guarded ROM at elbows, knees. Muscle atrophy in quadriceps. Extremities: no peripheral edema. Circ: good. Neuro: DTRs diminished +1. Motor/sensory intact. Rectal: no signs hemorrhage. No hemorrhoids. By digital exam—vault clean. No internal hemorrhoids palpated. Stool guaiac negative. Anoscopy not performed. Psych: good spirits other than for immediate complaints. Memory testing not administered at this time.

(continued)

Sample Documentation—99305 (Continued)

Labs: UA WNL. CBC w/diff ordered; chem profile; stool for WBC, O&P, C&S. Discussed patient's care and healthcare status with daughter who has power of attorney. As patient has exceeded the care available at assisted living facility, it was determined that it would be appropriate to admit the patient to the nursing facility for care of ongoing and acute health issues.

A: (1) R/O gastroenteritis. (2) Probable dizziness secondary dehydration by vomiting/diarrhea and n.p.o. status. (3) On Cognex—reassess efficacy; schedule testing after GI symptoms resolution. (4) Severe HTN. (5) OD blepharitis/conjunctivitis. (6) Psoriasis, active at elbows, bilat. (7) Arthritis, as described. Care plan includes plan below and is placed in chart.

P: (1) Tetracycline 250 mg t.i.d. for gastroenteritis; (2) Imodium capsules 4 mg and then 2 mg t.i.d. until stool forms; (3) Tigan 200 mg IM. If no improvement, another 200 mg in four hours; (4) Neosporin ophthalmic ung—apply t.i.d. to OD, affected area; (5) continue HCTZ/Cardizem; (6) continue Elocon; (7) continue Cognex; (8) hold Daypro until GI distress subsides. Labs pending—fax results to my office. (9) When nausea subsides, begin clear liquid diet, progress to light meals as directed in orders on chart.

(General multisystem)

QUICK TIP

The patient has multiple problems with an exacerbation as supported by the documentation.

99306

DOCUMENTATION REQUIREMENTS

Note: This code is to be used for an initial nursing facility assessment at the time of initial admission or readmission to the facility. Three of three components required.

Medical Decision Making: high
- Extensive number of diagnoses or management options considered
- Extensive amount or complexity of data reviewed
- High risk of complications or morbidity or mortality

Problem Severity: high
- Determined by initial admission or readmission assessment. The creation of a new medical plan of care is required.

History: comprehensive
- Chief complaint
- Extended history of present illness (four or more HPI elements or the status of three chronic problems)
- Complete system review (10 systems)
- Complete past, family, social history (at least one element from all history areas)

Examination: comprehensive
- 1995: eight or more organ systems
- 1997: multisystem exam must include all bullet (•) elements from at least nine organ systems or body areas unless specific instructions limit content of the exam; at least two bullet elements from each area/system reviewed are expected to be documented.
- 1997: single organ system/body area exam must include all bullet (•) elements in shaded boxes PLUS at least one element in each unshaded box.

Code Indicators (from tables of risk—including some AMA indicators in italic)

Presenting Problem(s)
- One or more chronic illness with severe exacerbation, progression, or side effects of treatment
- Acute or chronic illness or injury that poses a threat to life or bodily function, e.g., multiple traumas, acute MI, pulmonary embolism, severe respiratory distress, progressive severe rheumatoid arthritis, psychiatric illness, with potential threat to self or others, peritonitis, ARF
- An abrupt change in neurological status, e.g., seizure, TIA, weakness, sensory loss

Management Options
- Elective major surgery with identified risk factors or emergency major surgery (open, percutaneous, endoscopic)
- Parenteral controlled substances

- Drug therapy requiring intensive monitoring for toxicity
- Decision not to resuscitate or to deescalate care because of poor prognosis

Counseling and/or Coordination of Care
- As appropriate for the problem

Time Spent Bedside and on Floor/Unit (average)
- 45 minutes

Sample Documentation—99306

Level III Initial Nursing Facility

This is a patient who is well-known to me. She is 84-years-of-age, and lived alone with minimal ADL/medical assistance. On the day of admission to the hospital, she slipped and fell in her home and fractured her right femur, lying on the floor until her part-time medical aide found her several hours later. She was admitted to the hospital via the ER with an uneventful hospital course, undergoing right femoral pinning by Dr. Orthopaedic Surgeon. Please see note detailing pt.'s hospital course and hospital discharge on this date for additional information.

She is admitted to the NH at this time for continued care of her femoral fracture as well as for her other medical ailments including HTN, hypothyroidism, polyarthritis and refractory left otitis externa. Upon admission to the nursing facility, the patient states she is feeling physically well but is "depressed and not looking forward to being in a nursing home." She is in a right long-leg cast and is not ambulatory. She says her leg periodically throbs during the night, especially over the incision. She is on p.o. 100 mg Ultram PRN pain, which she takes continually, with good relief of pain but with some sedation.

ROS: General: feels fatigued at times. Eats three meals/day, all prepared by her without assistance. HEENT: Wears dentures. No complaints with the exception of the otitis externa, AS, with intense pruritus as the primary symptoms. Some otorrhea on pillow in a.m.'s—whitish in color; not on meds at this time. Chest/Resp: no complaints. CV: No SOB. Some lightheadedness. HTN as stated, controlled with Norvasc 5 mg p.o. q.d. GI: No complaints. GU: no incontinence. Musculoskeletal: mild degenerative arthritis in major joints including hips, knees, shoulders. Worse in a.m.'s. Takes an occasional Motrin with some relief prior to fall but otherwise prefers not to take meds for this. Right femoral fracture as described. Skin: no complaints except for incisional discomfort over right upper thigh. Says ankles and feet constantly feel cold. Endo: On Synthroid 88 mcg daily. Admits to not being very compliant with her thyroid medicine as she doesn't "see the need any-more."

PMH: Chronic conditions as listed. Noncontributory otherwise. NKDA.

SH: Widowed; lives alone with assistance coordinated through Social Services three days per week, for approximately four hours each day. Has three children, 10 grandchildren. Her family visits her every week and takes her to church each Sunday.

FH: Thyroid disease and hypertension.

O: General: well-developed, well-nourished female in no acute distress, lying passively in bed. BP: 138/86; P: 60; R: 20 and regular. T: 99.2. Height and weight will be recorded later today. Affect: Patient feels "very down" about being shifted to a nursing facility from the hospital, and wants to go home ASAP. Head: normocephalic. Patchy alopecia areata. No scalp lesions. Ears: AS canal erythemic with traces of frothy otorrhea. No signs of excoriations. TM thickened without perforation. AD: some cerumen. TM appears WNL. Pharynx: pale mucosa. Uvula appears long and brushes posterior pharynx and tongue (apparently this does not elicit the cough reflex). Dentition: patient is edentulous. Gingivae appear healthy. Neck: no lymphadenopathy. Thyroid palpable and without nodule or mass. Chest is clear to A/P. Heart: regular rate, rhythm. S4 gallop but no murmurs, rubs. Abdomen: no mass or tenderness. Spleen, liver without tenderness or organomegaly. Normal BS. Genitalia: normal female. Skin: clear, cool. Buttocks: no signs of decubitus ulcer. Musculoskeletal: right femoral fracture, in long-leg cast. No muscle atrophy noted. Pedal pulse good on right. Joints with full passive ROM with some guarded resistance. Motor/sensory intact. Left extremity WNL with intact neuro. DTRs delayed at left knee +1.

(continued)

Sample Documentation—99306 (Continued)

A: (1) S/P open reduction internal fixation, right femoral fracture. (2) Hypertension, controlled. Fall possibly due to orthostasis on Norvasc. (3) Hypothyroid, on Synthroid. (4) Otitis externa, chronic, refractory, left. (5) Osteoarthritis. (6) Mild reactive depression.

P: Patient's convalescence should take about six weeks, at which point she may be transitioned to another setting. Will coordinate with her family and SS to determine the best course. She will begin to ambulate in a few weeks. Will coordinate physical therapy at that time. Follow hypertension, continue on Norvasc 5 mg q.d. and check for orthostatic hypotension; follow hypothyroid, continue on Synthroid 88 mcg q.d. and follow on T4/TSH levels. Rx—begin (1) Domeboro otic solution two drops t.i.d.; (2) decrease Ultram to 50 mg p.o. q.6h. PRN pain. Add acetaminophen for pain, q.4 h. Monitor BMs—will switch to Duract two capsules q.6h. if constipation develops; (3) check Beck's depression scale when patient is on Ultram and euthyroid; consider antidepressant if no change. The patient's family will be coming by today. Have full disclosure consent and will apprise them of the details. Detailed new care plan to be placed in chart, Ortho will be by to see the patient in 10 days.

(General multisystem)

Subsequent Nursing Facility Care, Discharge, and Annual Nursing Assessment (99307–99318)

QUICK COMPARISON

Nursing Facility Services—Subsequent Nursing Facility Care

E/M Code	Medical Decision Making[1]	History[1]	Exam[1]	Counseling and/or Coordination of Care	Time Spent[2] Face to Face (avg.)
99307	Straightforward	Problem focused interval	Problem focused	Consistent with problems and patient's or family's needs	10 min.
99308	Low complexity	Expanded problem focused interval	Expanded problem focused	Consistent with problems and patient's or family's needs	15 min.
99309	Moderate complexity	Detailed interval	Detailed	Consistent with problems and patient's or family's needs	25 min.
99310	High complexity	Comprehensive interval	Comprehensive	Consistent with problems and patient's or family's needs	35 min.
99315	Nursing facility discharge day management				30 minutes or less[3]
99316	Nursing facility discharge day management				More than 30 minutes[3]
99318	Low to moderate complexity	Detailed interval	Comprehensive	Consistent with problems and patient's or family's needs	30 min.

1   Key component. For subsequent care, at least two of the three components (history, exam and medical decision making) are needed to select the correct code and must be adequately documented in the medical record to substantiate the level of service reported.

2   Time is not considered a key element; this information is provided here only as a guideline for assigning the appropriate level of service. Scenarios during which time becomes the critical factor in deciding the appropriate level of service include encounters for counseling and/or coordinating of care, when these services constitute more than 50 percent of the time spent with the patient and/or family. This includes time spent with patient family members or others who will assume responsibility for the care of the patient or decision making whether or not they are family members (e.g., foster parents, person acting in locum parentis, legal guardian).

3   These codes are not based on the three key elements of patient history, physical examination, and level of medical decision making. These codes are correctly assigned based on time, as the CPT code description indicates.

GENERAL GUIDELINES

- Use these codes to report services provided to a resident of a nursing facility, including reviewing diagnostic studies and noting changes in the patient's status.
- Use these codes to report subsequent E/M services provided in a psychiatric residential treatment center.
- Code 99318 is used to report the annual nursing facility assessment. Unlike other subsequent care codes, all three key components (history, exam, and medical decision making) are needed to select the correct code and must be adequately documented in the medical record to substantiate the service.
- For reporting these services, unit/floor intraservice time includes both bedside services and those services rendered while on the hospital unit.

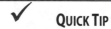 QUICK TIP

Report these services for subsequent nursing facility services. Note that some payers may evaluate frequency of services for coverage.

Unit/floor time includes chart review, patient examination, record documentation, and communication with the patient's family and facility staff.

- Consider assigning the appropriate consultation code instead of these codes when an opinion or advice was provided about a patient for a specific problem at the request of another physician or other appropriate source.

- Use a domiciliary, rest home, or home care plan oversight services (99339–99340) code when coordination of care involved other providers or agencies but did not involve a patient encounter on that day.

- Assign modifier 24 to indicate that an E/M service performed during the postoperative period was not related to the prior procedure. The claim should show a different diagnosis from that for the surgery.

- Append modifier 25 to report that a separately identifiable E/M service was performed by the same physician/qualified healthcare professional on the same day as a procedure or service. Only the content of work associated with the separate E/M service should be considered when assigning the correct E/M code.

- Use modifier 32 when the services are mandated, such as by a third-party payer, or as a result of a governmental, legislative, or regulatory requirement.

- For codes 99307–99310:

  Append modifier 95 to indicate that the E/M service was rendered to a patient at a distant site via a real-time interactive audio and video telecommunications system. The communication between the physician or other qualified healthcare professional and the patient should be commensurate with the same key components or requirements of those that would be required if the service had been rendered in a face-to-face setting.

- Report separately the codes for the diagnostic tests or studies performed.

- Codes 99315 and 99316 for nursing facility discharge services are appropriately assigned by the length of time devoted to performing the service (e.g., 99315 requires 30 minutes or less and 99316 requires more than 30 minutes).

ISSUES IN THIS CODE RANGE

- In this section we find one of only a few E/M codes where the level of medical decision making is expressed as a range. Normally these levels are clearly indicated though the nature of presenting problem may state "low-moderate severity." In 99318, the level of decision making is expressed as low to moderate.

- Medicare Part B will cover visits to evaluate and monitor the patient at least once every 30 days for the first 90 days and continuing at least once every 60 days. More frequent visits when medically necessary will also be covered.

99307

DOCUMENTATION REQUIREMENTS

Note: This code is for a new or established patient in a nursing facility being seen for evaluation and management of medical conditions.

Medical Decision Making: straightforward
- Minimal number of diagnoses or management options considered
- No or minimal amount or complexity of data reviewed
- Minimal risk of complications or morbidity or mortality

Problem Severity
- Stability, recovery or improvement

History: problem focused *interval*
- Chief complaint
- Brief history of present illness (one to three HPI elements)

Examination: problem focused
- 1995: one organ system or body area
- 1997: one to five bullet (•) elements in one or more organ systems/body areas

Code Indicators (from tables of risk—including some AMA indicators in italic)

Presenting Problem(s)
- Two or more self-limited or minor problem(s)
- One stable chronic illness (e.g., well controlled hypertension or non-insulin-dependent diabetes, cataract, BPH)
- Acute uncomplicated illness or injury (e.g., cystitis, allergic rhinitis, simple sprain)

Management Options
- Physical therapy, *rest or exercise, diet, stress management*
- Over the counter drugs, *medication management with minimal risk*
- Minor surgery, with no identified risk factors
- Occupational therapy
- IV fluids, without additives

Counseling and/or Coordination of Care
- As appropriate for the problem

Time Spent Bedside and on Floor/Unit (average)
- 10 minutes

99308

DOCUMENTATION REQUIREMENTS

Note: This code is for an established patient in a nursing facility being seen for evaluation and management of medical conditions.

Medical Decision Making: low
- Limited number of diagnoses or management options considered
- Limited amount and complexity of data reviewed
- Low risk of complications or morbidity or mortality

Problem Severity
- Inadequate response to treatment or development of a minor complication

History: expanded problem focused *interval*
- Chief complaint
- Brief history of present illness (one to three HPI elements)
- Problem pertinent system review (one or two systems)

Examination: expanded problem focused
- 1995: two to seven organ systems or body areas
- 1997: at least six bullet (•) elements in one or more organ systems/body areas

Code Indicators (from tables of risk-including some AMA indicators in italic)

Presenting Problem(s)
- One or more chronic illness with mild exacerbation, progression, or side effects of treatment
- Two or more stable chronic illnesses
- Undiagnosed new *illness, injury,* or problem with uncertain prognosis
- Acute illness, with systemic symptoms (pyelonephritis, pleuritis, colitis)
- Acute complicated injury, e.g., head injury, with brief loss of consciousness

Management Options
- Prescription drug management
- Closed treatment of fracture or dislocation, without manipulation
- IV fluids with additives
- Minor surgery, with identified risk factors
- Elective major surgery (open, percutaneous, endoscopic), with no identified risk factors
- Therapeutic nuclear medicine

Counseling and/or Coordination of Care
- As appropriate for the problem

Time Spent Bedside and on Floor/Unit (average)
- 15 minutes

99309

DOCUMENTATION REQUIREMENTS

Note: This code is for an established patient in a nursing facility being seen for evaluation and management of medical conditions.

Medical Decision Making: moderate
- Multiple number of diagnoses or management options considered
- Moderate amount or complexity of data reviewed
- Moderate risk of complications or morbidity or mortality

Problem Severity
- The patient may have developed a significant complication or significant new problem.

History: detailed *interval*
- Chief complaint
- Extended history of present illness (four or more HPI elements or the status of three chronic problems)
- Extended system review (two to nine systems)
- Pertinent past, family, and/or social history (one of the history areas)

Examination: detailed
- 1995: two to seven organ systems or body areas with an extended exam of the affected area(s)
- 1997: at least two bullet (•) elements from at least six organ systems or body areas, OR at least 12 bullet (•) elements from two or more organ systems or body areas. Eye and psychiatric single-system exams must include at last nine bullet (•) elements.

Code Indicators (from tables of risk—including some AMA indicators in italic)

Presenting Problem(s)
- One or more chronic illness with mild exacerbation, progression, or side effects of treatment
- Two or more stable chronic illnesses
- Undiagnosed new *illness, injury,* or problem with uncertain prognosis
- Acute illness, with systemic symptoms (pyelonephritis, pleuritis, colitis)
- Acute complicated injury, e.g., head injury, with brief loss of consciousness

Management Options
- Prescription drug management
- Closed treatment of fracture or dislocation, without manipulation
- IV fluids with additives
- Minor surgery, with identified risk factors
- Elective major surgery (open, percutaneous, endoscopic), with no identified risk factors
- Therapeutic nuclear medicine

 QUICK TIP

These services require documentation that a face-to-face encounter with the patient was provided by the provider. "Chart rounds" are not covered services and should not be reported.

Counseling and/or Coordination of Care
- As appropriate for the problem

Time Spent Bedside and on Floor/Unit (average)
- 25 minutes

99310

DOCUMENTATION REQUIREMENTS

Note: This code is for an established patient in a nursing facility being seen for evaluation and management of medical conditions.

Medical Decision Making: high
- Extensive number of diagnoses or management options considered
- Extensive amount or complexity of data reviewed
- High risk of complications or morbidity or mortality

Problem Severity
- The patient may have developed a significant complication or significant new problem requiring physician attendance.

History: comprehensive *interval*
- Chief complaint
- Extended history of present illness (four or more HPI elements or the status of three chronic problems)
- Complete system review (10 systems for 1995/1997 guidelines)
- Complete past, family, and/or social history (at least one element from all history areas)

Examination: comprehensive
- 1995: eight or more organ systems
- 1997: multisystem exam must include all bullet (•) elements from at least nine organ systems or body areas unless specific instruction limit content of the exam; at least two bullet elements from each area/system reviewed are expected to be documented
- 1997: single organ system/body area exam must include all bullet (•) elements in shaded boxes PLUS at least one element in each unshaded box

Code Indicators (from tables of risk—including some AMA indicators in italic)

Presenting Problem(s)
- One or more chronic illness with severe exacerbation, progression, or side effects of treatment
- Acute or chronic illness or injury that poses a threat to life or bodily function, e.g., multiple traumas, acute MI, pulmonary embolism, severe respiratory distress, progressive severe rheumatoid arthritis, psychiatric illness, with potential threat to self or others, peritonitis, ARF

- An abrupt change in neurological status, e.g., seizure, TIA, weakness, sensory loss

Management Options
- Elective major surgery with identified risk factors or emergency major surgery (open, percutaneous, endoscopic)
- Parenteral controlled substances
- Drug therapy requiring intensive monitoring for toxicity
- Decision not to resuscitate or to deescalate care because of poor prognosis

Counseling and/or Coordination of Care
- As appropriate for the problem

Time Spent Bedside and on Floor/Unit (average)
- 35 minutes

99315

DOCUMENTATION REQUIREMENTS

Nursing Facility Discharge Day Management
- 30 minutes or less
- Constitutes the total duration of time spent performing the discharge service, even if the time spent on that date was not continuous

Parameters
- Includes final physical examination
- Includes discussion regarding nursing facility stay and post-discharge patient care guidelines
- Includes preparation of discharge records, prescriptions, and referral forms, among other documents

Coding Exclusions
- Excludes services for patients admitted as a hospital inpatient
- Excludes annual nursing facility assessment

99316

DOCUMENTATION REQUIREMENTS

Nursing Facility Discharge Day Management
- 31 minutes or more
- Constitutes the total duration of time spent performing the discharge service, even if the time spent on that date was not continuous

Parameters
- Includes final physical examination
- Includes discussion regarding nursing facility stay and post-discharge patient care guidelines
- Includes preparation of discharge records, prescriptions, and referral forms, among other documents

Coding exclusions
- Excludes services for patients admitted as hospital inpatients
- Excludes annual nursing facility assessment

☞ KEY POINT

To report this code, the provider must document that the time spent was more than 30 minutes.

99318

DOCUMENTATION REQUIREMENTS

Note: This code is for a new or established patient involving an annual nursing facility assessment. Three of three components required.

Medical Decision Making: low to moderate
- Limited number of diagnoses or management options considered
- Limited amount and complexity of data reviewed
- Low risk of complications or morbidity or mortality

OR
- Multiple number of diagnoses or management options considered
- Moderate amount or complexity of data reviewed
- Moderate risk of complications or morbidity or mortality

Problem Severity
- Stability, recovery, or improvement

History: detailed *interval*
- Chief complaint
- Extended history of present illness (four or more HPI elements or the status of three chronic problems)
- Extended system review (two to nine systems)
- Pertinent past, family, and/or social history (one of the history areas)

Examination: comprehensive
- 1995: eight or more organ systems

- 1997: multisystem exam must include all bullet (•) elements from at least nine organ systems or body areas unless specific instruction limit content of the exam; at least two bullet elements from each area/system reviewed are expected to be documented
- 1997: single organ system/body area exam must include all bullet (•) elements in shaded boxes PLUS at least one element in each unshaded box

Code Indicators (from tables of risk-including some AMA indicators in italic)

Presenting Problem(s)
- Two or more self-limited or minor problem(s)
- One stable chronic illness (e.g., well-controlled hypertension or non-insulin-dependent diabetes, cataract, BPH)
- Acute uncomplicated illness or injury (e.g., cystitis, allergic rhinitis, simple sprain)
- One or more chronic illness with mild exacerbation, progression, or side effects of treatment
- Two or more stable chronic illnesses
- Undiagnosed new *illness, injury,* or problem with uncertain prognosis
- Acute illness, with systemic symptoms (pyelonephritis, pleuritis, colitis)
- Acute complicated injury, e.g., head injury, with brief loss of consciousness

Management Options
- Physical therapy, *rest or exercise, diet, stress management*
- Over the counter drugs, *medication management with minimal risk*
- Minor surgery, with or without identified risk factors
- Occupational therapy
- IV fluids, with or without additives
- Prescription drug management
- Closed treatment of fracture or dislocation, without manipulation
- Elective major surgery with no identified risk factors

Counseling and/or Coordination of Care
- As appropriate for the problem.

Time Spent Bedside and on Floor/Unit (average)
- 30 minutes

Domiciliary, Rest Home, or Custodial Care Services—New Patient (99324–99328)

QUICK COMPARISON

Domiciliary, Rest Home or Custodial Care Services—New Patient

E/M Code	Medical Decision Making[1]	History[1]	Exam[1]	Counseling and/or Coordination of Care	Time Spent Face to Face (avg.)
99324	Straight-forward	Problem focused	Problem focused	Consistent with problems and patient's or family's needs	20 min.
99325	Low complexity	Expanded problem focused	Expanded problem focused	Consistent with problems and patient's or family's needs	30 min.
99326	Moderate complexity	Detailed	Detailed	Consistent with problems and patient's or family's needs	45 min.
99327	Moderate complexity	Comprehensive	Comprehensive	Consistent with problems and patient's or family's needs	60 min.
99328	High complexity	Comprehensive	Comprehensive	Consistent with problems and patient's or family's needs	75 min.

1   Key component. For new patients, all three components (history, exam, and medical decision making) are crucial for selecting the correct code and must be adequately documented in the medical record to substantiate the level of service reported.

GENERAL GUIDELINES

- Use these codes to report E/M services provided to a new patient in a setting that generally includes room, board and other personal assistance services on a long-term basis with no medical component rendered in:
  - assisted living facilities
  - group homes
  - custodial care
  - intermediate care facilities
- Consider assigning the appropriate consultation code instead of these codes when an opinion or advice was provided about a patient for a specific problem at the request of another physician or other appropriate source.
- Use a case management code when coordination of care involved other providers or agencies but did not involve a patient encounter on that day.
- Append modifier 25 to report that a separately identifiable E/M service was performed by the same physician/qualified healthcare professional on the same day as a procedure or service. Only the content of work associated with the separate E/M service should be considered when assigning the correct E/M code.
- Use modifier 32 when the services were mandated, and must be adequately documented in the medical record to substantiate the level of service reported.

- Report separately the codes for the diagnostic tests or studies performed.

99324

DOCUMENTATION REQUIREMENTS

Medical Decision Making: straightforward
- Minimal number of diagnoses or management options considered
- No or minimal amount or complexity of data reviewed
- Minimal risk of complications or morbidity or mortality

Problem Severity: low
- Expectation of full recovery without functional impairment, or uncertain outcome or increased probability of prolonged functional impairment.
- Expectation of full recovery without functional impairment
- Low risk of morbidity without treatment

History: problem focused
- Chief complaint
- Brief history of present illness or problem (one to three HPI elements)

Examination: problem focused
- 1995: one organ system or body area
- 1997: one to five bullet (•) elements in one or more organ systems/body areas

Code Indicators (from tables of risk—including some AMA indicators in italic)

Presenting Problem(s)
- One self-limited or minor problem

Management Options
- Rest, gargles, elastic bandages, superficial dressings

Counseling and/or Coordination of Care
- As appropriate for the problem

Time Spent Face to Face (average)
- 20 minutes

99325

DOCUMENTATION REQUIREMENTS

Medical Decision Making: low
- Limited number of diagnoses or management options considered
- Limited amount or complexity of data reviewed
- Low risk of complications or morbidity or mortality

Problem Severity: moderate
- Moderate risk of morbidity without treatment
- Moderate risk of mortality without treatment
- Uncertain outcome or increased probability of prolonged functional impairment or increased probability of prolonged functional impairment

History: expanded problem focused
- Chief complaint
- Brief history of present illness (one to three HPI elements)
- Problem pertinent system review (one or two systems)

Examination: expanded problem focused
- 1995: two to seven organ systems or body areas
- 1997: at least six bullet (•) elements in one or more organ systems/body areas

Code Indicators (from tables of risk—including some AMA indicators in italic)

Presenting Problem(s)
- Two or more self-limited or minor problem(s)
- One stable chronic illness (e.g., well controlled hypertension or non-insulin dependent diabetes, cataract, BPH
- Acute uncomplicated illness or injury (e.g., cystitis, allergic rhinitis, simple sprain)

Management Options
- Physical therapy
- Over the counter drugs, medication management with minimal risk
- Minor surgery, with no identified risk factors
- Occupational therapy
- IV fluids, without additives

Counseling and/or Coordination of Care
- As appropriate for the problem.

Time Spent Face to Face (average)
- 30 minutes

99326

DOCUMENTATION REQUIREMENTS

Medical Decision Making: moderate
- Extensive number of diagnoses or management options considered
- Extensive amount or complexity of data reviewed
- High risk of complications or morbidity or mortality

Problem Severity: moderate to high
- Moderate to extreme risk of morbidity without treatment
- Moderate to high risk of mortality without treatment
- Uncertain outcome or increased probability of prolonged functional impairment or high probability of severe prolonged functional impairment.

History: detailed
- Chief complaint
- Extended history of present illness (four or more HPI elements or the status of three chronic problems)
- Extended system review (two to nine systems)
- Pertinent past, family, and/or social history (one of the history areas)

Examination: detailed
- 1995: two to seven organ systems or body areas with an extended exam of affected area(s)
- 1997: at least two bullet (•) elements from at least six organ systems or body areas, OR at least 12 bullet (•) elements from two or more organ systems or body areas. Eye and psychiatric single-system exams must include at least nine bullet (•) elements.

Code Indicators (from tables of risk—including some AMA indicators in italic)

Presenting Problem(s)
- One or more chronic illness with mild exacerbation, progression, or side effects of treatment
- Two or more stable chronic illnesses
- Undiagnosed new *illness, injury,* or problem with uncertain prognosis
- Acute illness, with systemic symptoms (pyelonephritis, pleuritis, colitis)
- Acute complicated injury, e.g., head injury, with brief loss of consciousness

Management Options
- Prescription drug management
- Closed treatment of fracture or dislocation, without manipulation
- IV fluids with additives
- Minor surgery, with identified risk factors
- Elective major surgery (open, percutaneous, endoscopic), with no identified risk factors
- Therapeutic nuclear medicine

 QUICK TIP

Note that the provider uses these services to report face-to-face encounters.

Counseling and/or Coordination of Care
- As appropriate for the problem.

Time Spent Face to Face (average)
- 45 minutes

99327

DOCUMENTATION REQUIREMENTS

Medical Decision Making: moderate
- Moderate number of diagnoses or management options considered
- Moderate amount and complexity of data reviewed
- Moderate risk of complications or morbidity or mortality

Problem Severity: high
- Extreme risk of morbidity without treatment
- High risk of mortality without treatment
- Uncertain outcome or increased probability of prolonged functional impairment or high probability of severe prolonged functional impairment

History: comprehensive
- Chief complaint
- Extended history of present illness (four or more HPI elements or the status of three chronic problems)
- Complete system review (10 systems)
- Complete past, family, social history (at least one element from all history areas)

Examination: comprehensive
- 1995: eight or more organ systems
- 1997: multisystem exam must include all bullet (•) elements from at least nine organ systems or body areas unless specific instruction limit content of the exam; at least two bullet elements from each area/system reviewed are expected to be documented
- 1997: single organ system/body area exam must include all bullet (•) elements in shaded boxes PLUS at least one element in each unshaded box

Code Indicators (from tables of risk-including some AMA indicators in italic)

Presenting Problem(s)
- One or more chronic illness with mild exacerbation, progression, or side effects of treatment
- Two or more stable chronic illnesses
- Undiagnosed new illness or problem with uncertain prognosis
- Acute illness, with systemic symptoms (pyelonephritis, pleuritis, colitis)
- Acute complicated injury, e.g., head injury, with brief loss of consciousness

Management Options
- Prescription drug management
- Closed treatment of fracture or dislocation, without manipulation
- IV fluids with additives
- Minor surgery, with identified risk factors
- Elective major surgery (open, percutaneous, endoscopic), with no identified risk factors
- Therapeutic nuclear medicine

Counseling and/or Coordination of Care
- As appropriate for the problem.

Time Spent Bedside and on Floor/Unit (average)
- 60 minutes

99328

DOCUMENTATION REQUIREMENTS

Medical Decision Making: high
- Extensive number of diagnoses or management options considered
- Extensive amount and complexity of data reviewed
- High risk of complications or morbidity or mortality

Problem Severity: requires immediate physician attention
- Extreme risk of morbidity without treatment
- High risk of mortality without treatment
- Conditions pose significant threat to life or risk of prolonged impairment
- Physician attention required

History: comprehensive
- Chief complaint
- Extended history of present illness (four or more HPI elements or the status of three chronic problems)
- Complete system review (10 systems)
- Complete past, family, social history (at least one element from all history areas)

Examination: comprehensive
- 1995: eight or more organ systems
- 1997: multisystem exam must include all bullet (•) elements from at least nine organ systems or body areas unless specific instruction limit content of the exam; at least two bullet elements from each area/system reviewed are expected to be documented
- 1997: single organ system/body area exam must include all bullet (•) elements in shaded boxes PLUS at least one element in each unshaded box

Code Indicators (from tables of risk-including some AMA indicators in italic)

Presenting Problem(s)

- One or more chronic illness with severe exacerbation, progression, or side effects of treatment
- Acute or chronic illness or injury that poses a threat to life or bodily function, e.g., multiple traumas, acute MI, pulmonary embolism, severe respiratory distress, progressive severe rheumatoid arthritis, psychiatric illness, with potential threat to self or others, peritonitis, ARF
- An abrupt change in neurological status, e.g., seizure, TIA, weakness, sensory loss

Management Options

- Elective major surgery with identified risk factors or emergency major surgery (open, percutaneous, endoscopic)
- Parenteral controlled substances
- Drug therapy requiring intensive monitoring for toxicity
- Decision not to resuscitate or to deescalate care because of poor prognosis

Counseling and/or Coordination of Care

- As appropriate for the problem.

Time Spent Bedside and on Floor/Unit (average)

- 75 minutes

Domiciliary, Rest Home, or Custodial Care Services—Established Patient (99334–99337)

QUICK COMPARISON

Domiciliary, Rest Home, or Custodial Care Services—Established Patient

E/M Code	Medical Decision Making[1]	History[1]	Exam[1]	Counseling and/or Coordination of Care	Time Spent Face to Face (avg.)
99334	Straight-forward complexity	Problem focused interval	Problem focused	Consistent with problems and patient's or family's needs	15 min.
99335	Low complexity	Expanded problem focused interval	Expanded problem focused	Consistent with problems and patient's or family's needs	25 min.
99336	Moderate complexity	Detailed interval	Detailed	Consistent with problems and patient's or family's needs	40 min.
99337	Moderate to high complexity	Comprehensive interval	Comprehensive	Consistent with problems and patient's or family's needs	60 min.

1 Key component. For established patients, at least two of the three components (history, exam and medical decision making) are needed to select the correct code and must be adequately documented in the medical record to substantiate the level of service reported.

GENERAL GUIDELINES

- Use these codes to report services provided to an established patient in a setting that generally includes room, board and other personal assistance services on a long-term basis with no medical component rendered in:
  - assisted living facilities
  - group homes
  - custodial care
  - intermediate care facilities
- Consider assigning the appropriate consultation code instead of these codes when an opinion or advice was provided about a patient for a specific problem at the request of another physician or other appropriate source.
- Use a case management code when coordination of care involved other providers or agencies but did not involve a patient encounter on that day.
- Assign modifier 24 to indicate that an E/M service performed during the postoperative period was not related to the prior procedure. The claim should show a different diagnosis from that for the surgery.
- Append modifier 25 to report that a separately identifiable E/M service was performed by the same physician/qualified healthcare professional on the same day as a procedure or service. Only the content of work associated with the separate E/M service should be considered when assigning the correct E/M code.

- Use modifier 32 when the services were mandated, such as by a peer review organization, third-party payer, or as a result of a governmental, legislative, or regulatory requirement.
- Report separately the codes for the diagnostic tests or studies performed.

99334

DOCUMENTATION REQUIREMENTS

Medical Decision Making: straightforward
- Minimal number of diagnoses or management options considered
- No or minimal amount or complexity of data reviewed
- Minimal risk of complications or morbidity or mortality

Problem Severity: self-limited or minor
- One self-limited or minor problem

History: problem focused *interval*
- Chief complaint
- Brief history of present illness or problem (one to three HPI elements)

Examination: problem focused
- 1995: one organ system or body area
- 1997: one to five bullet (•) elements in one or more organ systems/body areas

Code Indicators (from tables of risk—including some AMA indicators in italic)

Presenting Problem(s)
- One self-limited or minor problem

Management Options
- Rest, gargles, elastic bandages, superficial dressings

Counseling and/or Coordination of Care
- As appropriate for the problem. No time has been established for these codes

Time Spent Bedside and on Floor/Unit (average)
- 15 minutes

99335

DOCUMENTATION REQUIREMENT

Medical Decision Making: low
- Limited number of diagnoses or management options considered
- Limited amount or complexity of data reviewed
- Low risk of complications or morbidity or mortality

Problem Severity: low to moderate
- Low risk of morbidity without treatment
- Little, if any, risk of mortality without treatment
- Expectation of full recovery without functional impairment

OR
- Moderate risk of morbidity without treatment
- Moderate risk of mortality without treatment
- Uncertain outcome or increased probability of prolonged functional impairment or increased probability of prolonged functional impairment

History: expanded problem focused *interval*
- Chief complaint
- Brief history of present illness (one to three HPI elements)
- Problem pertinent system review (one or two systems)

Examination: expanded problem focused
- 1995: two to seven organ systems or body areas
- 1997: at least six bullet (•) elements in one or more organ systems/body areas

Code Indicators (from tables of risk—including some AMA indicators in italic)

Presenting Problem(s)
- Two or more self-limited or minor problem(s)
- One stable chronic illness (e.g., well controlled hypertension or non-insulin dependent diabetes, cataract, BPH
- Acute uncomplicated illness or injury (e.g., cystitis, allergic rhinitis, simple sprain)

Management Options
- Physical therapy
- Over the counter drugs, medication management with minimal risk
- Minor surgery, with no identified risk factors
- Occupational therapy
- IV fluids, without additives

Counseling and/or Coordination of Care
- As appropriate for the problem.

Time Spent Bedside and on Floor/Unit (average)
- 25 minutes

99336

DOCUMENTATION REQUIREMENTS

Medical Decision Making: moderate
- Multiple number of diagnoses or management options considered
- Moderate amount or complexity of data reviewed
- Moderate risk of complications or morbidity or mortality

Problem Severity: moderate to high
- Moderate risk of morbidity without treatment
- Moderate risk of mortality without treatment
- Uncertain outcome or increased probability of prolonged functional impairment or increased probability of prolonged functional impairment

History: detailed *interval*
- Chief complaint
- Extended history of present illness (four or more HPI elements or the status of three chronic problems)
- Extended system review (two to nine systems)
- Pertinent past, family and/or social history (one of the history areas)

Examination: detailed
- 1995: two to seven organ systems or body areas with an extended exam of affected area(s)
- 1997: at least two bullet (•) elements from at least six organ systems or body areas, OR at least 12 bullet (•) elements from two or more organ systems or body areas. Eye and psychiatric single-system exams must include at least nine bullet (•) elements.

Code Indicators (from tables of risk—including some AMA indicators in italic)

Presenting Problem(s)
- One or more chronic illness with mild exacerbation, progression, or side effects of treatment
- Two or more stable chronic illnesses
- Undiagnosed new illness or problem with uncertain prognosis
- Acute illness, with systemic symptoms (pyelonephritis, pleuritis, colitis)
- Acute complicated injury, e.g., head injury, with brief loss of consciousness

Management Options
- Prescription drug management
- Closed treatment of fracture or dislocation, without manipulation
- IV fluids with additives
- Minor surgery, with identified risk factors
- Elective major surgery (open, percutaneous, endoscopic), with no identified risk factors
- Therapeutic nuclear medicine

✓ **QUICK TIP**

Non-face-to-face services can be reported with a code for care plan oversight if appropriately documented and if they meet the required time guidelines.

Counseling and/or Coordination of Care
- As appropriate for the problem. No time has been established for these codes.

Time Spent Bedside and on Floor/Unit (average)
- 40 minutes

99337

DOCUMENTATION REQUIREMENTS

Medical Decision Making: high
- Extensive number of diagnoses or management options considered
- Multiple number of diagnoses or management options considered
- Moderate amount or complexity of data reviewed
- Moderate risk of complications or morbidity or mortality OR
- Extensive amount and complexity of data reviewed
- High risk of complications or morbidity or mortality

Problem Severity: moderate to high
- Moderate to extreme risk of morbidity without treatment
- Moderate to high risk of mortality without treatment
- Conditions pose significant threat to life or risk of prolonged impairment
- Physician attention required

History: comprehensive *interval*
- Chief complaint
- Extended history of present illness (four or more HPI elements or the status of three chronic problems)
- Complete system review (10 systems)
- Complete past, family, social history (at least one element from all history areas)

Examination: comprehensive
- 1995: eight or more organ systems
- 1997: multisystem exam must include all bullet (•) elements from at least nine organ systems or body areas unless specific instruction limit content of the exam; at least two bullet elements from each area/system reviewed are expected to be documented
- 1997: single organ system/body area exam must include all bullet (•) elements in shaded boxes PLUS at least one element in each unshaded box

Code Indicators (from tables of risk-including some AMA indicators in italic)

Presenting Problem(s)

- One or more chronic illness with severe exacerbation, progression, or side effects of treatment
- Acute or chronic illness or injury that poses a threat to life or bodily function, e.g., multiple traumas, acute MI, pulmonary embolism, severe respiratory distress, progressive severe rheumatoid arthritis, psychiatric illness, with potential threat to self or others, peritonitis, ARF
- An abrupt change in neurological status, e.g., seizure, TIA, weakness, sensory loss

Management Options

- Elective major surgery with identified risk factors or emergency major surgery (open, percutaneous, endoscopic)
- Parenteral controlled substances
- Drug therapy requiring intensive monitoring for toxicity
- Decision not to resuscitate or to deescalate care because of poor prognosis

Counseling and/or Coordination of Care

- As appropriate for the problem.

Time Spent Bedside and on Floor/Unit (average)

- 60 minutes

Domiciliary, Rest Home (e.g., Assisted Living Facility), or Home Care Plan Oversight Services (99339–99340)

QUICK COMPARISON

Care Plan Oversight Services (99339–99340)

E/M Code	Intent of Service	Place of Service	Time
99339	Individual physician supervision of a patient (patient not present) in home, domiciliary, or rest home (e.g., assisted living facility) requiring complex and multidisciplinary care modalities involving regular physician development and/or revision of care plans, review of subsequent reports of patient status, review of related laboratory and other studies, communication (including telephone calls) for purposes of assessment of care decisions with healthcare professional(s), family member(s), surrogate decision maker(s) (e.g., legal guardian) and/or key care giver(s) involved in patient's care, integration of new information into the medical treatment plan and/or adjustment of medical therapy, within a calendar month.	Physician office	15–29 min.
99340	Individual physician supervision of a patient (patient not present) in home, domiciliary, or rest home (e.g., assisted living facility) requiring complex and multidisciplinary care modalities involving regular physician development and/or revision of care plans, review of subsequent reports of patient status, review of related laboratory and other studies, communication (including telephone calls) for purposes of assessment of care decisions with healthcare professional(s), family member(s), surrogate decision maker(s) (e.g., legal guardian) and/or key care giver(s) involved in patient's care, integration of new information into the medical treatment plan and/or adjustment of medical therapy, within a calendar month.	Physician office	30 min. or more

GENERAL GUIDELINES

Care Plan Oversight Services

- These codes are reported separately from other E/M services.
- The inclusion of healthcare professional(s), family member(s), surrogate decision maker(s) (e.g., legal guardian), and/or key care giver(s) is consistent with current practice and care plan oversight services provided to hospice, home health, and nursing facility patients.
- For care plan oversight services provided to hospice, home health, and nursing facility patients, see codes 99374–99380.
- Total time for service provided within a 30-day period determines the code selection.
- Only one physician may report care plan oversight services for a given period of time.

Medicare has created HCPCS Level II codes G0180–G0182 to address care plan oversight because of CPT wording revisions for these codes. Refer to chapter 17 of this book and your HCPCS Level II guide for special coverage instructions.

KNOWLEDGE ASSESSMENT CHAPTER 9

See chapter 19 for answers and rationale.

1. What level of history and exam are required to report 99305 or 99306?
    a. Detailed
    b. Detailed or comprehensive
    c. Comprehensive
    d. Expanded problem focused

2. It is acceptable for a physician assistant to perform the initial nursing facility encounter as long as the physician reviews and signs the medical record.
    a. True
    b. False

3. Based on the sample documentation for a 99304 on page 234, which of the following organ systems was not examined by the physician?
    a. Genitourinary
    b. Eyes
    c. Lymphatic
    d. Cardiovascular

4. What code would be assigned when the physician documents a subsequent nursing facility visit where the physician spent 25 minutes with the patient and 15 of those minutes was spent counseling the patient on a recent hip fracture and depressive symptoms as a result of being in a nursing home?
    a. 99309
    b. 99304
    c. 99315
    d. 99308

5. Code 99318 is a subsequent care code. How many of the key components must be documented in order to bill 99318 for an annual nursing facility assessment?
    a. Two out of three
    b. None—this is a time-based code
    c. Only the physical exam
    d. All three must be documented

6. What code is reported when a detailed history and exam with low complexity MDM are documented for a new patient in an assisted living facility?
    a. 99324
    b. 99325
    c. 99326
    d. 99327

7. Codes 99339 and 99340 are used to report care plan oversight services for patients using home health or in a nursing facility.
   a. True
   b. False

Chapter 10: Home Services (99341–99350)

New Patient (99341–99345)

QUICK COMPARISON

Home Services—New Patient

E/M Code	Medical Decision Making[1]	History[1]	Exam[1]	Counseling and/or Coordination of Care	Time Spent Face to Face (avg.)
99341	Straight-forward complexity	Problem focused	Problem focused	Consistent with problems and patient's or family's needs	20 min.
99342	Low complexity	Expanded problem focused	Expanded problem focused	Consistent with problems and patient's or family's needs	30 min.
99343	Moderate complexity	Detailed	Detailed	Consistent with problems and patient's or family's needs	45 min.
99344	Moderate complexity	Comprehensive	Comprehensive	Consistent with problems and patient's or family's needs	60 min.
99345	High complexity	Comprehensive	Comprehensive	Consistent with problems and patient's or family's needs	75 min.

1   Key component. For new patients, all three components (history, exam, and medical decision making) are crucial for selecting the correct code and must be adequately documented in the medical record to substantiate the level of service reported.

GENERAL GUIDELINES

- Use these CPT® codes to report any E/M services provided to a new patient in a private residence, temporary lodging, or short-term accommodation such as hotel, campground, hostel, or cruise ship. Do not confuse these codes with those for services provided by home care nurses or other home health providers. These codes are for evaluation and management services being provided by physicians or other qualified nonphysician practitioners.

- For commercial payers, consider assigning the appropriate consultation code instead of these codes when an opinion or advice was provided about a patient for a specific problem at the request of another physician/qualified healthcare professional or other appropriate source.

- Use a case management code when coordination of care involved other providers or agencies but did not involve a patient encounter on that day.

- Assign modifier 24 to indicate that an E/M service performed during the postoperative period was not related to the prior procedure. The claim should show a different diagnosis from that for the surgery.

- Append modifier 25 to report that a separately identifiable E/M service was performed by the same physician/qualified healthcare professional on the same day as a procedure or service. Only the content of work associated with the separate E/M service should be considered when assigning the correct E/M code.
- User modifier 32 when the services were mandated, such as by a peer review organization, third-party payer, or as a result of a governmental, legislative, or regulatory requirement.
- Report separately the codes for the diagnostic tests or studies performed.

99341

DOCUMENTATION REQUIREMENTS

Medical Decision Making: straightforward
- Minimal number of diagnoses or management options considered
- No or minimal amount and complexity of data reviewed
- Minimal risk of complications or morbidity or mortality

Problem Severity: low
- Low risk of morbidity without treatment
- Little, if any, risk of mortality without treatment
- Expectation of full recovery without functional impairment

History: problem focused
- Chief complaint
- Brief history of present illness or problem (one to three HPI elements)

Examination: problem focused
- 1995: one organ system or body area
- 1997: one to five bullet (•) elements in one or more organ systems/body areas

Code Indicators (from tables of risk—including some AMA indicators in italic)

Presenting Problem(s)
- One self-limited or minor problem

Management Options
- Rest, gargles, elastic bandages, superficial dressings

Counseling and/or Coordination of Care
- As appropriate for the problem

Time Spent Face to Face (average)
- 20 minutes

✓ **QUICK TIP**

Report with the correct place-of-service (POS) code for electronic and paper claims submission.

99342

DOCUMENTATION REQUIREMENTS

Medical Decision Making: low
- Limited number of diagnoses or management options considered
- Limited amount and complexity of data reviewed
- Low risk of complications or morbidity or mortality

Problem Severity: moderate
- Moderate risk of morbidity without treatment
- Moderate risk of mortality without treatment
- Uncertain outcome or increased probability of prolonged functional impairment

History: expanded problem focused
- Chief complaint
- Brief history of present illness (one to three HPI elements)
- Problem pertinent system review (one or two systems)

Examination: expanded problem focused
- 1995: two to seven organ systems or body areas
- 1997: at least six bullet (•) elements in one or more organ systems/body areas

Problem Severity
- Moderate risk of morbidity without treatment
- Moderate risk of mortality without treatment
- Uncertain outcome or increased probability of prolonged functional impairment

Code Indicators (from tables of risk—including some AMA indicators in italic)

Presenting Problem(s)
- Two or more self-limited or minor problem(s)
- One stable chronic illness (e.g., well controlled hypertension or non-insulin-dependent diabetes, cataract, BPH)
- Acute uncomplicated illness or injury (e.g., cystitis, allergic rhinitis, simple sprain)

Management Options
- Physical therapy, *rest or exercise, diet, stress management*
- Over the counter drugs, *medication management with minimal risk*
- Minor surgery, with no identified risk factors
- Occupational therapy
- IV fluids, without additives

Counseling and/or Coordination of Care
- As appropriate for the problem
  (See "General Guidelines" for additional documentation considerations.)

Time Spent Face to Face (average)
- 30 minutes

99343

DOCUMENTATION REQUIREMENTS

Medical Decision Making: moderate
- Multiple number of diagnoses or management options considered
- Moderate amount or complexity of data reviewed
- Moderate risk of complications or morbidity or mortality

Problem Severity: moderate to high
- Moderate to high risk of morbidity without treatment
- Moderate to high risk of mortality without treatment
- Uncertain outcome or increased probability of prolonged functional impairment or high probability of severe prolonged functional impairment

History: detailed
- Chief complaint
- Extended history of present illness (four or more HPI elements or the status of three chronic problems)
- Extended system review (two to nine systems)
- Pertinent past, family, and/or social history (one of the history areas)

Examination: detailed
- 1995: two to seven organ systems or body areas with an extended exam of affected area(s)
- 1997: at least two bullet (•) elements from at least six organ systems or body areas, OR at least 12 bullet (•) elements from two or more organ systems or body areas. Eye and psychiatric single-system exams must include at least nine bullet (•) elements.

Code Indicators (from tables of risk—including some AMA indicators in italic)

Presenting Problem(s)
- One or more chronic illness with mild exacerbation, progression, or side effects of treatment
- Two or more stable chronic illnesses
- Undiagnosed new *illness, injury,* or problem with uncertain prognosis
- Acute illness, with systemic symptoms (pyelonephritis, pleuritis, colitis)
- Acute complicated injury, e.g., head injury, with brief loss of consciousnessp

Management Options
- Prescription drug management
- Closed treatment of fracture or dislocation, without manipulation
- IV fluids with additives

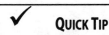

QUICK TIP

See codes 99241–99245 for examples of chart documentation.

- Minor surgery, with identified risk factors
- Elective major surgery (open, percutaneous, endoscopic), with no identified risk factors
- Therapeutic nuclear medicine

Counseling and/or Coordination of Care
- As appropriate for the problem

Time Spent Face to Face (average)
- 45 minutes

99344

DOCUMENTATION REQUIREMENTS

Medical Decision Making: moderate
- Multiple number of diagnoses or management options considered
- Moderate amount or complexity of data reviewed
- Moderate risk of complications or morbidity or mortality

Problem Severity: high
- Moderate to extreme risk of morbidity without treatment
- Moderate to high risk of mortality without treatment
- Uncertain outcome or increased probability of prolonged functional impairment or high probability of severe prolonged functional impairment

History: comprehensive
- Chief complaint
- Extended history of present illness (four or more HPI elements or the status of three chronic problems)
- Complete system review (10 systems)
- Complete past, family, social history (at least one element from all history areas)

Examination: comprehensive
- 1995: eight or more organ systems
- 1997: multisystem exam must include all bullet (•) elements from at least nine organ systems or body areas unless specific instructions limit content of the exam; at least two bullet elements from each area/system reviewed are expected to be documented.
- 1997: single organ system/body area exam must include all bullet (•) elements in shaded boxes PLUS at least one element in each unshaded box.

Code Indicators (from tables of risk—including some AMA indicators in italic)

Presenting Problem(s)
- One or more chronic illness with mild exacerbation, progression, or side effects of treatment

QUICK TIP

Documentation should indicate why this service was performed in the home setting and not in the office or other outpatient setting.

- Two or more stable chronic illnesses
- Undiagnosed new *illness, injury,* or problem with uncertain prognosis
- Acute illness, with systemic symptoms (pyelonephritis, pleuritis, colitis)
- Acute complicated injury, e.g., head injury, with brief loss of consciousness

Management Options
- Prescription drug management
- Closed treatment of fracture or dislocation, without manipulation
- IV fluids with additives
- Minor surgery, with identified risk factors
- Elective major surgery (open, percutaneous, endoscopic), with no identified risk factors
- Therapeutic nuclear medicine

Counseling and/or Coordination of Care
- As appropriate for the problem

Time Spent Face to Face (average)
- 60 minutes

99345

DOCUMENTATION REQUIREMENTS

Medical Decision Making: high
- Extensive number of diagnoses or management options considered
- Extensive amount or complexity of data reviewed
- High risk of complications or morbidity or mortality

Problem Severity
- Usually the patient has developed a significant new problem requiring immediate physician attention

History: comprehensive
- Chief complaint
- Extended history of present illness (four or more HPI elements or the status of three chronic problems)
- Complete system review (10 systems)
- Complete past, family, social history (at least one element from all history areas)

Examination: comprehensive
- 1995: eight or more organ systems
- 1997: multisystem exam must include all bullet (•) elements from at least nine organ systems or body areas unless specific instructions limit content of the exam; at least two bullet elements from each area/system reviewed are expected to be documented.

✓ QUICK TIP

Payers may require documentation of the level of medical decision making and why the service was performed in the home setting.

- 1997: single organ system/body area exam must include all bullet (•) elements in shaded boxes PLUS at least one element in each unshaded box.

Code Indicators (from tables of risk—including some AMA indicators in italic)

Presenting Problem(s)

- One or more chronic illness with severe exacerbation, progression, or side effects of treatment
- Acute or chronic illness or injury that poses a threat to life or bodily function, e.g., multiple traumas, acute MI, pulmonary embolism, severe respiratory distress, progressive severe rheumatoid arthritis, psychiatric illness, with potential threat to self or others, peritonitis, ARF
- An abrupt change in neurological status, e.g., seizure, TIA, weakness, sensory loss

Management Options

- Elective major surgery with identified risk factors or emergency major surgery (open, percutaneous, endoscopic)
- Parenteral controlled substances
- Drug therapy requiring intensive monitoring for toxicity
- Decision not to resuscitate or to deescalate care because of poor prognosis

Counseling and/or Coordination of Care

- As appropriate for the problem

Time Spent Face to Face (average)

- 75 minutes

Established Patient (99347–99350)

QUICK COMPARISON

Home Services—Established Patient

E/M Code	Medical Decision Making[1]	History[1]	Exam[1]	Counseling and/or Coordination of Care	Time Spent Face to Face (avg.)
99347	Straightforward complexity	Problem focused interval	Problem focused	Consistent with problems and patient's or family's needs	15 min.
99348	Low complexity	Expanded problem focused interval	Expanded problem focused	Consistent with problems and patient's or family's needs	25 min.
99349	Moderate complexity	Detailed interval	Detailed	Consistent with problems and patient's or family's needs	40 min.
99350	Moderate to high complexity	Comprehensive interval	Comprehensive	Consistent with problems and patient's or family's needs	60 min.

1   Key component. For established patients, at least two of the three components (history, exam, and medical decision making) are needed to select the correct code and must be adequately documented in the medical record to substantiate the level of service reported.

GENERAL GUIDELINES

- Use these codes to report any E/M services provided to an established patient in a private residence, temporary lodging, or short-term accommodation such as hotel, campground, hostel, or cruise ship, by a physician or appropriate qualified nonphysician practitioner.
- Consider assigning the appropriate consultation code instead of these codes when an opinion or advice was provided about a patient for a specific problem at the request of another physician/qualified healthcare professional or other appropriate source.
- Use a case management code when coordination of care involved other providers or agencies but did not involve a patient encounter on that day.
- Assign modifier 24 to indicate that an E/M service performed during the postoperative period was not related to the prior procedure. The claim should show a different diagnosis from that for the surgery.
- Append modifier 25 to report that a separately identifiable E/M service was performed by the same physician/qualified healthcare professional on the same day as a procedure or service. Only the content of work associated with the separate E/M service should be considered when assigning the correct E/M code.
- User modifier 32 when the services were mandated, such as by a third-party payer, or as a result of a governmental, legislative, or regulatory requirement.
- Report separately the codes for the diagnostic tests or studies performed.

ISSUES IN THIS CODE RANGE

Code 99350 is one of only a few E/M codes where the level of medical decision making is expressed as a range. Normally these levels are clearly indicated though the nature of presenting problem may state "low-moderate severity." In this case, the level of decision making is defined as moderate to high. The presenting problems are also defined as moderate-high. The additional statement "Usually the patient has developed a significant new problem requiring immediate physician attention" is also found in code 99345 where the decision making is defined as high. For this reason we have included the code indicators for high level decision making. This may simply be an anomaly in the CPT book.

99347

DOCUMENTATION REQUIREMENTS

Medical Decision Making: straightforward
- Minimal number of diagnoses or management options considered
- No or minimal amount or complexity of data reviewed
- Minimal risk of complications or morbidity or mortality

Problem Severity: self-limited or minor
- Little, if any, risk of morbidity without treatment
- Little, if any, risk of mortality without treatment
- Transient problem, low probability of permanently altered status
- Good prognosis

History: problem focused interval
- Chief complaint
- Brief history of present illness or problem (one to three HPI elements)

Examination: problem focused
- 1995: one organ system or body area
- 1997: one to five bullet (•) elements in one or more organ systems/body areas

Code Indicators (from tables of risk—including some AMA indicators in italic)

Presenting Problem(s)
- One self-limited or minor problem

Management Options
- Rest, gargles, elastic bandages, superficial dressings

Counseling and/or Coordination of Care
- As appropriate for the problem

Time Spent Face to Face (average)
- 15 minutes

99348

DOCUMENTATION REQUIREMENTS

Medical Decision Making: low
- Limited number of diagnoses or management options considered
- Limited amount and complexity of data reviewed
- Low risk of complications or morbidity or mortality

Problem Severity: low to moderate
- Expectation of full recovery without functional impairment, or uncertain outcome or increased probability of prolonged functional impairment.
- Low to moderate risk of morbidity, if any, without treatment

History: expanded problem focused interval
- Chief complaint
- Brief history of present illness (one to three HPI elements)
- Problem pertinent system review (one or two systems)

Examination: expanded problem focused
- 1995: two to seven organ systems or body areas
- 1997: at least six bullet (•) elements in one or more organ systems/body areas

Code Indicators (from tables of risk—including some AMA indicators in italic)

Presenting Problem(s)
- Two or more self-limited or minor problem(s)
- One stable chronic illness (e.g., well controlled hypertension or non-insulin-dependent diabetes, cataract, BPH)
- Acute uncomplicated illness or injury (e.g., cystitis, allergic rhinitis, simple sprain)

Management Options
- Physical therapy, *rest or exercise, diet, stress management*
- Over the counter drugs, *medication management with minimal risk*
- Minor surgery, with no identified risk factors
- Occupational therapy
- IV fluids, without additives

Counseling and/or Coordination of Care
- As appropriate for the problem

Time Spent Face to Face (average)
- 25 minutes

QUICK TIP

Documentation examples may be found with codes 99241–99245.

99349

DOCUMENTATION REQUIREMENTS

Medical Decision Making: moderate
- Multiple number of diagnoses or management options considered
- Moderate amount or complexity of data reviewed
- Moderate risk of complications or morbidity or mortality

Problem Severity: moderate to high
- Moderate to high risk of morbidity without treatment
- Moderate to high risk of mortality without treatment
- Uncertain outcome or increased probability of prolonged functional impairment or high probability of severe prolonged functional impairment

History: detailed interval
- Chief complaint
- Extended history of present illness (four or more HPI elements or the status of three chronic problems)
- Extended system review (two to nine systems)
- Pertinent past, family, and/or social history (one of the history areas)

Examination: detailed
- 1995: two to seven organ systems or body areas (safe harbor is five systems)
- 1997: at least two bullet (•) elements from at least six organ systems or body areas, OR at least 12 bullet (•) elements from two or more organ systems or body areas. Eye and psychiatric single-system exams must include at least nine bullet (n) elements.

Code Indicators (from tables of risk—including some AMA indicators in italic)

Presenting Problem(s)
- One or more chronic illness with mild exacerbation, progression, or side effects of treatment
- Two or more stable chronic illnesses
- Undiagnosed new *illness, injury, or* problem with uncertain prognosis
- Acute illness, with systemic symptoms (pyelonephritis, pleuritis, colitis)
- Acute complicated injury, e.g., head injury, with brief loss of consciousness

Management Options
- Prescription drug management
- Closed treatment of fracture or dislocation, without manipulation
- IV fluids with additives
- Minor surgery, with identified risk factors
- Elective major surgery (open, percutaneous, endoscopic), with no identified risk factors
- Therapeutic nuclear medicine

QUICK TIP

Report with the correct place-of-service (POS) code for electronic and paper copy claims submission.

Counseling and/or Coordination of Care
- As appropriate for the problem

Time Spent Face to Face (average)
- 40 minutes

99350

DOCUMENTATION REQUIREMENTS

Medical Decision Making: moderate to high
- Multiple number of diagnoses or management options considered
- Moderate amount or complexity of data reviewed
- Moderate risk of complications or morbidity or mortality

OR
- Extensive number of diagnoses or management options considered
- Extensive amount or complexity of data reviewed
- High risk of complications or morbidity or mortality

Problem Severity: moderate to high
- Moderate to high risk of morbidity without treatment
- Moderate to high risk of mortality without treatment
- Uncertain outcome or increased probability of prolonged functional impairment or high probability of severe prolonged functional impairment
- The patient may be unstable or may have developed a significant new problem requiring immediate physician attention.

History: comprehensive interval
- Chief complaint
- Extended history of present illness (four or more HPI elements or the status of three chronic problems)
- Complete system review (10 systems)
- Complete past, family, social history (at least one element from all history areas)

Examination: comprehensive
- 1995: eight or more organ systems
- 1997: multisystem exam must include all bullet (•) elements from at least nine organ systems or body areas unless specific instructions limit content of the exam; at least two bullet elements from each area/system reviewed are expected to be documented.
- 1997: single organ system/body area exam must include all bullet (•) elements in shaded boxes PLUS at least one element in each unshaded box.

Code Indicators (from tables of risk—including some AMA indicators in italic)

Presenting Problem(s)

- One or more chronic illness with severe exacerbation, progression, or side effects of treatment
- Acute or chronic illness or injury that poses a threat to life or bodily function, e.g., multiple traumas, acute MI, pulmonary embolism, severe respiratory distress, progressive severe rheumatoid arthritis, psychiatric illness, with potential threat to self or others, peritonitis, ARF
- An abrupt change in neurological status, e.g., seizure, TIA, weakness, sensory loss

Management Options

- Elective major surgery with identified risk factors or emergency major surgery (open, percutaneous, endoscopic)
- Parenteral controlled substances
- Drug therapy requiring intensive monitoring for toxicity
- Decision not to resuscitate or to deescalate care because of poor prognosis

Counseling and/or Coordination of Care

- As appropriate for the problem

Time Spent Face to Face (average)

- 60 minutes

KNOWLEDGE ASSESSMENT CHAPTER 10

See chapter 19 for answers and rationale.

1. What codes are used to report new patient encounters in the patient's home?
   a. 99341–99345
   b. 99241–99245
   c. 99347–99350
   d. 99202–99205

2. What home services code would be assigned for an established patient with a comprehensive history and exam and moderate MDM?
   a. 99349
   b. 99350
   c. 99344
   d. None of the above

3. What modifier should be appended to codes 99341–99350 when services were mandated by a court order?
   a. 25
   b. 52
   c. 59
   d. 32

4. Based on the 1995 E/M documentation guidelines, how many organ systems must be examined in order to bill a 99350?
   a. At least two
   b. Eight or more
   c. Ten or more
   d. Two to four

5. What home services code would be assigned for a new patient with moderate MDM, a comprehensive history and a detailed physical examination?
   a. 99344
   b. 99343
   c. 99349
   d. None of the above

Chapter 11: Prolonged Physician Services (99354–99359, 99415–99416, 99417, 99360)

Prolonged Service with Direct Patient Contact (99354–99357)

QUICK COMPARISON

Prolonged Services—with Direct Patient Contact

| E/M Code | Where the Service was Provided | | Time Spent Face to Face (avg.) |
	Office or Outpatient Facility	Inpatient or Observation Setting	
99354	Yes	No	First 30–74 min.
99355	Yes	No	Each additional 30 min.
99356	No	Yes	First 30–74 min.
99357	No	Yes	Each additional 30 min.

GENERAL GUIDELINES

- These codes are used to report direct, face-to-face patient contact for an unusually long period of time rendered by a physician or other qualified healthcare professional in either an inpatient or outpatient setting.
- These codes are only used in addition to other time based evaluation and management services provided; they are adjunctive codes and cannot be used alone.
- Appropriate code selection is based on the time the clinician spent with the patient face to face, as well as additional time spent on non-face-to-face activities on the patient's floor or unit in a hospital or nursing facility.
- Other services provided during these prolonged service periods should be reported separately. Time involved performing these activities should not count toward the prolonged services time.
- Services of less than 30 minutes beyond the usual service are not separately reported.
- Only report these codes once per date.
- Report 99354 with 90837, 90847, 99241–99245, 99324–99337, 99341–99350, and 99483.
- Codes 99354 and 99355 should not be reported with 99202–99205, 99212–99215, or 99415–99417.

 QUICK TIP

Time is not required to be continuous, but may be intermittent. For inpatient or observation, both face-to-face time and additional non-face-to-face services on the patient's floor or unit are considered part of the overall time.

- The federal Medicare program has strict protocol that must be followed when reporting prolonged service codes 99354–99357. The following table provides the threshold times necessary to report prolonged services. All times should be clearly documented in the patient's medical record. Carriers may request supporting documentation during a prepayment screen or a postpayment audit.
- For codes 99354–99355:

  Append modifier 95 to indicate that the E/M service was rendered to a patient at a distant site via a real-time interactive audio and video telecommunications system. The communication between the physician or other qualified health care professional and the patient should be commensurate with the same key components or requirements of those that would be required if the service had been rendered in a face-to-face setting.

Prolonged Service Thresholds

As the total time for prolonged service must exceed the basic service by at least 30 minutes to qualify for reporting, threshold times have been established for prolonged services. The following is a selection of the threshold times cited in the *Medicare Carriers Manual*, part 3, sec. 15511, "Prolonged Services." (See CMS web-based manual, *Medicare Claims Processing Manual*, Pub. 100-04, chapter 12, sections 30.6.15.1 to 30.6.15.2.)

To report CPT codes 99354 and 99355:

Basic Service	Typical Time	Threshold for 99354	Threshold for 99355
99326	45 min.	75 min.	120 min.
99327	60 min.	90 min.	135 min.
99334	15 min.	45 min.	90 min.
99335	25 min.	55 min.	100 min.
99349	40 min.	70 min.	115 min.
99350	60 min.	90 min.	135 min.

To report CPT codes 99356 and 99357:

Basic Service	Typical Time	Threshold for 99356	Threshold for 99357
99221	30 min.	60 min.	105 min.
99223	70 min.	100 min.	145 min.
99231	15 min.	45 min.	90 min.
99232	25 min.	55 min.	100 min.

 KEY POINT

CPT specifies that prolonged services are reported with codes that have a time component. They include:

99218–99220, 99221–99223, 99224–99226, 99231–99233. 99234–99236, 99241–99245, 99251–99255, 99304–99310, 99324–99337, 99341–99350, 99483, 90837, 90847

SPECIAL INSTRUCTIONS FOR PROLONGED PHYSICIANS SERVICES

Medicare contractors have performed many audits on prolonged physician services (99354–99357) in the past. Prolonged service codes are a consistent area of concern due to the continued errors. The common errors are as follows:

Error Type	Error Description
Missing/illegible provider signature	Medical documentation must be legible and contain the handwritten or electronic signature of the provider who rendered the service. Stamp signatures are not permitted.
Incomplete/missing beneficiary information	Medical record documentation must contain a legible beneficiary name for identification purposes as well as a clearly denoted date of service that corresponds to the date reported on the claim form.
Lack of documentation of total visit duration	The duration and content of the medically necessary E/M service as well as the additional prolonged services reported must be clearly detailed in the medical record documentation.
Lack of documentation to establish face-to-face contact by the provider	Only direct face-to-face contact with the patient, continuous or not, beyond the average time of the E/M visit code reported can be counted towards whether it is permissible to bill prolonged services in addition to the selected E/M code as well as to determine which prolonged service code is appropriate. Medical record documentation must clearly specify and support that the rendering provider personally provided direct face-to-face services.
Lack of an E/M companion code	Prolonged service codes are not billed as stand-alone codes; they must be reported with the appropriate level of E/M companion code. Further, two prolonged physician service codes, 99355 and 99357 are add-on codes to primary prolonged physician service codes, 99354 and 99356, respectively and must be billed in conjunction with the primary codes as well as the E/M companion code reported.
Lack of appropriate E/M companion code	In cases where an E/M service is dominated by counseling and/or coordination of care, the E/M code is chosen based on the average or typical time associated with the various code levels. Thus, when the E/M service is based on time, prolonged physician services codes may only be reported with the highest code level in that particular category of codes as the companion code.

99354

DOCUMENTATION REQUIREMENTS

Intent of Service
- Extended evaluation and management of a patient's specific problem

Presence of Patient
- Necessary (direct, face-to-face contact for a portion of the service)

Time Spent on Prolonged Service (average)
- First 30 to 74 minutes

Special Coding and Documentation Considerations
- Use this code to report E/M services that exceed the typical time defined in the code's narrative by 30 minutes. The service must have been rendered in the office or other outpatient setting.
- Use this code only once per date.

99355

DOCUMENTATION REQUIREMENTS

Intent of Service
- Extended evaluation and management of a patient's specific problem

Presence of Patient
- Necessary (direct, face-to-face contact for a portion of the service)

Time Spent on Prolonged Service (average)
- Each additional 30 minutes

Special Coding and Documentation Considerations
- Use this code to report each additional 30 minutes of E/M services after the first 74 minutes over the typical time defined in the code's narrative. The service must have been rendered in the office or other outpatient setting.
- Never report this code alone—it should always be reported with 99354.

Clinical Example: 99354–99355
An asthma patient is seen in the home for moderate respiratory distress and bronchospasms. Patient presents with difficulty breathing and wheezing in all lung fields. Treatment requires intermittent time with the patient over a three- to four-hour period and includes epinephrine administration and intermittent bronchial dilation.

QUICK TIP

Documentation needs to indicate the total time spent face to face with the patient, as well as the floor/unit time spent working on this patient's case. Other activities outside of this patient's care cannot be included in this patient's prolonged services time.

99356

DOCUMENTATION REQUIREMENTS

Intent of Service
- Extended evaluation and management of a patient's specific problem

Presence of Patient
- Necessary (direct, face-to-face contact for a portion of the service)

Time Spent on Prolonged Service (average)
- First 30 to 74 minutes

Special Coding and Documentation Considerations
- Use this code to report E/M services that exceed the typical time defined in the code's narrative by 30 minutes. The service must have been rendered in the inpatient setting.
- Use this code only once per date.

99357

DOCUMENTATION REQUIREMENTS

Intent of Service
- Extended evaluation and management of a patient's specific problem

Presence of Patient
- Necessary (direct, face-to-face contact for a portion of the service)

Time Spent on Prolonged Service (average)
- Each additional 30 minutes

Special Coding and Documentation Considerations
- Use this code to report each additional 30 minutes of E/M services after the first 74 minutes over the typical time defined in the code's narrative. The service must have been rendered in the inpatient setting.
- Never report this code alone—it should always be reported with 99356.

Prolonged Service Without Direct Patient Contact (99358–99359)

Quick Comparison

Evaluation and Management Service Before and/or After Direct Patient Care

E/M Code	Office or Outpatient Facility	Inpatient Facility	Time Spent Before/After Direct Patient Care
99358	Yes	Yes	First 30–74 min.
99359	Yes	Yes	Each additional 30 min.

General Guidelines

- Use these codes when a physician or qualified health care professional provides a prolonged service that does not involve direct care beyond the usual service in either an inpatient, observation, or outpatient setting. **Note:** These codes are not used to report additional floor/unit time in the hospital or nursing facility settings.

- These codes are reported in addition to the other evaluation and management service provided on the same date, except 99202–99205 and 99212–99215.

- For prolonged services in addition to office and other outpatient services on the same date of service without direct patient contact, see 99417.

- Services of less than 30 minutes beyond the usual service are not separately reported.

- These codes should not be used to report services that have more specific codes and no upper time limit, such as communication with other professionals and/or the patient family or review of extensive records and tests before and after direct patient care, such as care plan oversight services (99339, 99340, 99374–99380), chronic care management by a physician or other qualified healthcare professional (99491), home and outpatient INR monitoring (93792, 99793), medical team conferences (99366–99368), interprofessional telephone/Internet/electronic health record consultations (99446–99449, 99451–99452), or online digital evaluation and management services (99421–99423).

- Many third-party and commercial payers do not recognize these codes for payment.

- Prolonged services may be reported on a different date from the primary service to which they apply; however, they must relate to ongoing management of direct patient care on a separate service date.

- These codes report the total duration of non-face-to-face service time (including noncontiguous time) spent providing prolonged services.

- Codes 99358–99359 exclude other non-face-to-face services, which are reportable by more specific codes (e.g., online medical evaluations, anticoagulation management, and care plan oversight).

99358

DOCUMENTATION REQUIREMENTS

Intent of Service
- Extended evaluation of a patient's specific problem

Presence of Patient
- Not required

Time
- Document the time spent and content of services

Special Coding and Documentation Considerations
- Use this code only once per day.
- Time does not have to be continuous but should reflect the total time spent in providing prolonged service.
- Prolonged services of less than 15 minutes past the first hour or less than 15 minutes beyond the final 30 minutes are not reported separately.

99359

DOCUMENTATION REQUIREMENTS

Intent of Service
- Extended evaluation of a patient's specific problem

Presence of Patient
- Not required

Time
- Document the time spent and content of services.

Special Coding and Documentation Considerations
- Time does not have to be continuous but should reflect the total time spent in providing prolonged service.
- Prolonged services of less than 15 minutes past the first hour or less than 15 minutes beyond the final 30 minutes are not reported separately.
- Never report this code alone—it should always be reported with 99358.

QUICK TIP

Note that some payers may not cover non-face-to-face prolonged services.

Prolonged Clinical Staff Services with Physician or Other Qualified Health Care Professional Supervision (99415–99416)

QUICK COMPARISON

Clinical Staff Service during an Evaluation and Management Service with Direct Patient Contact

E/M Code	Office or Outpatient Facility	Inpatient Facility	Time Spent Face to Face (avg.)
99415	Yes	No	First 45–74 min.
99416	Yes	No	Each additional 30 min.

GENERAL GUIDELINES

- These CPT codes are used when the clinical staff provides direct patient care for a prolonged period of time in an office or other outpatient setting beyond the highest total time stated in the E/M code description.
- These codes are reported in addition to the other evaluation and management service provided on the same date.
- A physician or other qualified health care professional must be available to provide direct supervision of the clinical staff.
- These codes are reported once per date for the total duration of face-to-face time (including noncontiguous time) spent with the patient.
- Services of less than 30 minutes beyond the usual service are not reported separately.
- Do not report codes 99415–99416 for more than two concurrent patients.
- Use codes 99354–99355 for face-to-face prolonged services provided by the physician.

99415

DOCUMENTATION REQUIREMENTS

Intent of Service
- Extended evaluation and management of a patient's specific problem

Presence of Patient
- Required (direct, face-to-face contact)

Time Spent on Prolonged Service (average)
- First 30 to 74 minutes

Special Coding and Documentation Considerations

- Direct supervision of the clinical staff by the physician or other qualified health care professional is required.
- Use this code to report E/M services that exceed the highest total time defined in the code's narrative by 30 minutes. The service must be rendered in the office or outpatient setting.
- Time does not have to be continuous but should reflect the total time spent providing the prolonged service.
- Use this code only once per day.

Clinical Example: 99415

A patient presents with symptoms of clinical dehydration, the physician reports a 99203 and directs a member of his clinical staff to initiate IV hydration with normal saline. Prolonged clinical staff services would begin after 44 minutes, the typical service time included in 99203. Code 99415 would be reported when at least 74 minutes of total face-to-face time are provided by the clinical staff.

99416

DOCUMENTATION REQUIREMENTS

Intent of Service

- Extended evaluation and management of a patient's specific problem

Presence of Patient

- Required (direct, face-to-face contact)

Time Spent on Prolonged Service (average)

- Each additional 30 minutes

Special Coding and Documentation Considerations

- Never report this code alone—it should always be reported with 99415.
- Time does not have to be continuous but should reflect the total time spent providing the prolonged service.
- Prolonged services less than 15 minutes beyond the final 30 minutes are not reported.

Prolonged Service With or Without Direct Patient Contact (99417)

QUICK COMPARISON

Prolonged Services With or Without Direct Patient Contact

E/M Code	Office or Other Outpatient Facility	Inpatient or Observation Setting	Time Spent With and/or Without Patient Contact (Avg.)
99417	Yes	No	Each additional 15 min.

GENERAL GUIDELINES

- Use this code to report each additional 15 minutes of E/M services beyond the time indicated in the code description. (Refer to the documentation requirements below for additional guidance on which time to use, since time is listed as a range in the new descriptions for 99205 and 99215.)
- This code is only used in addition to time-based evaluation and management services 99205 and 99215.
- Use of this code is based on the total time the clinician spent on the day of the patient visit, including face-to-face and non-face-to-face activities.
- Other services provided during prolonged service periods may be reported separately. Time involved performing these activities should not count toward prolonged service times.
- Services of less than 15 minutes beyond the usual service are not reported separately.
- This code should not be reported with 99354–99355, 99358–99359, or 99415–99416 on the same date of service

99417

DOCUMENTATION REQUIREMENTS

Intent of Service
- Extended evaluation and management of a patient's specific problem

Presence of Patient
- Includes direct face-to-face contact and non-face-to-face activities

Time Spent on Prolonged Service (average)
- Each additional 15 minutes

Special Coding and Documentation Considerations
- This code is used to report total time spent on the date of the encounter, with or without direct patient contact, that extends beyond the time designated in the primary code description. **Note:** CPT states

to report 99417 for services at least 15 minutes beyond the minimum time required to report level 5 new or established office or other outpatient services. CMS states in the CY2021 PFS Proposed Rule to report for services when the *maximum* time for level 5 office/outpatient E/M visit is exceeded. The CY2021 PFS Final Rule was not available at the time of this publication. Go to https://www.cms.gov/Medicare/Medicare-Fee-for-Service-Payment/PhysicianFeeSched to review the CY2021 final rule.

- Document the total time (with and without direct patient contact) spent on the patient's case. Time does not have to be continuous but should reflect the total time spent on the day of the visit providing the prolonged service.

- Never report this code alone; it should be reported with 99205 or 99215.

Standby Services (99360)

QUICK COMPARISON

Standby Services

E/M Code	Intent of Service	Face-to-Face Visits	Time Spent on Standby
99360	Standby services are provided by a clinician at the request of another clinician and include prolonged attendance without face-to-face contact with the patient (i.e., operative high-risk delivery standby, EEG monitoring)	No	Each 30 min.

99360

DOCUMENTATION REQUIREMENTS

Intent of Service
- Professional services specifically requested by another clinician that involves extended attendance

Presence of Patient
- Not required

Time Spent on Prolonged Service (average)
- Each 30 minutes
- Report total duration of the standby time period; however, services of less than 30 minutes total duration should not be reported
- Report each additional 30 minutes of standby services beyond the initial time period only if a *full* 30-minute period was provided

Special Coding and Documentation Considerations
- Exclusive, no other care or services may be provided by the standby provider to other patients during this period.
- Do not use this code to report time spent proctoring another individual OR when the standby period ends with the performance of a global surgery package procedure by the same clinician who was on standby.

KNOWLEDGE ASSESSMENT CHAPTER 11

See chapter 19 for answers and rationale.

1. When coding prolonged services, what major element out of the following is the determining factor for when to use 99354–99357 vs. 99358–99359?
   a. New vs. established
   b. Office or outpatient facility
   c. With or without direct patient contact
   d. All of the above

2. Codes 99354, 99356, and 99358 may only be used once per date of service.
   a. True
   b. False

3. Codes 99354, 99355, 99356, 99357, and 99359 are all add-on codes and can be billed alone with sufficient documentation.
   a. True
   b. False

4. In order to bill prolonged services 99354–99357, the total time of the encounter must exceed the basic service by at least _____ minutes.
   a. 15
   b. 30
   c. 45
   d. 60

5. To report prolonged services provided by the clinical staff (99415–99416), direct supervision by a physician is required.
   a. True
   b. False

6. A clinician may not report standby services if the standby service period ends with the standby clinician performing a global surgery package procedure.
   a. True
   b. False

Chapter 12: Other E/M Services (99366–99457)

Medical Team Conferences (99366–99368)

QUICK COMPARISON

Medical Team Conferences

E/M Code	Intent of Service	Provider	Presence of Patient	Time
99366	To plan and coordinate	Nonphysician member of interdisciplinary team	Patient and/or family present	30 min.
99367	To plan and coordinate	Physician member of interdisciplinary team	Patient and/or family not present	30 min.
99368	To plan and coordinate	Nonphysician member of interdisciplinary team	Patient and/or family not present	30 min.

GENERAL GUIDELINES

- A minimum of three healthcare professionals of different specialties or disciplines who provide direct care to the patient must participate.
- Participants must have performed a face-to-face evaluation or treatment of the patient in the prior 60 days.
- Physician's report team conferences with the patient present using the appropriate E/M code and time as the key controlling factor if counseling and coordination of care dominate the service.
- Only one person per specialty may report participation in the team conference.
- Time is calculated based upon the review of the individual patient and ends at the conclusion.
- Time does not include record keeping or generation of reports.
- Time is not reported concurrently with any other billable service.
- The services are reported as face-to-face if the patient is present for any part of the service.
- Team conference services of less than 30 minutes are not reported.
- Team conferences are not reported if part of a contractual agreement of a facility or organization.
- Each participant must document his or her participation and care recommendations.

 QUICK TIP

Healthcare professionals may include PT, OT, speech-language pathologists, social workers, dietitians, nurse practitioners, physician assistants, discharge coordinators, and other appropriate ancillary healthcare providers.

Care Plan Oversight Services (99374–99380)

Quick Comparison

Care Plan Oversight Services

E/M Code	Intent of Service	Place of Service	Under Care of	Presence of Patient	Time
99374	Supervision of a patient requiring complex and multidisciplinary care modalities involving regular development and/or revision of care plans by that individual, review of subsequent reports of patient status, review of laboratory and other studies, communication (including telephone calls) for purposes of assessment or care decisions with healthcare professionals, family member(s), surrogate decision maker(s) (e.g., legal guardians) and/or key caregivers involved in the patient's care, integration of new information into the medical treatment plan and/or adjustment of medical therapy, within a calendar month	In home, a domiciliary or equivalent environment (e.g., Alzheimer's facility)	Home health agency	Patient not present	15–29 min.
99375	Supervision of a patient requiring complex and multidisciplinary care modalities involving regular development and/or revision of care plans by that individual, review of subsequent reports of patient status, review of laboratory and other studies, communication (including telephone calls) for purposes of assessment or care decisions with healthcare professionals, family member(s), surrogate decision maker(s) (e.g., legal guardians) and/or key caregivers involved in the patient's care, integration of new information into the medical treatment plan and/or adjustment of medical therapy, within a calendar month	In home, a domiciliary or equivalent environment (e.g., Alzheimer's facility)	Home health agency	Patient not present	30 min. or more
99377	Supervision of a patient requiring complex and multidisciplinary care modalities involving regular development and/or revision of care plans by that individual, review of subsequent reports of patient status, review of laboratory and other studies, communication (including telephone calls) for purposes of assessment or care decisions with healthcare professionals, family member(s), surrogate decision maker(s) (e.g., legal guardians) and/or key caregivers involved in the patient's care, integration of new information into the medical treatment plan and/or adjustment of medical therapy, within a calendar month	Hospice	Hospice	Patient not present	15–29 min.
99378	Supervision of a patient requiring complex and multidisciplinary care modalities involving regular development and/or revision of care plans by that individual, review of subsequent reports of patient status, review of laboratory and other studies, communication (including telephone calls) for purposes of assessment or care decisions with healthcare professionals, family member(s), surrogate decision maker(s) (e.g., legal guardians) and/or key caregivers involved in the patient's care, integration of new information into the medical treatment plan and/or adjustment of medical therapy, within a calendar month	Hospice	Hospice	Patient not present	30 min. or more

E/M Code	Intent of Service	Place of Service	Under Care of	Presence of Patient	Time
99379	Supervision of a patient requiring complex and multidisciplinary care modalities involving regular development and/or revision of care plans by that individual, review of subsequent reports of patient status, review of laboratory and other studies, communication (including telephone calls) for purposes of assessment or care decisions with healthcare professionals, family member(s), surrogate decision maker(s) (e.g., legal guardians) and/or key caregivers involved in the patient's care, integration of new information into the medical treatment plan and/or adjustment of medical therapy, within a calendar month	Nursing facility	Nursing facility	Patient not present	15–29 min.
99380	Supervision of a patient requiring complex and multidisciplinary care modalities involving regular development and/or revision of care plans by that individual, review of subsequent reports of patient status, review of laboratory and other studies, communication (including telephone calls) for purposes of assessment or care decisions with healthcare professionals, family member(s), surrogate decision maker(s) (e.g., legal guardians) and/or key caregivers involved in the patient's care, integration of new information into the medical treatment plan and/or adjustment of medical therapy, within a calendar month	Nursing facility	Nursing facility	Patient not present	30 min. or more

GENERAL GUIDELINES

Care Plan Oversight Services

- Care plan oversight (CPO) is physician, or other qualified healthcare provider, supervision of patients receiving either home health or hospice benefits where complex or multidisciplinary care modalities and the ongoing provider involvement are required.
- CMS extended Medicare coverage to allow separate payment for CPO services exceeding 30 minutes per month for patients who are receiving Medicare-covered home health or hospice benefits.
- Medicare does not pay for CPO services for nursing facility or skilled nursing facility patients.
- Code descriptors for these codes include communication with family member(s), surrogate decision maker(s) (e.g., legal guardians) and/or key caregivers as well as healthcare professionals. This broader definition is more consistent with current practice.
- These codes are reported separately from other E/M services.
- Total time for services provided within a 30-day period determine the code selection.
- Only one provider, per month, will be paid for CPO services for a patient .
- Care plan oversight for domiciliary, rest home (e.g., assisted living facility), or home care plan oversight services are reported with CPT® codes 99339–99340.

 QUICK TIP

Providers must include their own documentation and may not rely on the orders or chart notes of the care giver to support care plan oversight. Each contact should be documented and include date, contact, orders given or changed, and time spent providing the remote care of the patient.

CODING AXIOM

The following are activities that count toward the requirement for care plan oversight:

- Development or revision of care plans
- Review of subsequent charts, reports, treatment plans, or lab or study results
- Integration of new information into the treatment plan and/or therapy adjustment
- Communication with other healthcare professionals (not employed in the same practice) involved in the care of the patient

CODING AXIOM

Services that do not count towards the requirement for care plan oversight:

- Time spent discussing treatment and medication adjustments with the patient, his or her family, or friends
- Time spent by staff getting or filing charts
- Travel time
- Provider time spent calling prescriptions into the pharmacist unless the telephone conversation involves a discussion of pharmaceutical therapies

The following coverage requirements apply to CPO services:

- The patient must require complex or multidisciplinary care modalities requiring ongoing provider involvement in the plan of care
- The patient must be receiving Medicare covered home health or hospice services during the period in which the CPO services are furnished
- The provider who bills CPO must be the same individual who signed the home health or hospice plan of care
- The provider must have furnished a covered service that required face-to-face encounter with the patient within the six months immediately preceding the provision of the first CPO plan oversight service within that calendar month
- The provider must furnish at least 15 minutes of CPO within the calendar month for which payment is claimed and no other provider has been paid for CPO within that calendar month
- The CPO billed must not be routine postoperative care provided in the global surgical period of a surgical procedure billed by the provider
- For patients receiving Medicare-covered home health services, the provider must not have a significant financial or contractual interest in the home health agency (HHA)
- For patients receiving Medicare hospice services, the provider must not be the medical director or an employee of the hospice or providing services under arrangements with the hospice
- CPO services must personally be furnished by the provider who bills them
- Services provided "incident-to" a physician's service do not qualify as CPO and do not count toward the time requirement for CPO
- The provider may not bill CPO during the same calendar month in which he or she bills the Medicare monthly capitation payment (end-stage renal disease benefit) for the same patient
- The provider billing for the CPO must document in the patient's medical record those services that were furnished, as well as the date and length of time associated with those services

Inherent in the CPO concept is the expectation that the provider has coordinated some aspect of the patient's care with the home health agency or hospice during the month for which CPO services are billed. It is required that the provider who bills for CPO must be the same individual who signs the plan of care. As previously stated, only one provider, per month, will be paid for CPO for a patient. Other providers working with the individual who signed the plan of care are not permitted to bill for these services.

Sample Documentation

Meets Expected Requirements:

The managing physician documents all time spent over the past 30 days to supervise the care plan for the patient. The content and time spent on each phone call and conference as well as any test results, consultant reports, review of old records, etc., is documented. The managing physician documents the review of patient status reports and care plans, pertinent findings and the time spent. Documentation describes phone calls involving active management of a problem over the phone after hours, and telephone communication with a pharmacy, the outside reference lab, the patient's physical therapist, social worker, home care provider and consulting physicians. Documentation also indicates the time spent discussing and giving direction to office staff who interact with the patient and family in the patient's care. Total time spent over the past 30 days is calculated and noted in the documentation.

Does NOT Meet Expected Requirements:

The managing physician documents the date and time spent over the past 30 days to supervise the care plan for the patient, however, the content such as discussion of test results and pertinent time is not documented.

Guidelines for Nonphysician Practitioners

According to provisions of the Balanced Budget Act of 1997, nonphysician practitioners (NPP), nurse practitioners (NP), physician assistants (PA), and clinical nurse specialists (CNS) may bill for care plan oversight services as long as they are practicing within the scope of state law. These practitioners must be providing ongoing care through evaluation and management services. Although NPPs are not permitted to certify a patient for home healthcare services, NPPs can provide care plan oversight services only when the physician that signs the plan of care provides regular ongoing care under the same plan of care as the NPP billing for care plan oversight and either:

- The physician and NPP are part of the same group practice
- If the NPP is an NP or a CNS, the physician that signs the plan of care must also have a collaborative agreement with the NPP
- If the NPP is a PA, the physician signing the plan of care also provides general supervision of PA services for the practice

Billing may be made for care plan oversight services provided by an NPP when:

- The NPP providing care plan oversight services has seen and examined the patient
- The NPP providing care plan oversight services is not acting as a consultant with his or her participation limited to a single medical condition rather than multidisciplinary coordination of care
- The NPP providing care plan oversight services combines the care he or she provides with that provided by the physician who signed the plan of care

The attending physician or the nurse practitioner designated as the attending physician may bill for hospice CPO when they are acting in the capacity of an attending physician. An attending physician is defined as the one identified by an individual, at the time he or she elects hospice coverage, as having the most significant role in the determination and delivery of their medical care. Attending physicians are not employed or paid by the hospice.

QUICK TIP

Care plan oversight services documentation should describe the care plan oversight services furnished, the dates and exact duration of time spent on these services

QUICK TIP

Codes 99339 and 99340 for care plan oversight services provided to a patient in a home, domiciliary or rest home, including assisted living facilities, are noncovered Medicare services.

CODING AXIOM

No other service may be billed on the claim with CPO services. CPO should not be billed until after the end of the month in which the service is performed. Be sure the ICD-10-CM code is reported with the highest level of specificity and that the code used specifically identifies the reason for the service.

Special Instructions for CPO Services

Codes 99374–99378 are not covered under Medicare. For these services and for reporting physician certification and recertification for Medicare covered home health services, refer to "Chapter 17: HCPCS G Codes and Evaluation and Management Services."

Preventive Medicine Services (99381–99429)

QUICK COMPARISON

Preventive Medicine Services—New Patient

E/M Code	Patient Status	Age	History	Exam	Medical Decision Making[1]
99381	No complaints	Under 1 year	Age and gender appropriate	Age and gender appropriate	Ordering lab/diagnostic procedures
99382	No complaints	1–4 years	Age and gender appropriate	Age and gender appropriate	Ordering lab/diagnostic procedures
99383	No complaints	5–11 years	Age and gender appropriate	Age and gender appropriate	Ordering lab/diagnostic procedures
99384	No complaints	12–17 years	Age and gender appropriate	Age and gender appropriate	Ordering lab/diagnostic procedures
99385	No complaints	18–39 years	Age and gender appropriate	Age and gender appropriate	Ordering lab/diagnostic procedures
99386	No complaints	40–64 years	Age and gender appropriate	Age and gender appropriate	Ordering lab/diagnostic procedures
99387	No complaints	65 and over	Age and gender appropriate	Age and gender appropriate	Ordering lab/diagnostic procedures

1   Includes age appropriate immunizations, laboratory/diagnostic procedures and age appropriate counseling/anticipatory guidance and risk factor reduction intervention(s).

Preventive Medicine Services—Established Patient

E/M Code	Patient Status	Age	History	Exam	Medical Decision Making[1]
99391	No complaints	Under 1 year	Age and gender appropriate	Age and gender appropriate	Ordering lab/diagnostic procedures
99392	No complaints	1–4 years	Age and gender appropriate	Age and gender appropriate	Ordering lab/diagnostic procedures
99393	No complaints	5–11 years	Age and gender appropriate	Age and gender appropriate	Ordering lab/diagnostic procedures
99394	No complaints	12–17 years	Age and gender appropriate	Age and gender appropriate	Ordering lab/diagnostic procedures
99395	No complaints	18–39 years	Age and gender appropriate	Age and gender appropriate	Ordering lab/diagnostic procedures
99396	No complaints	40–64 years	Age and gender appropriate	Age and gender appropriate	Ordering lab/diagnostic procedures
99397	No complaints	65 and over	Age and gender appropriate	Age and gender appropriate	Ordering lab/diagnostic procedures

1   Includes age appropriate immunizations, laboratory/diagnostic procedures, and age appropriate counseling/anticipatory guidance and risk factor reduction intervention(s).

Preventive Medicine Services—Counseling and/or Risk Factor Reduction Intervention

E/M Code	Patient Status	Intent of Service	Time
Individual Counseling			
99401	No complaints	Promote health, prevent illness or injury	15 min.
99402	No complaints	Promote health, prevent illness or injury	30 min.
99403	No complaints	Promote health, prevent illness or injury	45 min.
99404	No complaints	Promote health, prevent illness or injury	60 min.
Behavior Change Interventions, Individual			
99406	Smoking or tobacco history	Promote health, smoking or tobacco cessation counseling	3–10 min.
99407	Smoking or tobacco history	Promote health, smoking or tobacco cessation counseling	> 10 min.
99408	Alcohol or substance screening	Promote health, alcohol or substance abuse screening with brief intervention	15–30 min.
99409	Alcohol or substance screening	Promote health, alcohol or substance abuse screening with brief intervention	> 30 min.
Group Counseling			
99411	No complaints	Promote health	30 min.
99412	No complaints	Promote health	60 min.
Other Preventive Medicine Services			
99429		Unlisted preventive medicine service	

KEY POINT

When a separate E/M service is reported with preventive medicine services, only the documentation specific to the separate problem may be considered when determining a separate E/M code. Usually, the additional E/M service is a low-level service as all other documentation is usually part of the comprehensive history and exam required for preventive medicine services.

GENERAL GUIDELINES

- Select a code from the preventive medicine services category based on whether the patient is new or established, and the age of the patient.

- Report the appropriate problem-oriented E/M code (e.g., 99202–99215) if a significant problem is encountered or a pre-existing problem is addressed and requires additional work during the course of the preventive medicine E/M service. Do not report a problem-oriented E/M code if a problem is encountered during the preventive medicine service but does not require additional work.

- Append modifier 25 to report that a separately identifiable E/M service was performed by the same physician/qualified healthcare professional on the same day as a procedure or service. Only the content of work associated with the separate E/M service should be considered when assigning the correct E/M code.

- Assign only the appropriate preventive medicine service code when E/M service and preventive medicine counseling is provided during the same visit.

- Report the appropriate code from the subcategory for counseling and/or risk factor reduction intervention when this service is provided at an encounter separate from the preventive medicine examination (codes 99401–99404).

- Report the appropriate code from the subcategory behavior change interventions, individual (99406–99409), when the behavior itself is considered an illness and specific interventions are suggested as part of the treatment of the condition related to the behavior, or to change the behavior before it results in an illness. These behaviors include; tobacco addiction, substance abuse, or obesity.

- For codes 99406–99409, append modifier 95 to indicate that the E/M service was rendered to a patient at a distant site via a real-time interactive audio and video telecommunications system. The communication between the physician or other qualified healthcare professional and the patient should be commensurate with the same key components or requirements of those that would be required if the service had been rendered in a face-to-face setting.

- Use code 99078 when reporting group counseling of patients with symptoms or established illnesses.

- Report separately the codes for the diagnostic tests or studies performed, including screening tests identified by specific CPT codes.

- Immunizations and administrations identified by a separate CPT code are reported separately and part of the preventive medicine service.

ISSUES IN THIS CODE RANGE

- Although these codes were never the subject of specific documentation criteria from CMS (likely because they are not covered)—compliance auditors have long sought to ensure that these services were appropriately documented when performed. The definitions of comprehensive history and physical exam are not the same as for other E/M services.

- The CPT book indicates that the history and exam for preventive medicine services should be "age and gender appropriate."

- Check with other commercial or third-party payers to see if there is a protocol or method of reporting combined services of this nature. Many carriers will not pay for two such services on the same day, or their computer systems will routinely deny one of the codes. Bring the situation to their attention.

- Medicare does not cover preventive medicine visits listed in this section.

- However, beginning in 2005, Medicare has offered and covered an initial preventive physical examination (IPPE) also commonly referred to as the welcome to Medicare examination. The IPPE is not a "routine physical checkup"; rather, the IPPE is more of an introduction to Medicare and enables new Medicare beneficiaries to receive important screenings and vaccinations. It also allows the providers to evaluate and review the patient's health. CMS also offers an annual wellness visit (AWV), which is an annual appointment for beneficiaries to discuss a plan for preventive care for the year ahead. While it is similar to the one-time only IPPE, the AWV is not a complete "head-to-toe" physical examination and the beneficiary cannot have an AWV during the first year of enrollment in the Medicare Program OR during the same year as an IPPE. There are also specific criteria associated with the AWV. **Note:** The IPPE and AWV services are represented with HCPCS Level II G codes and are further discussed in "Chapter 17: G Codes and Evaluation and Management Services."

QUICK TIP

These codes should be used to report counseling and risk factor reduction. Codes 96150–96155 are used to report health and behavior assessment and intervention for psychological, behavioral, emotional, cognitive, and social factors affecting health status.

QUICK TIP

Pediatric practitioners may follow *Recommendations for Preventive Pediatric Healthcare/Bright Futures/American Academy of Pediatrics* when rendering preventive care services to their patients. For more information on the guidance and pocket guide, visit: https://brightfutures.aap.org/materials-and-tools/guidelines-and-pocket-guide/Pages/default.aspx.

Non-Face-to-Face Physician Services (99441–99443, 99421–99423)

QUICK COMPARISON

Telephone Services (99441–99443)

E/M Code	Intent of Service	Type of Communication	Time
99441	E/M service at the request of established patient or care giver	Telephone	5–10 min
99442	E/M service at the request of established patient or care giver	Telephone	11–20 min.
99443	E/M service at the request of established patient or care giver	Telephone	21–30 min.

KEY POINT

For additional guidance on the use of these codes during the public health emergency due to COVID-19, go to https://www.cms.gov/files/document/03092020-covid-19-faqs-508.pdf.

GENERAL GUIDELINES

- Care must be initiated by patient or guardian of an established patient.
- The service cannot be reported if related E/M service has been provided in the prior seven days.
- The service cannot be reported if the provider sees the patient within 24 hours or soonest available appointment.
- The service cannot be reported if it falls within the postoperative period of a previously performed procedure, even if more than seven days.
- Telephone call code selection is based upon time of medical discussion, not including the time to document the service provided.
- Non-face-to-face nonphysician services are reported with codes 98966–98969.
- These services are not reportable when performed concurrently with other billable services, such as anticoagulation management.
- When home and outpatient INR monitoring is evaluated during a telephone do not report 93792 or 93793 separately.

QUICK COMPARISON

Online Digital Evaluation and Management Services (99421-99423)

E/M Code	Intent of Service	Type of Communication	Time
99421	Online E/M service at the request of established patient	Online digital	5–10 min.
99422	Online E/M service at the request of established patient	Online digital	11–20 min.
99423	Online E/M service at the request of established patient	Online digital	At least 21 min.

GENERAL GUIDELINES

- Care must be initiated through a HIPAA compliant platform by an established patient.
- The service cannot be reported if a related E/M service has been provided in the prior seven days.
- These services are for cumulative time over a seven-day period and include initial inquiry, records review, physician interaction with clinical staff regarding the patient's problem, development of management plans, generation of prescriptions, ordering tests, and subsequent communication with the patient online, via telephone, email, or other supported digital communication.
- Do not report cumulative services of less than five minutes.
- The service cannot be reported if it falls within the postoperative period of a previously performed procedure, even if more than seven days.
- Online digital E/M services require permanent storage of documentation (electronic or hard copy) of the encounter.
- When a separately reportable E/M service occurs within seven days of initiation of the online service, the work devoted to the online service is counted into the separately reportable E/M service.
- Online digital E/M services performed by nonphysician providers are reported with 98970–98972.
- These services are not reportable when performed concurrently with other billable services, such as anticoagulation management.
- When home and outpatient INR monitoring is evaluated during an online encounter, do not report these codes separately.

Interprofessional Telephone/Internet/Electronic Health Record Consultations (99446–99452)

Quick Comparison

Telephone, Internet or Electronic Health Record Consultations

E/M Code	Intent of Service	Time Spent
99446	Consultation, including verbal and written report, at the request of another provider via the telephone, internet, or EHR	5–10 min
99447	Consultation, including verbal and written report, at the request of another provider via the telephone, internet, or EHR	11–20 min.
99448	Consultation, including verbal and written report, at the request of another provider via the telephone, internet, or EHR	21–30 min.
99449	Consultation, including verbal and written report, at the request of another provider via the telephone, internet, or EHR	31 min. or more
99451	Consultation, including written report, at the request of another provider via the telephone, internet, or EHR	5 min. or more
99452	Interprofessional telephone, internet, or electronic health record referral services provided by a requesting or treating provider	30 min.

General Guidelines

In urgent or complex situations, an interprofessional telephone, internet, or electronic health record consultation (99446–99451) may be performed.

- Four levels, including a verbal and written report, are available depending on the time spent; time must be documented.
- Use code 99451 for consultation services of 5 minutes or more that include only a written report.
- In these consultations, a physician or other qualified healthcare provider requests an opinion from another provider who may have a specific specialty expertise.
- These codes do not require a face-to-face visit with the patient because the sole purpose is to help the treating physician diagnose or manage the patient's problem.
- As with other consultation codes, the verbal or written request and reason for the request must be documented in the patient chart. In addition, to report 99446–99449 the consultant must give a verbal opinion and written report back to the requesting provider. For 99451 only a written report is required.
- Additional time required to complete the consultation should be reported by adding together each segment of time spent in providing the service with the cumulative total used to determine the correct code assignment.
- The majority of time reported must be devoted to the verbal/internet discussion.
- Do not report 99446–99449 if more than 50 percent of the service time is spent reviewing and analyzing data.

- Do not report these services more than once within a seven-day interval.
- There is no designation between new or established patient.
- These services include the review of records pertinent to the diagnosis in question, laboratory/pathology studies, radiology studies, and medication profile via mail or fax prior to the consultation.
- It is inappropriate for the consultant to report these codes if the patient has been seen 14 days prior to the consult or the consult leads to a transfer of the patient's care or other face-to-face service within 14 days.
- It is inappropriate for the consultant to report this service if it is less than 5 minutes.
- The physician consultant may report non-face-to-face direct communication with the patient and/or family via telephone or by way of an online medical evaluation with codes 99441–99444; for non-face-to-face, nonphysician services, see codes 98966–98969. Note: This time would not be included in the time spent providing the consultation with the requesting provider as reported with codes 99446–99451.
- When the consultation leads to an immediate transfer of patient care (e.g., surgery, hospital visit, scheduled face to face examination of the patient, etc), to the consulting provider within the next 14-day period, do not report these codes.
- Interprofessional telephone, internet, or electronic health record referral services provided by a requesting or treating provider (99452):
  - May be reported when 16 to 30 minutes is spent arranging a referral and/or communicating with the consultant.
  - Can only be reported once in a 14-day period.
- In addition, if consultation exceeds 30 minutes beyond the typical time of the E/M service and the patient is physically present and available to the *requesting provider*, the provider may report prolonged services (99354–99357) for his/her time spent while on the telephone or internet with the consulting provider. If the patient is not present, the requesting provider may report non-face-to-face prolonged services (99358–99359).

Digitally Stored Data Services/Remote Physiologic Monitoring and Physiologic Monitoring Treatment Services (99453–99454, 99091, 99473–99474, 99457–99458)

QUICK COMPARISON

Digitally Stored Data Services/Remote Physiologic Monitoring and Treatment Services

E/M Code	Intent of Service	Face-to-Face Visit	Time Spent
99453	Setup and patient education on the use of remote monitoring equipment used by the patient that collects, monitors, and reports health-related data (e.g., weight, blood pressure, pulse oximetry) to the provider	No	N/A
99454	Daily recordings or program alert transmissions via the remote monitoring device, for each 30-day period	No	N/A
99091	Collection and interpretation of health-related data gathered via a remote patient monitoring system used to manage physiologic data (e.g., blood pressure, glucose), including education and training	No	At least 30 min.
99473	Patient education/training and device calibration for the patient to self-measure their blood pressure	Yes	N/A
99474	Collection of data reported to the provider of average systolic and diastolic pressures over a 30-day period (minimum of 12 readings) with subsequent treatment plan provided to the patient	No	N/A
99457	Remote patient monitoring by the provider/clinical staff utilizing data from an FDA-defined remote monitoring system to oversee the patient's treatment plan	No. Does require interactive communication with the patient	At least 20 min.
99458	Remote patient monitoring by the provider/clinical staff utilizing data from an FDA-defined remote monitoring system to oversee the patient's treatment plan	No. Does require interactive communication with the patient	Each additional 20 min.

GENERAL GUIDELINES

- Codes 99453, 99454, 99091, and 99457 are provided and reported once for each 30-day period. Code 99474 should be reported no more than once per calendar month.
- To report remote physiological monitoring, the device used must be a medical device as defined by the FDA.
- Services must be ordered by a physician or other qualified healthcare professional.
- Do not report 99453 or 99454 for monitoring services of less than 16 days.
- Time spent monitoring a more specific physiological condition, such as continuous glucose monitoring (95250), should not be included in time counted towards reporting 99453 or 99454.

- Do not report 99453 or 99454 in addition to codes for more specific physiologic conditions, such as 93296 (remote device monitoring of a pacemaker system).
- Report 99453 only once per episode of care.
- When the patient is seen for another E/M service, services provided in 99091 are included in that E/M service and should not be reported separately.
- Do not report 99091 in addition to 99339–99340, 99374–99380, 99457, or 99491 in the same calendar month.
- Report 99473 only once per device.
- Code 99457 requires live, interactive communication with the patient or caregiver and a minimum of 20 minutes of provider or staff time within a calendar month; report 99458 for each additional completed 20 minutes.
- Do not report remote physiologic monitoring treatment services (99457) of less than 20 minutes.
- Codes 99457 and 99458 may be reported in addition to 99439, 99487–99491, 99495, 99496, 99484, and 99492–99494, when performed during the same reporting period. However, time spent performing those services should not be included in the time used to count toward 99457 and 99458.
- Only report 99457 and 99458 when requirements for a more specific treatment management service have not been met.
- Do not count the time toward 99457 or 99458 on days when other separate and distinct services are provided, including: 99202–99215, 99324–99328, 99334–99337, 99341–99350, 99221–99233, and 99251–99255.
- Do not report 99457 in addition to 93264 or 99091 or in the same month as 99473 or 99474.

Special Evaluation and Management Services (99450–99456)

Quick Comparison

Special Evaluation and Management Services

E/M Code	Intent of Service	Specific Data Provided
99450	Evaluation of patient prior to or after issuance of basic life policy or for determination of disability	Vital statistics, including blood pressure, height, weight Medical history completed as identified on life insurance pro forma Urine and blood samples collected and "chain of custody" protocols Complete documentation and certificates according to requester
99455	Evaluation of patient by treating physician for work related or medical disability examination	Medical history, including record review, completed as appropriate with patient condition. Examination appropriate to the patient condition and disability(ies) Identification of the diagnosis Assessment of patient stability, capabilities, and impairment calculation according to accepted guidelines (state or AMA impairment guidelines) Future treatment identified or developed Complete documentation, certificates and reports according to requester specifics
99456	Evaluation of patient by non treating physician for work-related or medical disability examination	Medical history, including record, review, completed as appropriate with patient condition Examination appropriate to the patient condition and disability(ies) Identification of the diagnosis Assessment of patient stability, capabilities, and impairment calculation according to accepted guidelines (state or AMA impairment guidelines) Future treatment identified or developed Complete documentation, certificates, and reports according to requester specifics

 Quick Tip

Work-related or medical disability evaluation may require review of prior medical records to determine any pre-existing conditions when calculating disability.

General Guidelines

- Select a code to report the evaluation of a patient and completion of the special forms based upon basic life/disability evaluation or work-related/medical disability evaluation.
- Report the appropriate problem-oriented E/M code (e.g., 99202–99215) if provided separate from the special evaluation. Do not report a problem-oriented E/M code if a problem is encountered during the service but does not require additional work.
- Append modifier 25 to report that a separately identifiable E/M service was performed by the same physician/qualified healthcare professional on the same day as a procedure or service. Only the content of work associated with the separate E/M service should be considered when assigning the correct E/M code.

- Report separately the codes for diagnostic tests or studies performed, including screening tests, identified by specific CPT codes.
- Work-related or medical disability evaluation services are selected based upon the provider being the treating or non treating physician.
- Codes 99455–99456 should **NOT** be reported with code 99080 Special reports such as insurance forms, or for completing workmens' compensation forms.

ISSUES IN THIS CODE RANGE

- These services are not usually covered by government payers.
- Basic life and disability evaluation may be requested as a screening tool by special insurers (e.g., life, disability, long term care).
- Work-related or medical disability evaluations may be requested by workers' compensation carrier, state, or federal disability determination services.
- It is not appropriate to report a special report (99080) with these services.
- Special coverage of these services may require coordination with the requester prior to the services being rendered.
- Impairment guidelines are specified in state workers' compensation statute and may use the AMA impairment guidelines or state developed guidelines.

QUICK TIP

Calculation of disability for some state workers' compensation carriers is based on state specific guidelines and others use the AMA impairment guidelines.

KNOWLEDGE ASSESSMENT CHAPTER 12

See chapter 19 for answers and rationale.

1. How many healthcare professionals of different specialties must participate in order to bill for a medical team conference (99366–99368)?
   a. Two or more
   b. Four or more
   c. More than 10
   d. Three or more

2. Which of the following activities would not count toward total time when billing for care plan oversight services?
   a. Adding new information to the treatment plan
   b. Discussing treatment adjustments with the patient or a caregiver
   c. Revisions to the plan of care
   d. Reviewing treatment plans and lab results

3. What is the appropriate code for a well-visit/preventive service provided to a 20-year-old established patient?
   a. 99215
   b. 99385
   c. 99395
   d. 99396

4. To bill telephone services (99441–99443), the following guidelines must be met. (Select all that apply.)
   a. The service cannot be within the postoperative period of a previous procedure
   b. The service cannot result in the decision to see the patient within 24 hours or the next available appointment
   c. The service must be initiated by an established patient or his or her guardian
   d. All of the above

Chapter 13: Newborn and Pediatric Services (99460–99486)

Newborn Care Services (99460–99465)

QUICK COMPARISON

Newborn Care Services and Delivery/Birthing Room Attendance and Resuscitation Services

E/M Code	Patient Status	Site of Care	Intent of Service
99460	Normal newborn	Hospital or birthing room	Perform history and physical exam; initiate diagnostic and treatment programs; prepare records
99461	Normal newborn	Other than hospital or birthing room	Perform physical examination; confer with parents
99462	Normal newborn	Hospital	Provide E/M subsequent care service per day
99463	Normal newborn	Hospital or birthing room	Perform history and exam; prepare medical records. Use this code for newborns assessed and discharged on the same date
99464	Unstable newborn	Hospital or birthing room	Initial stabilization of newborn when requested by delivering physician
99465	High-risk newborn at delivery	Hospital or birthing room	Provide inhalation therapy, aspirate, administer medication for stabilization

GENERAL GUIDELINES

- These services are reported for the care of newborns in a variety of settings.
- Newborns are defined as birth through 28 days of age.
- Normal newborn services are to be used to report services to care of the newborn in the first days after birth.
- Review codes to determine the correct code based upon place of service.
- The provider should appropriately document newborn status and care required for unstable newborns and high-risk newborn infants.
- Initial stabilization codes may be reported the same date as initial evaluation of infant admitted to critical care.
- See codes 99468–99469 and 99477–99480 for newborns requiring additional care and supervision
- For newborns seen for follow-up in the office or outpatient setting following discharge, refer to 99202–99215, 99381, or 99391.

ISSUES IN THIS CODE RANGE

- Newborns admitted and discharged in the hospital or birthing center on the same date should be reported with code 99463.
- Newborn care spanning more than one day should be reported with the appropriate codes, even if the patient was discharged before he or she was 24 hours old.
- Circumcision and other procedures are reported in addition to the admission and evaluation of the newborn.

Pediatric Critical Care Patient Transport (99466–99467 and 99485–99486)

QUICK COMPARISON

E/M Code	Patient Status	Site of Care	Intent of Service
99466	Critically ill or critically injured, under 24 months	Constant during transport	First 30–74 min.
99467	Critically ill or critically injured, under 24 months	Constant during transport	Each additional 30 minutes beyond the first 74 min.
99485	Critically ill or critically injured, under 24 months	Two-way communication	First 16–45 min.
99486	Critically ill or critically injured, under 24 months	Two-way communication	Each additional 30 min.

GENERAL GUIDELINES

- Assign the appropriate outpatient visit or subsequent hospital care code if critical care services took less than 30 minutes on a given day.
- Record in the patient's record the time spent with the patient and the service provided.
- A critical illness or injury acutely impairs one or more vital organ systems such that there is a high probability of imminent or life-threatening deterioration in the patient's condition.
- Critical care involves high-complexity decision making to assess, manipulate, and support vital system functions to treat single or multiple vital organ system failure and/or to prevent further life-threatening deterioration of the patient's condition.
- Examples of vital organ system failure include but are not limited to central nervous system failure, circulatory failure, shock, and renal, hepatic, metabolic, and/or respiratory failure. Although critical care typically requires interpretation of multiple physiologic parameters and/or application of advanced technologies, critical care may be provided in life-threatening situations when these elements are not present.
- Codes 99466 and 99467 represent physician attendance for a critically ill or injured pediatric patient (less than 24 months of age) being transported to or from a facility or hospital. Codes 99291 and 99292 should be used for physician attendance during a transport of a critically ill patient older than 24 months.
- For total body and selective head cooling of neonates, use 99184.
- The first hour of critical care transport can be reported only once per day. Assign the correct code for critical care provided to a hospital inpatient according to the following guidelines:
  - less than 30 minutes assign appropriate E/M code
  - 30–74 minutes 99466 x 1
  - 75–104 minutes 99466 x 1 and 99467 x 1
  - 105–134 minutes 99466 x 1 and 99467 x 2

- 135–164 minutes 99466 x 1 and 99467 x 3
- 165–194 minutes 99466 x 1 and 99467 x 4

Codes 99485–99486 represent the physician's role in interfacility transport of a critically ill or injured patient, (less than 24 months of age). These codes are for non-face-to-face contact; the physician is directing the transport services during an interfacility transport. The control physician uses a two-way radio to communicate treatment advice to the transport team providing the patient care. The first hour of critical care transport can be reported only once per day. Assign the correct code for critical care provided to a hospital inpatient according to the following guidelines:

- less than 15 minutes assign appropriate E/M code
- 16–45 minutes 99485 x 1
- 46–75 minutes 99485 x 1 and 99486 x 1
- 76–105 minutes 99485 x 1 and 99486 x 2
- 106–135 minutes 99485 x 1 and 99486 x 3
- 136–165 minutes 99485 x 1 and 99486 x 4

There are no absolute limits on the amount of critical care transport time that can be reported per day or hospital stay as long as the medical records can support the need for all critical care services provided. However, time spent performing separately reportable procedures or services should not be included in the time reported as critical care transport time. The following services should not be reported separately when performed during the transport of a critical care pediatric patient:

36000	Introduction of needle or intracath, vein
36400	Venipuncture, younger than age 3 years, necessitating physician's skill, not to be used for routine venipuncture; femoral or jugular vein
36405	Venipuncture, younger than age 3 years, necessitating physician's skill, not to be used for routine venipuncture; scalp vein
36406	Venipuncture, younger than age 3 years, necessitating physician's skill, not to be used for routine venipuncture; other vein
36415	Venipuncture
36591	Collection of blood specimen from a completely implantable venous access device
36600	Arterial puncture
43752	Naso- or oro-gastric tube placement, necessitating physician's skill
43753	Therapeutic gastric intubation and aspiration(s), necessitating physician's skill
71045	Radiologic examination, chest; single view
71046	Radiologic examination, chest; 2 views
92953	Temporary transcutaneous pacing
93562	Indicator dilution studies, subsequent measurements
94002	Ventilation assist and management, initiation of pressure or volume preset ventilators for assisted or controlled breathing; hospital inpatient/observation, initial day

94003	Ventilation assist and management, initiation of pressure or volume preset ventilators for assisted or controlled breathing; hospital inpatient/observation, each subsequent day
94660	Continuous positive airway pressure ventilation (CPAP) initiation and management
94662	Continuous negative pressure ventilation initiation and management
94760	Noninvasive ear or pulse oximetry for oxygen saturation; single determination
94761	Noninvasive ear or pulse oximetry for oxygen saturation; multiple determinations (e.g., during exercise)
94762	Noninvasive ear or pulse oximetry for oxygen saturation; by continuous overnight monitoring (separate procedure)

Inpatient Neonatal and Pediatric Critical Care (99468–99476)

QUICK COMPARISON

E/M Code	Patient Status	Type of Visit
99468	Critically ill neonate, aged 28 days or less	Initial inpatient
99469	Critically ill neonate, aged 28 days or less	Subsequent inpatient
99471	Critically ill infant or young child, aged 29 days to 24 months	Initial inpatient
99472	Critically ill infant or young child, aged 29 days to 24 months	Subsequent inpatient
99475	Critically ill infant or young child, two to five years	Initial inpatient
99476	Critically ill infant or young child, two to five years	Subsequent inpatient

GENERAL GUIDELINES

- The same definitions for critical care services apply, regardless of the age of the patient. See "General Guidelines" for codes 99291–99292 for additional information. Note that codes 99291–99292 should not be reported by the same provider or different provider of the same specialty and group when neonatal or pediatric critical care services are reported for the same patient on the same date of service; however, these codes may be reported when the services are reported by a provider of a different specialty whether that provider is part of the same group or not, on the same date of service as neonatal or pediatric critical care services were reported.

- Critical care face-to-face transport or supervisory services may be reported by the same or different provider on the same date of service as neonatal or pediatric critical care services are reported for the same patient.

- Critical care services provided to a pediatric patient who is six years of age or older are reported using the time-based, critical care codes 99291–99292.

- Unlike the adult critical care codes, these codes are not measured in time but by day. Report "initial" care for the first day of services and "subsequent" care for the following day or days.

- Codes 99468–99476 include the following management, monitoring, and treatment services, which cannot be billed separately:
  - respiratory
  - pharmacologic control of the circulatory system
  - enteral and parenteral nutrition
  - metabolic and hematologic maintenance
  - parent/family counseling
  - case management services

- Codes 99468 and 99469 are used to represent care starting with the date of admission (99468) to a critical care unit and subsequent day(s) (99469) that the neonate or infant remains critical. They may only be reported by one physician and only once per day, per patient.

 KEY POINT

Use 99184 to report selective head or total body hypothermia in critically ill neonates.

- If a neonate or infant is readmitted to the critical care unit during the same day or same stay, report the subsequent day code 99469 for the first day of readmission, and 99469 for each subsequent day following readmission.
- Codes 99471–99476 may only be reported by one physician and only once per day, per patient. If readmitted to the pediatric critical care unit during the same day or same stay, report the subsequent day code, 99472 or 99476, for the first day of readmission and for each subsequent day following readmission.
- Report codes 99468, 99471, and 99475 only once per hospital stay.
- Personal direct supervision of the healthcare team in the performance of cognitive and procedural activities.
- In addition to the services included in critical care codes 99291–99292, these codes include the following procedures:

31500	Intubation, endotracheal, emergency procedure
36000	Introduction of needle or intracatheter, vein
36140	Introduction of needle or intracatheter; extremity artery
36400	Venipuncture, younger than age 3 years, necessitating physician's skill, not to be used for routine venipuncture; femoral or jugular vein
36405	Venipuncture, younger than age 3 years, necessitating physician's skill, not to be used for routine venipuncture; scalp vein
36406	Venipuncture, younger than age 3 years, necessitating physician's skill, not to be used for routine venipuncture; other vein
36420	Venipuncture, cutdown; under age 1 year
36430	Transfusion, blood or blood components
36440	Push transfusion, blood, 2 years or under
36510	Catheterization of umbilical vein for diagnosis and therapy, newborn
36555	Insertion of non-tunneled centrally inserted central venous catheter; younger than 5 years of age
36600	Arterial puncture, withdrawal of blood for diagnosis
36620	Arterial catheterization or cannulation for sampling, monitoring, or transfusion; percutaneous
36660	Catheterization, umbilical artery, newborn, for diagnosis or therapy
43752	Naso or orogastric tube placement, necessitating physician's skill
51100	Aspiration of bladder by needle
51701	Insertion of non indwelling bladder catheter
51702	Insertion of temporary indwelling bladder catheter; simple
62270	Spinal puncture, lumbar, diagnostic
94002	Ventilation assist and management, initiation of pressure or volume preset ventilators for assisted or controlled breathing; hospital inpatient/observation, initial day
94003	Ventilation assist and management, initiation of pressure or volume preset ventilators for assisted or controlled breathing; hospital inpatient/observation, each subsequent day

94004	Ventilation assist and management, initiation of pressure or volume preset ventilators for assisted or controlled breathing; nursing facility, per day
94375	Respiratory flow volume loop
94610	Intrapulmonary surfactant administration by a physician through endotracheal tube
94660	Continuous positive airway pressure ventilation (CPAP), initiation and management
94760	Noninvasive ear or pulse oximetry for oxygen saturation; single determination
94761	Noninvasive ear or pulse oximetry for oxygen saturation; multiple determinations
94762	Noninvasive ear or pulse oximetry for oxygen saturation; by continuous overnight monitoring
94780	Car seat/bed testing for airway integrity, neonate, with continual nursing observation and continuous recording of pulse oximetry, heart rate and respiratory rate, with interpretation and report; 60 minutes
94781	each additional full 30 minutes (List separately in additional to code for primary procedure)

These services are considered bundled into codes 99468–99476 and are therefore not separately billable:

- Any services performed that are not shown in the above listings should be reported separately.
- Unlike codes 99291 and 99292, Medicare considers codes 99468–99476 as "inpatient only" codes, and no APC payment will be made for them in an outpatient setting.
- For initiation of selective head or total body hypothermia in a critically ill neonate, report 99184. Included services may be reported separately by the facility.

Initial and Continuing Intensive Care Services (99477–99480)

QUICK COMPARISON

E/M Code	Patient Status	Type of Visit
99477	Neonate, aged 28 days or less	Initial inpatient care for the neonate requiring intensive observation, frequent interventions, and other intensive care services who is not critically ill
99478	Infant with present body weight of less than 1500 grams, no longer critically ill	Subsequent inpatient
99479	Infant with present body weight of 1500 - 2500 grams, no longer critically ill	Subsequent inpatient
99480	Infant with present body weight of 2501-5000 grams, no longer critically ill	Subsequent inpatient

GENERAL GUIDELINES

- These services are not used to report the care of a normal newborn.
- These services are not used to report the care of a critically ill neonate.
- Inpatient care of a neonate not requiring intensive observation, interventions, or other services, weighing more than 5,000 grams, is reported with the inpatient treatment codes 99221–99233.
- Do not use 99477 to report services for an infant older than 28 days.
- Subsequent intensive care codes are reported based upon patient weight.
- These patients may require:
  - cardiac monitoring
  - respiratory monitoring
  - vital sign monitoring
  - heat maintenance
  - nutritional management
  - oxygen monitoring
  - laboratory evaluations
  - constant observations
- These codes include the same procedures that are listed under the critical codes (99291–99292) and the neonatal and pediatric inpatient critical care codes (99468–99476).

KNOWLEDGE ASSESSMENT CHAPTER 13

See chapter 19 for answers and rationale.

1. Patients from birth to 28 days of age are considered newborns when assigning codes 99460–99486.
    a. True
    b. False

2. What codes would be used to report physician attendance of a critically ill infant less than 24 months of age being transported to the hospital?
    a. 99485–99486
    b. 99466–99467
    c. 99291–99292
    d. None of the above

3. What codes are used to report critical care services of a 3-year-old patient?
    a. 99291 and 99292
    b. 99468 and 99469
    c. 99475 and 99476
    d. 99471 and 99472

4. Subsequent *intensive* critical care codes (99478–99480), are determined based on the patient's body weight.
    a. True
    b. False

5. What code is reported when a newborn is admitted and discharged in the hospital or birthing center on the same date of service?
    a. 99460
    b. 99461
    c. 99462
    d. 99463

6. Adult critical care codes are reported based on the amount of time spent with the patient. What factors determine which neonatal or pediatric critical care code is appropriate?
    a. Type of visit (initial or subsequent)
    b. Time
    c. Age
    d. a and c

Chapter 14: Care Plan and Care Management Services (99483–99494)

Cognitive Assessment and Care Plan Services (99483)

QUICK COMPARISON

Cognitive Assessment and Care Plan Services

E/M Code	Intent of Service	Face-to-Face Visit	Time Spent
99483	Assessment of and care planning for a patient with cognitive impairment, requiring an independent historian, in the office or other outpatient, home or domiciliary or rest home, with several required elements	Patient and/or family/caregiver	50 min. on average

GENERAL GUIDELINES

- These services are provided for new or existing patients that display signs of cognitive impairment that require a comprehensive assessment to determine a specific diagnosis, etiology, and severity of the impairment.
- All of the following elements must be performed in order to report this code.
  - cognition-focused evaluation that includes a relevant history and physical exam
  - medical decision making of moderate to high complexity
  - assessment of performance of activities of daily living, including decision-making capabilities
  - use of standardized tests (e.g., FAST, CDR) to determine the stage of dementia
  - medication reconciliation and review of high-risk medications
  - evaluation, including standardized tests, for neuropsychiatric and behavioral symptoms, such as depression
  - evaluation of patient safety in the home and operating a motor vehicle
  - identification of caregiver, the caregivers abilities, needs, support, and willingness to take on caregiving tasks
  - review, develop, update, or revise an advance care plan
  - creation of a written care plan that includes:
    — initial plans to address neuropsychiatric issues, neurocognitive issues, and functional limitations
    — referral to community resources as needed
    — initial education and support provided to the patient and/or caregiver

- Provider typically spends 50 minutes face to face with the patient and/or caregiver.
- A single provider can only report 99483 once every 180 days for a given patient.
- This service includes assessment of medical and psychosocial issues that may contribute to increased morbidity.
- This code further defines what cognition-relevant history may be considered, as well as other factors contributing to the patient's cognitive impairment that this service includes:
  - psychoactive medication
  - infection
  - chronic pain syndromes
  - depression
  - tumor
  - stroke
  - normal pressure hydrocephalus
  - other brain disease
- Code 99483 should not be reported on the same date of service as the following services: 99202–99205, 99211–99215, 99241–99245, 99324–99328, 99334–99337, 99341–99345, 99347–99350, 99366–99368, 99497–99498, 90785, 90791–90792, 96127, 96146 96160–96161 or 99605–99607.

ISSUES IN THIS CODE RANGE

- This code should not be reported if all of the required elements listed above are not performed or are considered unnecessary to assess the patient's condition. In these circumstances, an appropriate evaluation and management service should be reported instead.

Care Management Services (99490, 99439, 99491, 99487, 99489)

QUICK COMPARISON

Chronic and Complex Chronic Care Management Services

E/M Code	Intent of Service	Face-to-Face Visit	Time Spent
99490	Chronic care management services, first 20 minutes of clinical staff time directed by a physician or other qualified healthcare professional, per calendar month	No	20 min.
99439	Chronic care management services, each additional 20 minutes of clinical staff time directed by a physician or other qualified healthcare professional, per calendar month	No	Each additional 20 min.
99491	Chronic care management services, provided personally by a physician or other qualified health care professional, at least 30 minutes of physician or other qualified health care professional time, per calendar month	No	A minimum of 30 min.
99487	Complex chronic care management services directed by a physician or other qualified healthcare professional, per calendar month	No	60–89 min.
99489	Complex chronic care management services directed by a physician or other qualified healthcare professional, per calendar month	n/a	Each additional 30 min.

GENERAL GUIDELINES

- These services are generally provided for chronically ill patients with continuous or episodic health conditions.
- These patients live at home or in an assisted living facility, domiciliary, or rest home. The services are not reported by location like other coordination services and are in part performed by clinical staff.
- For 99490, 99439, 99487, and 99489, the clinical staff develops, implements, and many times substantially revises and monitors the care plan under the direction of the physician or other qualified healthcare professional.
- Use 99491 to report chronic care management services provided directly by the physician or other qualified healthcare professional.
- Patients typically require coordination of multiple medical specialties and services. In addition, they have multiple illnesses and medications, are unable to perform daily activities, require a caregiver, and have repeat visits to the emergency room and hospital admissions.
- These codes further define what a typical adult patient and a pediatric patient would require to support the use of these codes.
- An adult patient:
  - takes or receives three or more prescription medications
  - may receive therapeutic interventions such as physical or occupational therapy

 KEY POINT

To report face-to-face visits by the physician that are performed in the same month as 99487, use the appropriate E/M code(s).

- has two or more chronic continuous or episodic health conditions. The duration of their conditions is expected to be at least 12 months or until the death of the patient, or the conditions place the patient at a significant risk of death, acute exacerbation/decompensation, or functional decline.
- A pediatric patient:
  - takes or receives three or more prescription medications or therapeutic interventions (e.g., medications, nutritional support, respiratory therapy)
  - has two or more chronic continuous or episodic health conditions. The duration of their conditions is expected to be at least 12 months or until the death of the patient, or the conditions place the patient at a significant risk of death, acute exacerbation/decompensation, or functional decline.
- The services are provided by a physician, other qualified healthcare professional, or clinical staff when directed by a physician or other qualified healthcare professional.
- Services that may be provided by the clinical staff include:
  - assessment and support for treatment regimen adherence and medication management
  - collection of health outcomes data and registry documentation
  - communication with home health agencies and other community services the patient may utilize
  - communication and engagement with patient, family members, caretaker or guardian, surrogate decision makers, and/or other professionals regarding aspects of care
  - development, communication and maintenance of a comprehensive care plan
  - facilitating access to care and services needed by the patient and/or family
  - identification of available community and health resources
  - patient and/or family/caretaker education to support self-management, independent living, and activities of daily living
  - ongoing review of patient status, including review of laboratory and other studies not reported as part of an E/M service
  - continuing review of the patient's status to include reviewing laboratory and other studies not reported as part of an E/M service as noted above
- A care plan should be designed around the physical, mental, cognitive, social, functional, and environmental needs of the patient after an assessment or reassessment as well as an inventory of resources and supports available.
- Care plan elements should be addressed when applicable for the patient, these include, but are not limited to, the following:
  - problem list
  - prognosis
  - expected outcome
  - measurable treatment objectives
  - management of patient symptoms
  - medical management

- planned interventions
- community/social services provided and the management thereof
- identification of providers of each service ordered
- cognitive assessment
- functional assessment
- advance directives summary
- environmental evaluation
- assessment of caregivers
- The following services may not be reported in addition to 99439, 99487, 99489, or 99490 in the same 30-day period by a physician or other qualified healthcare professional:
  - care plan oversight (99339–99340, 99374–99380)
  - chronic care management (99491)
  - ESRD related services (90951–90970)
  - medication therapy management (99605–99607)
- Do not report 99439 or 99490 with 99487 or 99489.
- A care management office or practice is required to have the following capabilities:
  - 24/7 access for physicians or other qualified healthcare professionals or clinical staff to provide patients and/or caregivers the ability to connect with healthcare professionals in order to address immediate needs, regardless of the time of day or day of the week
  - continuing care with a specified care team member with whom the patient can schedule consecutive, routine appointments
  - timely access and management for follow-up care upon discharge from an emergency department or facility
  - electronic health record system usage to ensure timely access to clinical information
  - standardized methodologies in place to readily identify patients requiring care management services
  - internal care management processes and functions which ensure patients identified as meeting care requirements begin receiving said services in as expeditious a manner as possible
  - standardized forms and formats implemented in the EHR system and throughout the practice
  - ability to engage and educate patients and caregivers in addition to coordinating care among all appropriate service professionals for each patient
  - reporting provider to supervise activities of the care team
  - clinical integration of all care team members that provide services to the patient
- Care management services codes factor in both face-to-face and non-face-to-face time spent by the clinical staff in communicating with the patient and/or the patient's family, caregiver, as well as other professionals and agencies to determine the total amount of time. Additionally, documentation and implementation of the care plan and the teaching of self-management, when appropriate are also required components to report these services.
- Report these services once per calendar month. Only count the time of one clinical staff member when two or more clinical staff members are

discussing the patient. Do not count any clinical staff time for a particular day if the physician or other qualified healthcare professional reports an E/M service.

- It is not appropriate to report these services when the care plan remains unchanged or required only minimal revisions such as a change in medication.
- If the physician or other qualified healthcare professional provides face-to-face visits in the month, these visits should be reported with the appropriate E/M code.
- These codes should not be reported by the surgeon if the services he or she rendered are within a global surgery period of the surgical procedure performed.
- In the event that a physician or qualified healthcare professional performs any of the clinical staff activities described in these codes, his/her time may be counted towards the clinical staff time to meet the requirements of the elements of the code.
- For chronic care management, assign the correct code according to the following guidelines:
  - less than 20 minutes not reported separately
  - 20–39 minutes 99490
  - 40–59 minutes 99490 and 99439 x 1
  - 60 minutes or more 99490 and 99439 x 2
- For complex chronic care management assign the correct code according to the following guidelines:
  - less than 60 minutes not reported separately
  - 60–89 minutes 99487
  - 90–119 minutes 99487 and 99489 x 1
  - 120 minutes or more 99487 and 99489 x 2 or more for each additional 30 minutes
- Code 99490 is reported for the first 20 minutes of clinical staff time spent in care coordination activities during the calendar month.
- Code 99439 is reported for each additional 20 minutes of clinical staff time spent in care coordination activities during the calendar month.
- Code 99439 should not be reported more than twice per calendar month.
- Code 99491 is reported when at least 30 minutes of physician or other qualified healthcare professional time is spent in care coordination activities during the calendar month.
- Chronic care coordination services of less than 20 minutes, in a calendar month, are not reported separately.
- Care management services are reportable in any month when clinical staff time requirements have been satisfied.
- Care management services which restart following a discharge during a *new* month begin a new period or the provider may use the transitional care management codes (99495–99496), as appropriate.
- For a discharge that occurs in the *same* month, continue the reporting period or use the transitional care management codes (99495–99496).
- Code 99439, 99490, and 99491 should not be reported together or with 99487 or 99489, in the same calendar month.

QUICK TIP

Previously, HCPCS Level II add-on code G2058 was reported for Medicare beneficiaries with 99490 for each additional 20 minutes of clinical staff time spent performing chronic care management services. This code has been replaced with CPT code 99439.

Behavioral Health Intervention Services (99492–99494, 99484)

QUICK COMPARISON

Psychiatric Collaborative Care Management and General Behavioral Health Integration Care Management Services

E/M Code	Intent of Service	Face-to-Face Visit	Time Spent
99492	Initial psychiatric collaborative care management, first 70 minutes in the first calendar month of behavioral healthcare manager activities, in consultation with a psychiatric consultant, and directed by the treating provider	No	36–85 min.
99493	Subsequent psychiatric collaborative care management, first 60 minutes in a subsequent month of behavioral healthcare manager activities, in consultation with a psychiatric consultant, and directed by the treating provider	No	31–75 min.
99494	Initial or subsequent psychiatric collaborative care management, each additional 30 minutes in a calendar month of behavioral healthcare manager activities, in consultation with a psychiatric consultant, and directed by the treating provider	N/A	Each additional 30 min.
99484	Care management services for behavioral health conditions, at least 20 minutes of clinical staff time, directed by a physician or other qualified healthcare professional, per calendar month	Face to face or non-face-to-face	A minimum of 20 min.

GENERAL GUIDELINES

- Codes 99492, 99493, and 99494 are used for patients with common psychiatric conditions, such as depression, anxiety disorders, post-traumatic stress disorders, and substance use disorders, that are treated in a primary care or other specialty setting by a care team.
- Codes 99492, 99493, and 99494 are reported by the treating provider for a calendar month and include the services of the treating physician or other qualified healthcare professional, a behavioral care manager and a psychiatric consultant.
- The initiating encounter must be performed face to face by the treating provider and the behavioral healthcare manager must be available to provide face-to-face visits if necessary. There are no other requirements for in-person encounters.
- The behavioral healthcare manager is a designated individual with formal education or specialized training in behavioral health that provides coordination services, assesses needs, develops a plan of care, maintains the registry, must be available to provide face-to-face services with the patient, and has a collaborative, integrated relationship with the treating physician and psychiatric consultant.
- The psychiatric consultant must be trained in psychiatry or behavioral health and be qualified to prescribe the full range of medication. The psychiatric consultant advises and makes treatment recommendations

to the behavioral healthcare manager and/or the treating provider, including:

- referrals to specialty services
- psychiatric and other medical diagnoses
- medical management of complications due to treatment of psychiatric disorders
- medication management

- To report 99492, the following services must be performed:
  - outreach to and engagement in treatment of a patient directed by the treating provider
  - initial patient assessment, including administration of validated rating scales, with the development of an individualized treatment plan
  - review by a psychiatric consultant with plan changes if recommended
  - entering the patient in a registry and using the registry to track the patient's progress and follow-up, with appropriate documentation, and participation in weekly caseload consultation with the psychiatric consultant
  - providing brief interventions using evidence-based methods such as behavioral activation, motivational interviewing, and other focused treatment plans
- To report 99493, the following services must be performed:
  - using the registry to track patient progress and follow-up, with appropriate documentation
  - participation in weekly caseload consultation with the psychiatric consultant
  - ongoing collaboration and coordination of the patient's mental wellbeing with the treating provider and any other treating mental health providers
  - additional review of progress and recommendations of changes in treatment, as necessary, including medication changes, based on recommendations provided by the psychiatric consultant
  - using validated rating scales to monitor patient outcomes
  - providing brief interventions using evidence-based methods, such as behavioral activation, motivational interviewing, and other focused treatment plans
  - relapse prevention planning with patients who achieve remission of symptoms or other treatment goals and are ready for discharge from active treatment

---

- The time thresholds are based on total time over a calendar month.
- For psychiatric collaborative care coordination services, assign the correct code according to the following guidelines:
  - initial services less than 36 minutes are not reported separately
  - initial services 36–85 minutes — 99492
  - initial services 86–115 minutes — 99492 and 99494 x 1
  - subsequent services less than 31 minutes are not reported separately
  - subsequent services 31–75 minutes — 99493

- – subsequent services 76–105 minutes — 99493 and 99494 x 1
- – report 99494 for each additional increment up to 30 minutes for initial and subsequent services
- The treating provider supervises the patient's care, including referring the patient to specialty care when applicable, prescribing medication, and providing treatment for medical conditions.
- The treating provider may report evaluation and management (E/M) and other services separately within the same calendar month.
- Do not report 99492 and 99493 in the same calendar month.
- Code 99484 is used to report general behavioral health integration (BHI) care coordination services reported by the supervising physician or other qualified healthcare professional.
- The supervising/reporting provider for the BHI service must perform the initial evaluation and management service.
- BHI services are typically performed by the clinical staff but may be provided solely by the reporting provider. Services require face-to-face and non-face-to-face care coordination services that must total 20 minutes or more in a calendar month.

KEY POINT

Typically 99492–99494 would not be reported by a psychiatrist because the psychiatrist's work is defined as a subcomponent of these behavioral services codes.

> - To report 99484, the following services must be performed:
>   - – initial assessment or follow-up monitoring, including the use of applicable validated rating scales
>   - – behavioral healthcare planning in relation to behavioral/psychiatric health problems, including revising plans for patients who are not improving or whose status change
>   - – facilitating and coordinating treatment such as psychotherapy, pharmacotherapy, counseling, and/or psychiatric consultation
>   - – continuity of care with a designated member of the care team

- Code 99484 is reported when at least 20 minutes of clinical staff time is spent in general behavioral healthcare coordination activities during the calendar month.
- General behavioral health integration care coordination activities of less than 20 minutes in a calendar month are not reported separately.
- Code 99484 may be used in any outpatient setting, as long as the clinical staff is available for face-to-face encounters with the patient, and the reporting provider has an ongoing relationship with the patient and clinical staff.
- The same provider should not report 99484 in addition to 99492, 99493, and 99494 in the same calendar month.
- All bulleted items listed for 99484, 99492, and 99493 must be performed and documented and the specific time thresholds met in order to report these codes.
- Time spent in the emergency department coordinating care may be counted toward the time elements for 99484, 99492, 99493, and 99494. However, time spent while the patient is an inpatient or admitted to observation status may not be reported using 99484, 99492, 99493, and 99494.
- When the treating/supervising provider performs the activities of the behavioral healthcare manager and is not counting these activities toward another service, this time may be added to the total time thresholds used to report 99484, 99492, 99493, and 99494.

KNOWLEDGE ASSESSMENT CHAPTER 14

See chapter 19 for answers and rationale.

1. A patient's chart indicates that 15 minutes of chronic care management services were provided for the month. What code would be reported for this service?
   a. 99490
   b. 99487
   c. 99489
   d. The service is not reportable

2. Care management services include both face-to-face and non-face-to-face time spent by clinical staff with the patient, caregiver, or other professionals and agencies involved in the patient's care.
   a. True
   b. False

3. Which of the following would be included in the care plan documentation for chronic care management?
   a. Expected outcomes
   b. Medication management
   c. Planned interventions
   d. All of the above

4. Care management services may only be provided by a physician or other qualified healthcare professional.
   a. True
   b. False

5. There are 10 required elements listed in the description for code 99483. For this patient only eight were performed. What code should be reported for the services provided?
   a. 99483-52
   b. 99483
   c. Another appropriate E/M code
   d. None of the above

6. Behavioral health intervention codes 99484, 99492, and 99493, may only be reported once by the same provider in a calendar month.
   a. True
   b. False

7. A patient's chart indicates that a total of 1 hour and 30 minutes of subsequent psychiatric collaborative care management services was provided for the calendar month. Which code(s) would be reported for these services?
   a. 99492 and 99494 x 1
   b. 99493
   c. 99492 and 99493
   d. 99493 and 99494 x 1

8. Psychiatric collaborative care management services are provided by a care team that includes a treating provider, a behavioral healthcare manager, and a psychiatric consultant. Which care team member reports codes 99492, 99493, and 99494 for the services provided?
   a. Behavioral healthcare manager
   b. Treating provider
   c. Psychiatric consultant
   d. Each provider reports his or her own services

9. General behavioral health integration management services of less than 20 minutes are not reportable.
   a. True
   b. False

Chapter 15: Transitional Care Management Services (99495–99496)

QUICK COMPARISON

Transitional Care Management (TCM) Services

E/M Code	Medical Decision Making	Intent of Service	Patient Presence	Medical Decision Making	Face-to-Face Visit Within 7 Days	Face-to-Face Visit Within 8 to 14 Days
99495	Moderate complexity	Transitional care management services with these required elements: communication (direct contact, telephone, electronic), within 2 business days of discharge	Patient or caregiver present	Moderate complexity	99495	99495
99496	High complexity	Transitional care management services with these required elements: communication (direct contact, telephone, electronic), within 2 business days of discharge	Patient or caregiver present	High complexity	99496	99495

GENERAL GUIDELINES

- Transitional care management (TCM) services are provided to new and established patients that are transitioning from an inpatient facility, partial hospital, observation status, or skilled nursing facility to an assisted living facility, home, domiciliary, or a rest home. The medical and psychological issues these patients may have necessitate a moderate or high level of medical decision making.
- TCM requires a face-to-face visit (first visit is included in the TCM service and is not reported separately), initial patient contact, and medication reconciliation within a specific time frame.
- The services are provided by a physician, other qualified healthcare professional, or clinical staff when directed by a physician or other qualified healthcare professional.
- Code 99495 requires one face-to-face visit within 14 calendar days of discharge.
- Code 99496 requires one face-to-face visit within seven calendar days of discharge.
- The required face-to-face visit must be performed by the physician or other qualified healthcare professional.
- The 30-day transitional care management (TCM) period begins on the date the beneficiary is discharged from the inpatient hospital setting and continues for the next 29 days. During the 30-day period, the following three TCM components must be furnished, per CMS:
  - interactive contact—The provider is required to make an interactive contact with the beneficiary and/or caregiver, as appropriate, within

CODING AXIOM

The Centers for Medicare and Medicaid Services (CMS) established a facility and nonfacility payment for transitional care management services. Practitioners should report these services with the appropriate place of service code for the face-to-face visit.

two business days following the patient's discharge. The contact may be via telephone, email, or face to face. If two or more separate attempts to communicate with the patient or caregiver are made but are unsuccessful and all other criteria for TCM codes are met, the service may be reported. Per CMS guidelines, providers may not bill the TCM codes if there was not a successful communication within the 30-day period between the facility discharge and the date of service for the post-discharge TCM code.

– non-face-to-face services—The provider must furnish non-face-to-face services to the patient unless the services are determined to be not medically indicated or necessary. Certain non-face-to-face services may be furnished by licensed clinical staff under the provider's direction.

– face-to-face visit—One face-to-face visit must be furnished within certain timeframes as described by codes 99495 (14 days) and 99496 (7 days)

- If the physician or other qualified healthcare professional provides more than one face-to-face visit in a month, additional visits should be reported with the appropriate E/M code.

- Services that may be provided by the physician or other qualified healthcare professional include:

  – assistance in scheduling any required follow-up with community providers and services

  – education of the patient, family, caregiver, and/or guardian.

  – establishment or re-establishment of referrals and arranging for needed community resources

  – interaction with other providers who will assume or reassume care of the patient's system-specific problems

  – obtaining and reviewing the discharge information (discharge summary or continuity of care documents)

  – reviewing the need for or follow-up on pending diagnostic tests and treatments

- Services that may be provided by the clinical staff include:

  – assessment and support for treatment regimen adherence and medication management

  – communication with home health agencies and other community services the patient may use

  – communication with patient, family members, caretaker or guardian, surrogate decision makers, and/or other professionals regarding aspects of care

  – facilitating access to care and services needed by the patient and/or family

  – identification of available community and health resources

  – patient and/or family/caretaker education to support self-management, independent living, and activities of daily living (ADL)

- When these services are reported by a physician or other qualified healthcare professional, codes 99441–99443 or 99497–99498 may not be reported during the period covered by TCM services. Additionally, TCM should not be reported during the same service.

  – telephone services (99441–99443)

- Do not report these services with 99421–99423 for the same time period.
- These codes should not be reported by the surgeon if the services he or she rendered are within a global surgery period of the surgical procedure performed.
- If another provider reports these services during a postoperative period of a surgical procedure, modifier 54 is not required.
- Append modifier 95 to indicate that the E/M service was rendered to a patient at a distant site via a real-time interactive audio and video telecommunications system. The communication between the physician or other qualified healthcare professional and the patient should be commensurate with the same key components or requirements of those that would be required if the service had been rendered in a face-to-face setting.
- These services may be reported only one time within 30 days of discharge and by only one provider.

KNOWLEDGE ASSESSMENT CHAPTER 15

See chapter 19 for answers and rationale.

1. Transitional care services may only be reported when a face-to-face visit by a physician or other qualified healthcare professional has been performed.
   a. True
   b. False

2. When does the 30-day transitional care management period begin?
   a. The day after the patient is discharged from the inpatient setting
   b. The day the patient is discharged from the inpatient setting
   c. The day the physician performs the face-to-face visit
   d. The first Monday following discharge

3. If the physician or other qualified healthcare professional provides more than one face-to-face visit in a month, these services are included in the transitional care codes and are not separately reportable.
   a. True
   b. False

4. Transitional care management services require interactive contact with the patient or caregiver within how many business days of discharge?
   a. Seven
   b. Two
   c. One
   d. Five

5. Which of the following are acceptable methods of communication for the required interactive contact? Select all that apply.
   a. Telephone
   b. Mail
   c. Face to face
   d. E-mail

Chapter 16: Advance Care Planning (99497–99498)

QUICK COMPARISON

Advance Care Planning (ACP)

E/M Code	Intent of Service	FacHealthcaree-to-Face Visit	Time Spent
99497	Advance care planning including the explanation and discussion of advance directives such as standard forms (with completion of such forms, when performed), by the physician or other qualified healthcare professional	Yes	Initial 30 min.
99498	Advance care planning including the explanation and discussion of advance directives such as standard forms (with completion of such forms, when performed), by the physician or other qualified healthcare professional	Yes	Each additional 30 min.

GENERAL GUIDELINES

- These codes describe counseling and discussion of advance care directives with the patient, family members, and/or surrogate that may or may not include completion of pertinent legal documents.
- No active management of the patient's problems is undertaken for the time period reported when these codes are used.
- Codes 99497–99498 should not be reported on the same date of service as the following E/M services: 99291–99292, 99468–99469, 99471–99472, 99475–99480, and 99483. However, these codes may be separately reported when performed on the same date of service in conjunction with the following E/M services: 99202–99215, 99217–99226, 99231–99236, 99238–99239, 99241–99245, 99251–99255, 99281–99285, 99304–99310, 99315–99316, 99318, 99324–99328, 99334–99337, 99341–99345, 99347–99350, 99381–99397, and 99495–99496.
- An advance directive is described as a written document that the patient uses to appoint a representative as well as to record his or her wishes as they relate to future medical treatment in the event the patient is incapacitated and unable to make decisions on his or her own.
- Types of written advance directives include, but are not limited to:
  - healthcare proxy
  - durable power of attorney for healthcare
  - living will
  - medical orders for life-sustaining treatment (MOLST)

QUICK TIP

Advance care planning codes 99497 and 99498 may be reported separately when performed on the same day as another E/M service.

FOR MORE INFO

Information pertaining to the ACP change may be found at: https://www.cms.gov/Outreach-and-Education/Medicare-Learning-Network-MLN/MLNMattersArticles/Downloads/MM9271.pdf.

Effective January 1, 2016, CMS made voluntary advance care planning (ACP) services separately payable by Medicare when the ACP is provided on the same date of service and by the same provider that performs the annual wellness visit (AWV). When the ACP and the AWV are provided on the same day, the ACP is considered a preventive service and the coinsurance and deductible are waived. Providers would report code 99497 and 99498, if applicable, for the advance care planning, along with code G0438 or G0439 for the annual wellness visit. Both services must be reported on the same claim with modifier 33 appended to the ACP service. **Note:** When the ACP is performed on a different date of service than the AWV or by a different provider, the coinsurance and deductible would apply. For more information on HCPCS Level II G codes, see chapter 17.

KNOWLEDGE ASSESSMENT CHAPTER 16

See chapter 19 for answers and rationale.

1. Which range of E/M codes should not be reported with 99497–99498 on the same date of service?
   a. 99202–99215
   b. 99304–99310
   c. 99381–99397
   d. 99475–99480

2. The physician provides active management of the patient's problems as part of the advance care planning.
   a. True
   b. False

Chapter 17: HCPCS G Codes and Evaluation and Management Services

Medicare Covered Care Plan Oversight Services (G0179–G0182)

QUICK COMPARISON

Care Plan Oversight Services

HCPCS Code	Medicare Covered CPO Services	Place of Service	Under Care of	Presence of Patient	Time
G0179	Physician recertification for Medicare-covered home health services under a home health plan of care (patient not present), including contacts with home health agency and review of reports of patient status required by physicians to affirm the initial implementation of the plan of care that meets patient's needs, per recertification period	In home, a domiciliary or equivalent environment (e.g., Alzheimer's facility)	Home health agency	Patient not present	N/A
G0180	Physician certification for Medicare-covered home health services under a home health plan of care (patient not present), including contacts with home health agency and review of reports of patient status required by physicians to affirm the initial implementation of the plan of care that meets patient's needs, per recertification period	In home, a domiciliary or equivalent environment (e.g., Alzheimer's facility)	Home health agency	Patient not present	N/A
G0181	Physician supervision of a patient receiving Medicare-covered services provided by a participating home health agency (patient not present) requiring complex and multidisciplinary care modalities involving regular physician development and/or revision of care plans, review of subsequent reports of patient status, review of laboratory and other studies, communication (including telephone calls) with other healthcare professionals involved in the patient's care, integration of new information into the medical treatment plan and/or adjustment of medical therapy, within a calendar month, 30 minutes or more	In home, a domiciliary or equivalent environment (e.g., Alzheimer's facility)	Home health agency	Patient not present	30 min. or more
G0182	Physician supervision of a patient under a Medicare-approved hospice (patient not present) requiring complex and multidisciplinary care modalities involving regular physician development and/or revision of care plans, review of subsequent reports of patient status, review of laboratory and other studies, communication (including telephone calls) with other healthcare professionals involved in the patient's care, integration of new information into the medical treatment plan and/or adjustment of medical therapy, within a calendar month, 30 minutes or more	Hospice	Hospice	Patient not present	30 min. or more

GENERAL GUIDELINES

Care Plan Oversight Services

QUICK TIP

Providers must include their own documentation and may not rely on the orders or chart notes of the care giver to support care plan oversight. Each contact should be documented and include date, contact, orders given or changed, and time spent providing the remote care of the patient.

- Care plan oversight (CPO) is physician, or other qualified healthcare provider, supervision of patients receiving either home health or hospice benefits where complex or multidisciplinary care modalities and ongoing provider involvement are required.
- CMS extended Medicare coverage to allow separate payment for CPO services of or exceeding 30 minutes per month for patients who are receiving Medicare-covered home health or hospice benefits.
- Medicare does not pay for CPO services for nursing facility or skilled nursing facility patients.
- Code descriptors for these codes include communication with family member(s), surrogate decision maker(s) (e.g., legal guardians) and/or key caregivers as well as healthcare professionals.
- Only one provider, per month, will be paid for CPO services for a patient.
- Codes 99374–99378 are not covered under Medicare. These services should be reported to Medicare with codes G0181 and G0182.
- Care plan oversight provided to Medicare patient's for home health or hospice care plan oversight services are reported with HCPCS Level II codes G0181–G0182.
- Care plan oversight for certification and recertification of home health services are reported with HCPCS Level II codes G0179–G0180.
- Home health certification includes creation of a plan of care and verification that the home health agency complies with the written plan of care.
- The physician must maintain awareness of a patient's ongoing needs and of changes in the patient's condition or medications.
- Code G0180 can only be reported when the patient has not received any Medicare covered home health services for a period of at least 60 days.
- The recertification code G0179 can be reported only when a patient has received services for at least 60 days.
- Code G0179 is to be reported only once every 60 days except in the rare instance whereby a patient starts a new episode of care prior to the end of 60 days and a new plan of care is needed to start the new episode of care.
- Codes G0179–G0182 are reported separately from other E/M services.

The following coverage requirements apply to CPO services G0181 and G0182:

- The patient must require complex or multidisciplinary care modalities requiring ongoing provider involvement in the plan of care.
- The provider will review subsequent reports regarding patient status, labs, and other studies during the calendar month, as well as communicate with other healthcare professionals involved in the patient's care.
- The patient must be receiving Medicare-covered home health or hospice services during the period in which the CPO services are furnished.

- The provider who bills CPO must be the same individual who signed the home health or hospice plan of care.
- CPO services should be reported after the end of the month in which the services were provided.
- No other services should be reported on the same claim form with the CPO service.
- The provider must furnish at least 30 minutes of CPO within the calendar month for which payment is claimed.
- For patients receiving Medicare-covered home health services, the provider must not have a significant financial or contractual interest in the home health agency (HHA).
- For patients receiving Medicare hospice services, the provider must not be the medical director or an employee of the hospice or providing services under arrangements with the hospice.
- The provider billing for the CPO must document in the patient's medical record those services that were furnished, as well as the date and length of time associated with those services.

CODING AXIOM

Services that do not count towards the 30-minute required threshold include:

- Time spent discussing treatment and medication adjustments with the patient, his or her family, or friends
- Time spent by staff getting or filing charts
- Travel time
- Provider time spent calling prescriptions into the pharmacist unless the telephone conversation involves a discussion of pharmaceutical therapies

Preventive Medicine Services (G0402, G0438–G0439)

QUICK COMPARISON

Medicare Preventive Medicine Services

E/M Code	Patient Status	Intent of Service	Time
G0402	No complaints	Welcome to Medicare evaluation and management service	Preventive-within first 12 months of coverage effective date
G0438	No complaints	Annual wellness visit with prevention plan services	Initial visit
G0439	No complaints	Annual wellness visit with prevention plan services	Subsequent visit

GENERAL GUIDELINES

- Code G0402 initial preventive physical exam (IPPE) is a preventive evaluation and management service provided to Medicare beneficiaries within the first 12 months of their coverage effective date. If a patient does not receive an IPPE within the first 12 months from their effective date, the patient may receive an annual wellness visit (AWV) with personalized prevention plan services (PPPS) instead.
- Medicare does not cover routine physicals. The IPPE is provided as an introduction to Medicare and enables new beneficiaries to receive important screenings and vaccinations.
- Physicians may measure the patient's body mass index (BMI) and discuss end-of-life planning when necessary.
- Neither the IPPE or AWV are subject to a deductible; however, the IPPE is subject to coinsurance.
- The IPPE face-to-face exam comprises seven individual components:
  - Review the patient's medical and social history
  - Review the patient's potential risk factors for depression and other mood disorders
  - Review the patient's functional ability and level of safety
  - Physical examination that includes height, weight, BP, visual acuity, BMI, and other factors as applicable depending on the patient's medical and social history and current clinical standards
  - End-of-life planning
  - Education, counseling, and referral based on the results of the review and evaluation services described above
  - Education, counseling, and referral, including a brief written plan or checklist, for obtaining the appropriate screening or other Part B preventive services

    Note: Each component must be provided or referred to another physician in order to appropriately submit this benefit to Medicare.
- HCPCS Level II code G0438 Annual wellness visit; includes a personalized prevention plan of service (PPPS), initial visit
- HCPCS Level II code G0439 Annual wellness visit, includes a personalized prevention plan of service (PPPS), subsequent visit

The AWV can be performed by a physician, physician's assistant, nurse practitioner, or clinical nurse specialist or other medical professional as defined by CMS regulations and consists of the following services for the first AWV:

- Health risk assessment
- Establishment of the patient's health history, including family history
- Establishment of the patient's current list of providers and suppliers routinely providing care to the individual
- Measurement of the patient's height, weight, BMI, blood pressure, and other routine measurements as appropriate
- Detection of any cognitive impairment
- Review of any potential risk factors for depression, including current or past experiences with depression or other mood disorders, based on the use of an appropriate screening instrument for persons without a current diagnosis of depression
- Review of the patient's functional ability and level of safety based on direct observation or the use of an appropriate screening questionnaire
- Establishment of a written screening schedule for the individual; i.e., a checklist for the next 5–10 years, as appropriate, based on recommendations of the United States Preventive Services Task Force (USPSTF) and the Advisory Committee on Immunization Practices (ACIP) as well as the patient's health history, screening history, and age appropriate preventive services covered by Medicare
- Establishment of a list of risk factors and conditions for which primary, secondary, or tertiary interventions are recommended or are underway for the patient; including any mental health conditions, or any such risk factors that have been identified through an IPPE, and a list of treatment options and their associated risks and benefits
- Furnishing personalized health advice to the patient and referrals, as appropriate, to health education or preventive counseling services or programs aimed at reducing identified risk factors and improving self-management or community based lifestyle interventions to reduce health risks, encourage self-management and wellness, including weight loss, increasing physical activity, smoking cessation, preventing falls, and good nutrition
- Other service element(s) as determined appropriate by the HHS secretary through national coverage determinations (NCD)

The following are elements to be included in a subsequent AWV:

- Update of Health Risk Assessment
- Update of medical and family history
- Measurement of the patient's height, weight, BMI, blood pressure, and other routine measurements, as appropriate
- Update to the patient's current list of providers and suppliers routinely providing care to the individual
- Detection of any cognitive impairment
- Update of the list of risk factors and conditions for which primary, secondary, or tertiary interventions are recommended or are underway for the patient

- Personalized health advice furnished to the patient and a referral, as applicable, to health education or preventive counseling services or programs
- Update of the written screening schedule for the patient

CMS created "quick reference" tools that function as a checklist for providers to ensure that all of the details of the specific elements of each visit type are documented appropriately. Copies of these documents can be downloaded from the following URLS: https://www.cms.gov/Outreach-and-Education/Medicare-Learning-Network-MLN/MLNProducts/downloads/MPS_QRI_IPPE001a.pdf.

https://www.cms.gov/Outreach-and-Education/Medicare-Learning-Network-MLN/MLNProducts/downloads/AWV_Chart_ICN905706.pdf

Additional information on both the IPPE and AWV can be found at: https://www.cms.gov/Medicare/Prevention/PrevntionGenInfo/ProviderResources.html.

For prolonged preventive services provided to Medicare beneficiaries, G0513 may be reported separately for the first 30 minutes beyond the usual service time and G0514 may be reported for each additional 30 minutes of service.

Telehealth Follow-up Inpatient Consultation Services (G0406–G0408)

QUICK COMPARISON

Telehealth Follow-up Consultations—Inpatient, New or Established Patient

HCPCS Level II Code	Medical Decision Making	History	Exam	Counseling and/or Coordination of Care	Time Spent Communicating with the Patient via Telehealth
G0406	Straight-forward or low complexity	Problem-focused interval history	Problem-focused exam	Consistent with problems and patient's or family's needs	15 min.
G0407	Moderate complexity	Expanded interval history	Expanded problem-focused exam	Consistent with problems and patient's or family's needs	25 min.
G0408	High complexity	Detailed interval history	Detailed	Consistent with problems and patient's or family's needs	35 min.

GENERAL GUIDELINES

- Note that the general guidelines described in the next section for codes G0425–G0427 up to and including the Special Note on Coverage Criteria are also applicable to follow-up telehealth consultative services.
- A follow-up telehealth consultation is one requested by the attending physician and subsequent to an initial inpatient consultation whether provided in person or via telehealth.
- Follow-up inpatient telehealth consultations are defined by CMS as when a provider requests the opinion or advice of another physician or qualified healthcare provider to evaluate and/or manage a specific problem in the hospital or skilled nursing facility to follow up on an initial consultation or subsequent consultative visit requested by the attending physician and includes the following services:
  - monitoring progress
  - recommending management modifications
  - advising on a new plan of care based upon the patient's response to changes in status or no changes on the consulted health matter
- These consultations include monitoring the patient's progress, as well as making recommendations and/or modifications to the patient's management or instituting a new plan of care based on changes in the patient's condition including no changes on the health issue for which the provider was consulted. Any counseling or coordination of care with other healthcare providers or agencies consistent with the nature of the problem and the patient's needs is also included in the follow-up consultation service.
- As with the emergency department and initial inpatient consultations, all consultation-related services rendered before, during, and after communicating with the patient are included in the payment. This may include, but is not limited to, review of patient diagnostic and/or

imaging studies and interim lab work, as well as communications with family members or other healthcare professionals, completing medical records, and documentation or communication of results and care plans to the requesting provider.

- Initial inpatient consult may have been provided in person or via telehealth.
- The follow-up telehealth consultation would be distinct from the follow-up care provided by the physician of record or the attending physician.
- When the consultation has been provided, the consultant prepares a written report containing his or her findings and recommendations to the referring provider.
- When counseling and coordination of care with other providers are included, consistent with the nature of the presenting problem, as well as the patient's needs.
- While these follow-up telehealth consultation service codes are specific to telehealth, CMS still requires that these codes be reported with one of the following modifiers to identify the type of telehealth technology used to report the service:

GT   Via interactive audio and video telecommunication systems

      OR

GQ   Via asynchronous telecommunications system

- Beginning January 1, 2018, providers submitting codes for telehealth services to Medicare administrative contractors (MAC) are not required to append modifier GT to the CPT or HCPCS code. The use of telehealth POS code 02 is sufficient to certify that the reported service meets the telehealth requirements.

Telehealth ED or Initial Inpatient Consultation Services (G0425–G0427)

QUICK COMPARISON

Telehealth Follow-up Consultations—Inpatient, New or Established Patient

HCPCS Level II Code	Medical Decision Making	History	Exam	Counseling and/or Coordination of Care	Time Spent Communicating with the Patient via Telehealth
G0425	Straight-forward	Problem-focused	Problem-focused	Consistent with problems and patient's or family's needs	30 min.
G0426	Moderate complexity	Detailed	Detailed	Consistent with problems and patient's or family's needs	50 min.
G0427	High Complexity	Comprehensive	Comprehensive	Consistent with problems and patient's or family's needs	70 min.

GENERAL GUIDELINES

- Teleconsultations most often involve a primary care practitioner with a patient at a remote, rural (spoke) site and a consulting medical specialist at an urban or referral (hub) facility with the primary care practitioner requesting advice from the consulting physician about the patient's condition or treatment.
- As a result of the Balanced Budget Act (BBA) of 1997, physicians and other appropriate practitioners providing professional consultations via telecommunication systems to Medicare beneficiaries residing in rural areas that have been designated as health professional shortage areas can receive payment for their services. The Benefits Improvement and Protection Act (BIPA) of 2000 greatly expanded many aspects of coverage and billing of telehealth services. In addition to coverage for teleconsultations, the legislation mandates coverage of many services using telecommunications systems including office visits, psychotherapy, and drug management. Telehealth services have also been extended to Medicare beneficiaries beyond the boundaries of HPSAs.
- The following are approved origination sites for telehealth services:
  - physician or practitioner offices
  - hospitals
  - community access hospitals (CAH)
  - rural health centers (RHC)
  - federally qualified health centers (FQHC)
  - hospital-based or critical access hospital-based renal dialysis centers (including satellites)
  - skilled nursing facilities (SNF)
  - community mental health centers (CMHC)

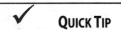

QUICK TIP

There has been a temporary expansion of telehealth services due to the COVID-19 Public Health Emergency (PHE). More details can be found starting on page 5.

- The following list identifies approved telehealth services:
  - ED or initial inpatient consultations
  - follow-up inpatient consultations
  - office or other outpatient visits
  - subsequent hospital care services (limit to one telehealth visit every three days)
  - subsequent inpatient nursing facility visits
  - individual and group kidney disease education services
  - individual and group diabetes self-management training services (minimum of 1 hour in-person instruction furnished within the initial year training period to ensure effective injection training)
  - individual psychotherapy
  - pharmacologic management
  - psychiatric diagnostic interview examination
  - end stage renal disease (ESRD) related services
  - individual and group medical nutrition therapy (MNT)
  - neurobehavioral status exam
  - individual and group health and behavior assessment and intervention (HBAI)
  - smoking cessation services
  - alcohol and/or substance (other than tobacco) abuse assessment and intervention services
- The following list identifies approved distant site practitioners:
  - physician
  - physician assistant (PA)
  - nurse practitioner (NP)
  - clinical nurse specialist (CNS)
  - nurse midwife
  - clinical psychologist
  - clinical social worker
  - certified registered nurse anesthetists
  - registered dietitian or nutrition professional
- It is also important to note that current deductible and coinsurance policies apply to these services.
- The originating site should report services with Q3014 Telehealth originating site facility fee. Submission of a claim with Q3014 attests that the originating site is a rural HPSA or non-MSA county or an entity that participates in a federal telemedicine demonstration project.
- Professional services commonly furnished remotely using telecommunications technology, but that do not require the patient to be present in person with the practitioner when they are furnished, are covered and paid in the same way as services delivered without the use of telecommunications technology when the practitioner is in-person at the medical facility furnishing care to the patient.

Special Instructions Regarding Coverage Criteria

To qualify as a teleconsultation, the patient encounter must meet criteria for a consultation service as defined by CPT code descriptors, as well as include the following requirements:

- Clinical assessment is performed via medical examination directed by the consultant (specialist)
- Audiovisual communications equipment is used that allows real-time communication between the beneficiary, primary care practitioner, and the specialist; this does not include the use of telephones, electronic mail, or facsimile machines
- If a practitioner other than the referring practitioner presents the patient, he or she is an employee of the referring practitioner
- The presenting practitioner's participation is appropriate for the needs of the patient and for providing information to the consultant and at the consultant's direction
- Feedback of the consultation is provided to the referring practitioner

In the majority of cases, it is expected that the referring practitioner will be present for the teleconsultation to satisfy the face-to-face examination requirement that is a prerequisite of a consultation under Medicare. The teleconsultation is subject to review if the referring practitioner is not present.

Physicians and other practitioners are instructed by CMS to report new or established patient office/other outpatient services codes, nursing facility care codes, or initial hospital visit codes. The first inpatient encounter by any physician is reported with initial hospital care codes 99221–99223, and subsequent inpatient encounters using codes 99231–99233. Knowing that only one physician may be the admitting physician, CMS created HCPCS Level II modifier AI Principal physician of record, that is to be reported with the initial hospital care code by the attending physician.

CMS also redistributed the value of the consultation codes across the other E/M codes for Medicare services. CMS retained values for codes 99241–99255 in the Medicare physician fee schedule for those private payers who use the data for reimbursement. Note that private payers may choose to follow CMS or CPT guidelines and the use of consultation codes should be verified with the individual payers.

Medicare requires the use of interactive audio and video telecommunications that allow for real-time communication between the physician or other practitioner at the distant site and the beneficiary. This may include x-rays, EKGs, MRIs, laboratory results, audio clips, photographs specific to the patient's condition that are capable of rendering or supporting a diagnosis, and text. It does not include telephone calls, electronic mail, or images transmitted via facsimile. CMS developed modifier GQ Via asynchronous telecommunications system, to identify the use of store-and-forward technology.

The following criteria necessitate the use of a telehealth consultation code for the emergency department or an initial inpatient consultative service:

- When a provider requests the opinion or advice of another physician or qualified healthcare provider to evaluate and/or manage a specific problem in the emergency department or as an inpatient service.

- When the reason for the telehealth consultation is clearly documented in the patient's medical record and included in the requesting provider's plan of care for the patient.
- When the consultation has been provided, the consultant prepares a written report containing his or her findings and recommendations to the referring provider.
- When counseling and coordination of care with other providers is included, consistent with the nature of the presenting problem as well as the patient's needs.
- All consultation related services rendered before, during, and after communicating with the patient is included in the payment. This may include but is not limited to review of patient diagnostic and/or imaging studies and interim lab work, as well as communications with family members or other healthcare professionals, completing medical records, and documenting or communicating results and care plans to the requesting provider.
- While these emergency department or initial inpatient telehealth consultation service codes are specific to telehealth, CMS still requires that these codes be reported with one of the following modifiers to identify the type of telehealth technology used to report the service:

  GT   Via interactive audio and video telecommunication systems

           OR

  GQ   Via asynchronous telecommunications system
- Beginning January 1, 2018, providers submitting codes for telehealth services to MAC's are not required to append modifier GT to the CPT or HCPCS code. The use of telehealth POS code 02 is sufficient to certify that the reported service meets the telehealth requirements.

Behavioral Screenings and Intervention (G0442–G0444)

QUICK COMPARISON

Behavioral Evaluations

E/M Code	Patient Status	Intent of Service	Time
G0442	Alcohol screening	Promote health, alcohol misuse screening	15 min.
G0443	Alcohol use	Promote health, alcohol misuse counseling	15 min.
G0444	Depression screening	Promote health, depression screening	15 min.

GENERAL GUIDELINES

- Medicare covers annual alcohol screening and up to four, brief face-to-face behavioral counseling sessions per year to reduce alcohol misuse.
- Deductible and coinsurance do not apply to these services.
- Counseling must be furnished by a qualified primary care physician or other primary care practitioner in a primary care setting.
- Medicare does not require use of a specific alcohol misuse screening tool. The provider in the primary care setting may choose the specific screening tool(s) he or she prefers.
- Counseling is covered for those patients that misuse alcohol, but do not meet the criteria for alcohol dependence, and are competent and alert when the counseling is provided.
- Annual screening and counseling for alcohol misuse in adults is recommended with a grade of B by the U.S. Preventive Services Task Force (USPSTF)
- The behavioral counseling intervention should follow the 5A's approach adopted by the USPSTF: assess, advise, agree, assist, and arrange.
- Medicare will cover a screening for depression provided in a primary care setting that has staff-assisted support in place to help ensure accurate diagnosis, as well as effective treatment plans, and patient follow-up.
- Staff-assisted support should at least consist of clinical staff that can advise the provider of screening results and who can coordinate referrals to mental health treatment when necessary.
- Medicare does not require use of a specific depression screening tool. The provider in the primary care setting may choose the specific screening tool(s) he or she prefers.
- Coverage for G0444 includes a screening service only it does not include treatment options for depression.
- Medicare covers an annual depression screening up to 15 minutes.

 KEY POINT

For reporting and payment for alcohol and substance abuse not provided as a screening service but performed in the context of diagnosis and treatment of illness or injury, CMS created HCPCS Level II codes G0396 and G0397.

ISSUES IN THIS CODE RANGE

- Alcohol screening (G0442) is only covered one time in a 12-month period.
- Brief face-to-face behavioral counseling interventions (G0443) are only covered once per day.
- Brief face-to-face behavioral counseling interventions (G0443) are only covered four times in a 12-month period.
- Screening for depression (G0444) is only covered one time in a 12-month period.

Care Management Services (G0506)

QUICK COMPARISON

Care Management Services

E/M Code	Intent of Service	Face-to-Face Visit
G0506	Add-on code for reporting comprehensive assessment of and care planning for patients that require chronic care management services	Yes

GENERAL GUIDELINES

- HCPCS Level II code G0506 is an add-on code and must be reported with a primary E/M service.
- This code may be applicable when the billing provider initiating CCM services personally performs extensive assessment and care planning outside the usual effort described by the primary procedure.
- Initial chronic care management (CCM) services including, the IPPE, AWV, and other qualifying face-to-face E/M services, are primary E/M services that may be reported with G0506. These include:

    G0402

    G0438

    G0439

    99202–99205

    99212–99215

    99495–99496

- Code G0506 cannot be used as an add-on code for behavioral health initiative services.
- The provider must create a written care plan centered on physical, mental, cognitive, psychosocial, functional, and environmental assessment, and the patient's available resources and support.
- Work and time used to report G0506 should not also be counted toward any other reported services, including CCM services.
- Code G0506 is only billable once, at the time of the CCM services.

Critical Care Telehealth Consultations (G0508–G0509)

QUICK COMPARISON

Telehealth Consultations-Critical Care

E/M Code	Type of Visit	Intent of Service	Time Spent Communicating with the Patient via Telehealth
G0508	Initial	Critical care consultation provided using telehealth technology	60 min.
G0509	Subsequent	Critical care consultation provided using telehealth technology	50 min.

GENERAL GUIDELINES

- HCPCS Level II codes G0508 and G0509 represent critical care consultations furnished via an interactive real-time telecommunication system.
- Report G0508 for the initial consultation requiring critical care services, such as stroke.
- Report G0509 for subsequent consultations requiring critical care services.
- The provider may communicate with either the patient or the patient's caregiver.
- Do not report these services more than one time per day.
- As a condition of Medicare payment for telehealth services, the provider at the distant site must be licensed to provide the services.
- The following list identifies approved distant site practitioners:
  - physician
  - physician assistant (PA)
  - nurse practitioner (NP)
  - clinical nurse specialist (CNS)
  - nurse midwife
  - clinical psychologist
  - clinical social worker
  - registered dietitian or nutrition professional
  - certified registered nurse anesthetists
- The requirement of reporting these codes with modifier GT has changed beginning January 1, 2018; providers submitting codes for telehealth services to MACs are not required to append modifier GT to the CPT or HCPCS code. The use of telehealth POS code 02 is sufficient to certify that the reported service meets the telehealth requirements.

KNOWLEDGE ASSESSMENT CHAPTER 17

See chapter 19 for answers and rationale.

1. What code is reported for a Medicare patient who received 30 minutes of physician supervised care plan oversight services in the calendar month under a Medicare-approved hospice program?
   a. G0181
   b. G0182
   c. 99378
   d. The service is not reportable

2. Code G0180 for physician certification for Medicare-covered, home health services can only be reported if the patient has not received any Medicare-covered, home health services for a period of at least 31 days.
   a. True
   b. False

3. Medicare does not cover preventive medicine services (99381–99429); however, the agency does cover a welcome to Medicare visit or initial preventive physical exam (IPPE). What code is used to report this visit?
   a. G0402
   b. 99387
   c. 99397
   d. G0438

4. How do providers reporting telehealth services to Medicare administrative contractors (MAC) indicate that the service was provided via telehealth real-time telecommunication systems?
   a. Report only the G code if the word telehealth is part of the code description
   b. Append modifier GT to the G code
   c. Submit using place of service (POS) code 02
   d. Both b and c

5. Which of the following are approved distant site telehealth practitioners?
   a. Nurse practitioner
   b. Clinical psychologist
   c. Nurse midwife
   d. All of the above

6. Codes G0425–G0427 and G0406–G0408 are only used to report telehealth consultations provided to Medicare beneficiaries.
   a. True
   b. False

Chapter 18: Coding and Compliance

QUICK COMPARISON

Ongoing Compliance Investigations

E/M Service	Compliance Issue	Investigating Agency
E/M codes reported during the global period	E/M services bundled into the global surgical package not provided	Office of Inspector General (OIG), recovery audit contractors (RAC)
Use of modifiers during the global surgery period	Modifiers used inappropriately to report E/M services that are bundled into the global surgical package	Office of Inspector General (OIG),
Inappropriate E/M code level selection	Selecting codes that do not have appropriate supporting documentation for that level of service	Centers for Medicare and Medicaid Services (CMS), Comprehensive Error Rate Testing (CERT) Program
Initial preventive physical examination (IPPE)	Misuse due to the likelihood that non-Medicare patients may have already received the preventive services listed under the IPPE	Office of Inspector General (OIG), recovery audit contractors (RAC)
Assigning new patient E/M codes	More than one new patient E/M service reported for the same beneficiary within a three-year period	Recovery audit contractors (RAC)
High level subsequent nursing facility care codes	Higher levels of care reported but not supported by documentation	Centers for Medicare and Medicaid Services (CMS), Medicare Administrative Contractor (MAC)—National Government Services (NGS)
Anesthesia care package and billing E/M codes separately	Unbundling of E/M services in anesthesia claims	Recovery audit contractors (RAC)
Critical care and emergency department (ED) services	Inappropriate use of critical care codes	Office of Inspector General (OIG), Recovery audit contractors (RAC)
Observation services	Duplication of observation codes and other E/M services	Recovery audit contractors (RAC)
Pulmonary diagnostic procedures with E/M services	Overpayments associated with E/M services and diagnostic pulmonary procedures	Recovery audit contractors (RAC)

E/M CODES REPORTED DURING THE GLOBAL PERIOD

General Guidelines
- CMS established a national definition for a global surgical package to ensure consistent payment for the same services across all carrier regions.
- CMS defined the global surgical package to include:
  - preoperative visits
  - intraoperative services
  - complications following surgery
    - — does not require a return trip to the operating room
  - postoperative visits related to recovery
  - postsurgical pain management provided by the surgeon

- certain supplies
- miscellaneous services, including:
    — dressing changes
    — local incisional wound care
    — removal of packing material
    — removal of sutures, staples, wires, lines, tubes, drains, casts, and splints
    — insertion, irrigation, and removal of urinary catheters, routine peripheral intravenous lines, nasogastric and rectal tubes
    — changes and removal of tracheostomy tubes
- In determining global surgery fees, CMS estimates the number of E/M services a physician provides to a typical beneficiary during the surgery period; physicians are compensated for the surgical service and related E/M services regardless of the number of E/M services actually provided during the global surgery period.
- Postoperative periods that apply to each surgical procedure are provided in the Medicare Physician Fee Schedule Data Base (MPFSDB). Payment rules for surgical procedures apply to codes with postoperative periods of 000, 010, 090, and sometimes YYY.
- Major surgeries include one day preceding the day of surgery, the day of surgery, and the 90 days immediately following the day of surgery.
- Minor surgeries include the day of surgery and the appropriate number of days immediately following the day of surgery.

Explanation of Investigation

- OIG has sought to determine whether payments were made to physicians for E/M services not provided during the global surgery period.
- One study showed the number of office visits were counted and compared to the number of E/M services included in the global surgery fee. Out of 300 claims reviewed, 201 of the surgeries performed showed that physicians provided fewer visits than those included in the global surgery fee.
    - OIG concluded that Medicare paid almost $98 million for E/M services bundled in to global surgery fees that were never provided.
- OIG recommendations to CMS included making an adjustment to the estimated number of E/M services included in the global surgery fee for surgeries that would reflect the actual number of services being provided, OR update the annual Medicare physician fee schedule (MPFS) to apply the audit results and other information.
    - CMS would not make changes to the codes in the MPFS stating the changes would simply end up being redistributed to all services and not result in savings to the Medicare program due to a requirement in the Medicare statute that mandated all changes must be done in a budget-neutral manner.
    - CMS did indicate the agency would work with the AMA Relative Value Scale Update Committee (RUC) and relevant physician specialty societies to identify and change services where the number of E/M services provided in the global period has changed.

Strategies for Risk Prevention

- Educate staff members on National Correct Coding Initiative (CCI) edits and demonstrate how to look up codes and determine the global period associated with the procedure code.

- Understand what is—and is not—included in the Medicare global surgery package vs. a commercial carrier global surgery fee. Many commercial carriers use CMS guidelines, but not all; therefore, it is important to note any differences. One example of differences in the global surgery package description is often reflected in complications. Medicare includes all complications except those requiring a return trip to the operating room in the global fee for the surgery; however, many commercial carriers pay for procedures such as incision and drainage performed in the physician office.

- Implement a process or mechanism, manual or automated, to indicate the start and stop dates for the global surgery period. This is helpful in knowing whether the type of visit is a preoperative visit and also to track the number of postoperative visits.
  - If the patient is being seen for reasons other than those related to the surgical service reminders should be given to the billing staff that a modifier may be appropriate and should be appended to the applicable E/M or other service; such as:
    — Modifier 24 Significant, Separately Identifiable E/M Service during a Postoperative Period
    — Modifier 79 Unrelated Procedure or Service by the Same Physician or Other Qualified Healthcare Professional during the Postoperative Period in cases where the patient is scheduled for an unrelated procedure during the postoperative period of another procedure
    — Modifier 58 Staged or Related Procedure or Service by the Same Physician or Other Qualified Healthcare Professional during the Postoperative Period

  Note: Modifier 24 is used to bypass carrier edits and, as such, should be used only when appropriate. The inappropriate use of any modifier to receive payment without following the necessary guidelines and documentation requirements can subject the provider to scrutiny and possible audits. In addition, as previously stated, append modifier 24 only to the evaluation and management service, not to the surgical procedure. Modifiers 58 and 79 may be used in conjunction with the procedure or other service codes.

- Download or print out a copy of the MPFS. Each surgery code shows the global period associated with it. Knowing whether the surgery has a 0-, 10-, or 90-day postoperative period can ensure that the proper number of visits are provided.

- Implement periodic spot checks of surgical claims to verify that any services reported during the global period have been reported in compliance with the carrier guidelines.
  - In many cases, when an E/M service is related to the surgery and inappropriately reported, carrier edits reject the claim.
  - Proactive review of claims prior to submission, as well as processed claims, allows identification of any recurrent errors or issues and provides an opportunity for corrections.

 QUICK TIP

Regular and ongoing review of the CMS Pub. 100-04, *Medicare Claims Processing Manual* sections on global surgery guidelines and commercial payer contract requirements will help ensure that coding staff members are informed and aware of any revisions or changes to current policies.

- Address billing issues with all staff members and providers as an educational tool to ensure that the problem has been remedied for future claims.

USE OF MODIFIERS DURING THE GLOBAL SURGERY PERIOD

General Guidelines
- CMS established a national definition for a global surgical package to ensure consistent payment for the same services across all carrier regions.
- CMS defined the global surgical package to include:
  - preoperative visits
  - intraoperative services
  - complications following surgery
    — does not require a return trip to the operating room
  - postoperative visits related to recovery
  - postsurgical pain management provided by the surgeon
  - certain supplies
  - miscellaneous services, including:
    — dressing changes
    — local incisional wound care
    — removal of packing material
    — removal of sutures, staples, wires, lines, tubes, drains, casts, and splints
    — insertion, irrigation, and removal of urinary catheters, routine peripheral intravenous lines, nasogastric and rectal tubes
    — changes and removal of tracheostomy tubes
- Major surgeries include one day preceding the day of surgery, the day of surgery, and the 90 days immediately following the day of surgery.
- Minor surgeries include the day of surgery and the appropriate number of days immediately following the day of surgery.
- Modifier 24 allows for an E/M service to be reported if the service was provided during the postoperative period of a surgical procedure by the same physician or other qualified healthcare professional who performed the procedure.
  - Documentation must support that the evaluation and management service is not related to the postoperative care of the procedure.
- Modifier 25 is used when the E/M service is separate from a procedure performed at the same encounter and signifies a clearly documented, distinct, and significantly identifiable service was rendered.
- Medicare and other payers require modifier 57 to be appended to the E/M service code only when the decision for surgery was made during the preoperative period of a surgical procedure with a 90-day postoperative period (i.e., major surgery). The preoperative period is defined as the day before and the day of the surgical procedure.

Explanation of Investigation
- The OIG has previously reported that inappropriate use of modifiers during the global surgical period has resulted in erroneous payments.

- Reporting E/M services related to the surgical procedure during the global period is a form of unbundling.

Strategies for Risk Prevention

- Maintain the most current version of the CCI edits; integrate these edits directly into the practice management system, if possible.
- Educate staff members on CCI edits and demonstrate how to look up codes and determine the global period associated with the procedure code.
- Understand what is—and is not—included in the Medicare global surgery package vs. a commercial carrier global surgery fee.
  - Many commercial carriers use CMS guidelines, but not all; therefore, it is important to note any differences.
  - One example of differences in the global surgery package description is often reflected in complications. Medicare includes ALL complications, except those requiring a return trip to the operating room in the global fee for the surgery. However, many commercial carriers pay for procedures such as incision and drainage performed in the physician office.
- Implement a process or mechanism, manual or automated, to indicate the start and stop dates for the global surgery period. This is helpful in knowing whether the type of visit is a preoperative visit and also to track the number of postoperative visits.
- Educate staff and clinicians on the appropriate use of E/M modifiers:
  - Modifier 24 permits an E/M service to be reported (other than inpatient hospital care before discharge from the hospital following surgery) if the service was provided during the postoperative period of a surgical procedure by the same physician or other qualified healthcare professional who performed the procedure. Documentation must support that the evaluation and management service is not related to the postoperative care of the procedure.
  - Modifier 25 should only be appended to codes describing E/M services and only when the services are provided by the same physician (or same qualified nonphysician practitioner) to the same patient on the same day as another procedure or service. It is not necessary to have a different diagnosis when reporting the E/M service on the same date as the procedure or other service.
    - Append modifier 25 to the E/M code only.
    - Both the E/M service and the procedure must be appropriately and sufficiently documented by the physician (or qualified nonphysician practitioner) in the patient's medical record demonstrating the medical necessity of the services reported; however, documentation is not required to be submitted with the claim.
  - Modifier 57 indicates an evaluation and management service provided on the day of or the day before surgery for codes assigned a 90-day global surgical period.
    - Modifier 57 indicates the E/M service provided resulted in the decision for surgery
    - It is not appropriate to report E/M services with a 0- or 10-day global surgical period with modifier 57.

Note: The modifiers discussed above are reported to bypass carrier edits; therefore, it is very important to only use when appropriate. Inappropriate use of any modifier to receive payment without following the necessary guidelines and documentation requirements can subject the provider to scrutiny and possible audits.

- Download or print out a copy of the Medicare physician fee schedule (MPFS).
  - Each surgery code shows the global period associated with it. Knowing whether the surgery has a 0-, 10-, or 90-day postoperative period can ensure that the proper number of visits are provided.
- Review regularly the CMS IOM Pub.100-04 sections on global surgery guidelines and commercial payer contract requirements to ensure staff and clinicians remain informed and aware of any revisions or changes to policies.
- Implement periodic spot checks of surgical claims to verify that any services reported during the global period have been reported in compliance with the carrier guidelines.
  - In many cases, when an E/M service is related to the surgery and inappropriately reported, carrier edits reject the claim, but not always.
  - Proactive review of claims prior to submission, as well as processed claims, allows identification of any recurrent errors or issues and provides an opportunity for corrections.
- Address billing issues with all staff members and providers as an educational tool to ensure that the problem has been remedied for future claims.

INAPPROPRIATE E/M CODE SELECTION

General Guidelines

- E/M services are covered when they are deemed to be medically necessary.
- The levels of E/M services define the wide variations in skill, effort, time, and medical knowledge required for preventing or diagnosing and treating illnesses or injuries. They also include services promoting optimal health and prevention of health conditions.
- The final E/M code is selected based upon a combination of the following factors:
  - location of the service
  - patient status (new or established)
  - level of key component documentation
    — history
    — physical examination
    — medical decision making
  - contributory components
  - status of the medical visit

 FOR MORE INFO

For detailed instruction on selecting the appropriate E/M code, refer to chapter 2, "The Building Block of E/M Coding."

Explanation of Investigation

- The "Medicare Fee-for-Service 2019 Improper Payments Report" indicates that five out of the top 10 highest improper payments are errors in assignment of E/M codes.
- Review of physician paid claims over the past decade indicates that evaluation and management code selection remains troublesome for many providers.
  - A Comprehensive Error Rate Testing (CERT) report revealed a common error involves over- or under-coding of E/M services by one level.
- CMS continues to investigate E/M services as an ongoing and preventive step in reducing over- or under-coding in the future. Specific E/M services are also cited in the OIG work plan every year.
- Nearly all medical record and claims audits include the review of E/M services.

Strategies for Risk Prevention

- Careful attention to educating clinical and administrative staff about the coding, documentation, and billing requirements associated with all E/M codes.
- Ongoing audits of E/M services and sharing results with staff. (See appendix A for sample physician E/M audit forms.)
- Continued training and educational opportunities in E/M coding.
- Designation of a clinical documentation improvement specialist to assist providers and staff in accurate and compliant documentation of patient encounters.

INITIAL PREVENTIVE PHYSICAL EXAM (IPPE)

General Guidelines

- The IPPE is a preventive evaluation and management service first allowed under section 611 of the Medicare Prescription Drug Improvement and Modernization Act (MMA) of 2003
- Considered to be an introduction to Medicare and covered benefits.
- The IPPE is not a "routine physical checkup" that seniors may receive every one to two years from their provider as Medicare does not cover routine physical exams.
- This is a one-time benefit and beneficiaries have 12 months from their effective date to receive this, as it's commonly referred to, Welcome to Medicare visit.
- Each component of the IPPE must be provided or referred to another physician in order to appropriately submit this benefit to Medicare. The IPPE face-to-face exam consists of the following seven distinct components:
  - review of patient's medical and social history
  - review the patient's potential risk factors for depression
  - review the patient's functional ability and level of safety
  - physical examination that includes height, weight, blood pressure, visual acuity, and BMI
  - end-of-life planning

– education, counseling, and referral based on the results of the review and evaluation services described above

– education, counseling, and referral, including a brief written plan or checklist, for obtaining the appropriate screening or other Part B preventive services

- Providers must use the appropriate screening tools typically used in routine physician practices and document all pertinent clinical information in the medical record, including any referrals and a medical plan.

Explanation of Investigation

- The OIG reviews claims and evaluates billing practices and payments as they relate to the initial preventive physician examination (IPPE).

- Some of the services included in the IPPE may have already been performed in a previous evaluation and management service previously reported yet the full IPPE service is billed by the provider.

- The OIG has focused on the IPPE as an area of possible fraud and abuse due to the higher reimbursement for this service and due to the likelihood that non-Medicare patients may have already received preventive services similar to those listed under the IPPE.

Strategies for Risk Prevention

- Have a well-designed compliance program in place.

- Ensure all seven components of the IPPE are provided or referred to another physician and that these preventive services were not provided before the patient became Medicare eligible.

- Refer to the CMS quick reference checklist that details the specific elements that must be documented for each of the seven components within the IPPE.

ASSIGNING NEW PATIENT E/M CODES

General Guidelines

- A new patient is defined by the American Medical Association (AMA) as a patient who is receiving face-to-face care from the provider or other qualified healthcare professional of the exact same specialty/subspecialty within the same practice for the first time in three years.

  – new patient examples include:

  — a patient sees the physician/qualified healthcare professional for the first time

  — a patient previously seen by a cardiologist 18 months prior sees an endocrinologist in the same group practice

  — a patient who has not seen the physician/qualified healthcare professional for 40 months returns complaining of abdominal pain

- Providers should not report a new patient E/M service for the same beneficiary more than once in a three-year period.

- For many of the E/M codes, correct code assignment is dependent upon whether the patient is new or established.

FOR MORE INFO

A quick reference checklist for appropriately billing the IPPE may be found at: https://www.cms.gov/Outreach-and-Education/Medicare-Learning-Network-MLN/MLNProducts/downloads/MPS_QRI_IPPE001a.pdf

---

CODING AXIOM

New patient visits typically require all three key components be met or exceeded. New patient visits frequently involve higher decision making ranges than the amount of history or exam performed. History and exam components are higher for new patients at a given level of decision making than they are for established patients at the same decision-making level. The requirement that all three components be met for new patients may mean that, on occasion, a code be assigned that is more consistent with history and exam than with medical decision making.

Explanation of Investigation

- The 2019 Medicare Improper Payment Report indicated that 18.4 percent of new patient office visits were paid erroneously resulting in $383,093,483 in improper payments.
  - This number included established patients billed with a new patient E/M code and incorrect level of new patient visits reported.

Strategies for Risk Prevention

- Ensure appropriate administrative and clinical staff members understand the guidelines for reporting new patient E/M codes.
- Perform provider and staff education.
- Develop a policy and procedure for determining patient status and include the policy as part of the compliance manual.
- Perform internal pre- and postprovider education audits to determine the prevalence, if any, of inappropriately reporting a patient's status.
- Develop a short questionnaire that the appointment clerk can use to help determine if a patient may be billed with a new patient status at the time the appointment is made.
- Use a decision tree to determine new vs. established patient status.

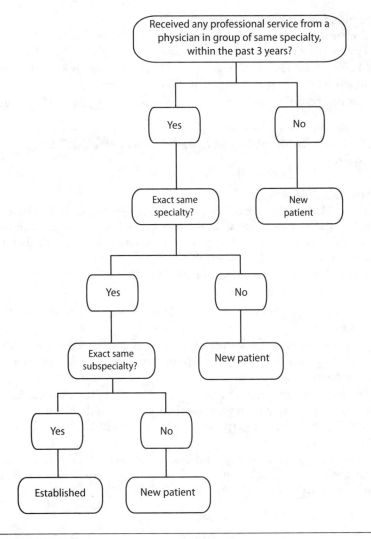

HIGH-LEVEL SUBSEQUENT NURSING FACILITY CARE CODES

General Guidelines
- Codes 99309–99310 represent per day, subsequent nursing facility care that requires a detailed to comprehensive history, detailed to comprehensive exam, and/or moderate to high complexity medical decision making.
- Reporting of these codes typically indicates the patient:
  - will have developed a significant complication or significant new problem
  - be unstable
  - require immediate physician attention
- It is not appropriate to bill a higher level of evaluation and management service when a lower level of service is warranted.

Explanation of Investigation
- A prepayment review of claims reported with codes 99309 and 99310.
- On average, 44 percent of claims were reported with a higher level of care than was supported by medical record documentation.

Strategies for Risk Prevention
- Ensure all coding staff is appropriately trained in the use 1995 and/or 1997 documentation guidelines for accurate coding of E/M services.
- Ongoing audits of E/M services and sharing results with staff. (See appendix A for sample physician E/M audit forms.)
- Continued training and educational opportunities in E/M coding.

ANESTHESIA CARE PACKAGE AND BILLING E/M CODES SEPARATELY

General Guidelines
- The CMS and American Society of Anesthesiologists (ASA) base unit value (BUV) represents all of the usual anesthesia services, with the exception of the time actually spent in anesthesia care, as well as any modifying factors that may occur.
- The following are included in the BUV:
  - pre- and postoperative visits
  - administration of fluids and/or blood as incident to the anesthesia care
  - interpretation of noninvasive monitoring such as electrocardiogram, temperature, blood pressure, oximetry, capnography, and mass spectrometry
- The basic documentation requirements include the preoperative evaluation, presurgery review, patient question and answer discussion, attendance during surgery, postanesthesia care unit evaluation, and attendance, as necessary.
- Pre-anesthesia examination and evaluation include a review of the patient's past medical, family, and social history; medications; and adverse reactions to previous anesthesia.

- To bill an anesthesia service AND an E/M service, review medical record documentation to determine that the E/M service performed was a significant, separately identifiable service that was not related to the condition for which anesthesia was performed.

Explanation of Investigation

- Review of anesthesia claims to determine if E/M services have been unbundled.

Strategies for Risk Prevention

- Inform and educate providers regarding services and procedures that are considered standards of anesthesia care, including pre- and postexamination of the patient.
- Review anesthesia coding and billing guidelines with clinicians.
- Determine if any claims have been billed with both anesthesia and E/M codes.
- Review documentation for these claims to verify the medical necessity of both services.
- Educate staff on CCI edits as they pertain to anesthesia services.

CODING AXIOM

Per CCI, E/M services (99202–99499) related to the anesthesia service (i.e., pre-anesthesia examination and evaluation) are bundled into the anesthesia codes.

CRITICAL CARE AND EMERGENCY DEPARTMENT (ED) SERVICES

General Guidelines

- CMS defines critical care services as medical care directly delivered by a physician to a critically ill or injured patient.
- For a patient to be deemed critically ill or injured, the illness or injury should represent grave harm to one or more vital organ systems and thereby present a worsening of the patient's condition including a strong likelihood of death.
- CMS guidance clearly states that providers should not report both critical care services and emergency department services on the same date of service. When both services are provided, only the critical care services may be billed.
- When an inpatient hospital service or office or other outpatient service is provided to the patient who subsequently requires critical care on the same date of service, both the critical care and the E/M service may be reimbursed.
- Physicians should submit documentation to substantiate the use of critical care services and separate E/M services on the same date of service by the same physician or physicians of the same specialty in the same group practice.
- For group practices, critical care services can be provided by providers of different specialties as long as those services are not duplicated by other members of the same specialty in the same group practice.
- Providers delivering critical care services to the same patient on the same date of service representing the same specialty and group practice are required to report their services as a single provider.
- Initial critical care time reported with code 99291 must be reached by a single provider, either in a single period of time or cumulatively on the same date.
- Subsequent critical care beyond the initial time period may be reported by a single provider or multiple providers of the same specialty in the

FOR MORE INFO

To review Medicare guidance regarding the use of critical care services see *Medicare Claims Processing Manual*, Pub. 100-04, chapter 12, section 30.6.12.

same group practice in order to meet the total number of minutes required by code 99292.

Explanation of Investigation

- RAC auditors investigated whether critical care services were billed and paid when rendered to the same patient, by the same physician, on the same day as emergency department services.

- RAC auditors also sought to determine whether physicians of the same specialty, in the same group practice, were billing for services separately. By doing so, physicians would have clearly been in violation of Medicare policy that required physicians representing the same specialty and group practice to function as a single physician for the purposes of billing and reimbursement.

Strategies for Risk Prevention

- Providers and staff should be made aware of CMS policies regarding appropriate reporting of critical care services in conjunction with other evaluation and management services.

- Particular emphasis should be made to advise providers that emergency department services are not reportable with critical care services despite these codes being categorized in the E/M section of the CPT code book.

- Providers within the same group of the same specialty offering call service should be counseled as to appropriate billing of critical care codes to ensure reporting services as a single provider representing the entire group rather than individual providers as per Medicare payment policy.

- Implementing a review of services prior to billing may be one way to ensure compliance and understanding of CMS guidelines:

  - Conduct a random review of claims containing critical care services to ensure that emergency department service codes were not also inadvertently submitted for the same date of service.

  - Consider checking with the practice management vendor to determine if it is possible to program the practice management system to provide a flag or alert when critical care codes are billed on the same patient claim with the same date of service as an emergency department service code, thereby allowing billing and coding staff to make the appropriate corrections prior to claims submission.

- Upon determining that a claim containing both critical care services and an emergency department service code was paid inappropriately, take the following steps:

  - Inform the Medicare administrative contractor (MAC) that processed the claim of the error.

  - Remit payment for the incorrectly paid ED service.

    — appropriate adjustments should be made in the practice management system

  - Ensure appropriate education is provided to staff members responsible for submitting the claim.

  - Proactively run a report to identify claims submitted with both critical care codes and ED codes to identify any further outstanding claims.

    — if more claims have been submitted, contact the MAC to see if the claims can be denied or pended for a corrected claim

— Discuss all identified claims with providers and staff.

— Implement a review of claims containing critical care services prior to billing.

OBSERVATION SERVICES

General Guidelines

- Patients are admitted to observation status in order for the provider to evaluate their condition and make the decision as to whether inpatient admission is required.

- Observation status does not require a designated area of the hospital; in fact many hospitals do not have separate areas for observation patients.

- Observation care less than eight hours is reported with a code from the Initial observation care code range 99218–99220.

- Observation care greater than eight hours but less than 24 hours with discharge on the same date of service is reported with a code from the observation and inpatient care services code range 99234–99236.

- Observation care provided to a patient admitted on one day and discharged on a different date is provided with a code from the Initial observation care code range 99218–99220 and the observation care discharge code 99217.

- When the physician who admitted the patient to observation care services subsequently admits the patient to inpatient status prior to the end of the date on which the patient was assigned to observation status, report the appropriate initial inpatient hospital visit code.

- Do not report observation care codes and initial inpatient hospital visit codes on the same date of service.

Explanation of Investigation

- RACs are focusing efforts on determining whether there was overlap or duplication between the use of observation codes and other E/M services. They are determining:

  — whether providers were billing observation care codes on the same date of service that a patient had also been admitted to the hospital as an inpatient

  — whether providers were reporting other E/M codes for services that totaled less than eight hours rather than an observation code

- RACs are evaluating the coding of observation services to ensure the appropriate codes are being reported based on the documentation in the patient's medical record. This includes issues such as the amount of time the patient is under care would dictate which E/M code(s) should be reported.

- Other areas under consideration involve occasions when the provider who admitted the patient to observation care subsequently decided to admit the patient to an inpatient status prior to the end of the date of service on which the patient began observation care. Initial inpatient hospital care codes include ALL E/M services provided to the patient on the day of admission regardless of the site of service.

Strategies for Risk Prevention

- Ensure that all providers and staff have been trained and educated on the Medicare policies regarding observation care and provide ongoing education as necessary.
- Include the Medicare Internet Only Manual (IOM) resource documents, RAC information, transmittals, and *Medicare Learning Network (MLN)* articles pertaining to the appropriate use of observation codes in the office policy and procedure manual.
- Create a flow chart or matrix to help physicians and nonphysician providers (NPP) easily ascertain which observation care service codes should be reported under the various circumstances.
- Conduct periodic, random sampling reviews of observation claims to ensure compliance with carrier policies.
  - Use patient information taken from the scheduling staff or the medical assistant/nurse to track those patients who have been seen in the ED, hospital, and other facilities.
    - If this is not currently being done, enact a policy and assign a staff member to maintain records on patients seen in the ED, hospital, and/or ambulatory surgery centers. This can be a simple document that lists:
      - patient's name
      - DOB
      - date of admission
      - status (IP, OP/OBS, ED)
      - date of discharge
      - procedures performed with CPT code
      - any hospital visits with CPT code or level of service identified
      - ICD-10-CM codes
- Advise providers to state clearly in placement orders "admit to inpatient" or "admit to observation status" to avoid any ambiguity.
- Also indicate where the patient was treated when the providers use more than one facility. Maintaining such patient records helps create a "checks and balances" system.
- Regardless of the process (manual tracking system or a report pulled from the practice management system), a review of observation care codes should be periodically conducted and claims monitored for appropriate coding.
- Avoid the use of standing orders for observation after an outpatient surgery or procedure as this is not considered appropriate use of observation services.
- Review Medicare-provided clarification regarding the use of hours for routine postsurgery/procedure care classified as recovery room hours.
  - Observation care services should only be used after a procedure when/if the care is no longer routine and the physician is deciding whether the patient would benefit from inpatient status.

PULMONARY DIAGNOSTIC PROCEDURES WITH E/M SERVICES

General Guidelines

- The *National Correct Coding Initiative Policy Manual*, chapter 11, section J.2 states that if "the physician in attendance during the course of a pulmonary function study obtains a limited history and performs a limited physical examination related to the pulmonary function testing, it is *not* appropriate to report a separate E/M service as this would be considered part of the service." Clearly, an unrelated E/M service performed can and should be reported separately with modifier 25 appended.

- Documentation for the E/M service must meet the requirements for the appropriate level selected and should be unrelated to the pulmonary diagnostic procedure performed.

- Laboratory procedures performed during the course of diagnostic pulmonary testing, as well as the provider's interpretation of results from those laboratory services, is included in the description of those codes.

  - It would not be appropriate to further factor in the results from those tests during the medical decision making process when the lab services were both ordered and performed by the same provider.

  - Note that in the event the lab services were performed at a different laboratory and the results were then delivered to the treating provider, any information obtained as a result of reviewing the laboratory values could be used as a determining factor while deciding the level of medical decision making.

Explanation of Investigation

- Recovery audit contractors initiated an automated review to identify overpayments associated with E/M services billed without modifier 25 on the same date of service as a pulmonary diagnostic procedure reported with CPT codes 94010–94799.

Strategies for Risk Prevention

- Identify all billed services in code range 94010–94799.

  - If the practice management system being used permits, runs a report that also identifies additional services billed with the aforementioned code range, particularly E/M service codes 99211–99215.

  - Note whether modifier 25 was appended to the E/M service.

  - Review the medical record documentation supporting the medical necessity of the two services for accuracy and appropriateness.

  - Ensure that any E/M service reported with the pulmonary diagnostic procedure is separate and distinct.

- Updates to the *National Correct Coding Initiative Policy Manual* should be downloaded quarterly.

  - Ensure the updates have been reviewed by all staff members each quarter.

  - Specific policies that relate to the specialty of the practice, such as those relating to pulmonary services should be printed and all staff members should sign off on that policy indicating an understanding of, and agreement to comply with, the guidelines.

 – Designate a specific individual, perhaps a coding or billing representative, to check for updates to the *National Correct Coding Initiative Policy Manual* and ensure each staff member has been made aware of any new versions released.

 – Some of the commercial payers with which the practice is in network may have specific language within the contract or terms that does not permit an E/M service on the same date as a pulmonary diagnostic procedure, regardless of whether modifier 25 was appended. Always know which contracts the provider is under and the terms of those contracts. In addition, determine the circumstances as to when an E/M service can be reported in conjunction with this type of procedure.

• Verify the patient's insurance coverage prior to the procedure being performed and determine the circumstances as to when an E/M service can be reported in conjunction with diagnostic pulmonary procedures.

• Ensure that policies are enacted and implemented regarding appropriate use of modifier 25 for an E/M billed in conjunction with diagnostic pulmonary procedures.

KNOWLEDGE ASSESSMENT CHAPTER 18

See chapter 19 for answers and rationale.

1. Out of the following, which are considered part of a global surgery package?
   a. Postoperative visits
   b. Postsurgical pain management
   c. Preoperative visits
   d. All postoperative complications not requiring a return to the operating room
   e. All of the above

2. Where is Medicare's official list of the number of postoperative days included in each surgical procedure found?
   a. *Medicare Claims Processing Manual*
   b. Medicare Physician Fee Schedule Database
   c. *Medicare Program Integrity Manual*
   d. National Correct Coding Initiative

3. Preoperative visits for major procedures begin the day before a major procedure.
   a. True
   b. False

4. How many distinct components must be provided or referred to another physician, in order to bill for Medicare's initial preventive physician examination (IPPE)?
   a. Four
   b. Seven
   c. The number varies based on preventive services already provided to the patient
   d. 10

5. How should providers delivering critical care services to the same patient on the same date of service representing the same specialty and group practice report their services?

    a. As a single provider

    b. One provider would report 99291 and the other providers would report 99292 for each additional 30 minutes of critical care time provided

    c. Each provider reports services separately

    d. None of the above

6. When a patient is admitted under observation status but before the end of the day is subsequently admitted as an inpatient, what category of code(s) is used?

    a. Office/outpatient code

    b. Inpatient code only

    c. Observation code only

    d. Both an inpatient code and observation code

Chapter 19: Knowledge Assessments with Answers

CHAPTER 1 QUESTIONS AND ANSWERS

1. What are the methods of documentation mentioned?
   a. Subjective, Objective, Assessment, Plan (SOAP) format
   b. Subjective, Nature of presenting problem, Objective, Counseling and/or coordination of care, Assessment, Medical decision making, and Plan (SNOCAMP)
   c. Who, What, When, Where, Why, and How (5 W and H) format
   d. <u>Both a and b</u>

   Rationale: See chapter 3 for more information on these two formats.

2. How is using a documentation method beneficial?
   a. Using a standardized documentation format expedites the revenue cycle process
   b. Using a standardized documentation format ensures a lower medical malpractice premium
   c. <u>Using a standardized documentation format can help decrease audit liability</u>
   d. Using a standardized documentation format has not been proven to be beneficial

   Rationale: Standardized documentation formats not only decrease audit liability by consistently and uniformly establishing medical necessity and ensuring that all of the appropriate elements are documented but they also help to promote continuity of care and quality of care. When all elements are regularly and reliably documented, the likelihood of omissions and errors greatly diminish and, furthermore, clinicians become more confident and comfortable in their documentation. More detailed, consistent, thorough documentation ensures more appropriate, accurate, and timely billing.

3. What are the primary differences between the 1995 and the 1997 documentation guidelines?
   a. There are no differences
   b. The 1995 guidelines do not outline history requirements and the 1997 history component is well defined
   c. <u>The 1997 guidelines use a detailed bullet point format for exam and the 1995 focuses on body areas and organ systems</u>
   d. The decision making for 1997 is determined solely on the table of risk

   Rationale: The 1995 guidelines are more generous in the requirements for documenting an exam component. The 1997 guidelines require a more detailed/bullet point approach to documenting the exam.

4. Why are E/M services considered the dominant source of revenue for most providers?
   a. <u>They are among the most frequently billed services</u>
   b. They have high reimbursement values
   c. Providers can bill all high levels of care
   d. These services are not monitored

   Rationale: Although the reimbursement amount for E/M services is considered relatively low in comparison to surgical services, the volume of E/M services performed makes them a significant source of revenue for most providers.

5. What can providers use to assess overall coding patterns?
   a. Reimbursement rates from payers
   b. Coder productivity
   c. Payer requests for documentation
   d. <u>Benchmark data</u>

   Rationale: Using E/M benchmark data can help providers analyze patterns of use for specific E/M codes.

6. Which modifier should be reported to indicate to a payer that service was provided via synchronous telemedicine?
   a. 25
   b. 57
   c. <u>95</u>
   d. 97

   Rationale: CPT modifier 95, effective January 1, 2017, is to be appended to certain CPT codes designated as synchronous telemedicine services, identified in the CPT book with a star symbol [★]. A list of applicable CPT codes for reporting real time telehealth services with modifier 95 can be found in appendix P of the CPT book.

CHAPTER 2 QUESTIONS AND ANSWERS

1. History, exam, and medical decision making are the key components in an E/M service?
   a. <u>True</u>
   b. False

   Rationale: There are seven components: history, examination, medical decision making, counseling, coordination of care, nature of presenting problem, and time; six of which are used to define levels of E/M service. The first three are considered the key components in selecting a level of E/M service.

2. Time is connected only to counseling and coordination of care and is not the only consideration in code selection.
   a. <u>True</u>
   b. False

   Rationale: In cases where counseling and coordination of care dominate more than half of the face-to-face time in the office or other outpatient setting with the patient and/or family, then time is considered to be the key or controlling factor in qualifying for a particular level of E/M service. The amount of time spent in counseling and coordination of care must be thoroughly and clearly documented in the patient's medical record.

3. Why is the medical decision making component so important?
    a. The medical decision making component is the only component completed entirely by the physician or other qualified healthcare provider, alone
    b. The medical decision making component is the only key component that is required for every E/M service
    c. <u>The medical decision making component will most often determine the true complexity of the management involved. The history and exam are best viewed as supporting components in terms of work performed and documented</u>
    d. None of the above

    Rationale: Medical decision making is the one key component which represents the amount of actual work and cognitive labor exerted by the clinician and is mostly based on the number of diagnoses or management options; the amount and complexity of data to be reviewed; and risk, morbidity, and mortality.

4. When can you use time as a controlling factor for selecting the appropriate level of E/M code?
    a. <u>When the provider has spent at least 50 percent of the time counseling the patient and coordinating care</u>
    b. When the provider has spent the specified time in face-to-face contact with the patient
    c. When the provider has documented that face-to-face counseling was provided to the patient
    d. When the provider documents 100 percent of the time spent with the patient and that some counseling was given

    Rationale: Time is considered the key or controlling factor in selecting the level of E/M service when counseling and/or coordination of care represents more than 50 percent of the physician/patient and/or family encounter. This should be clearly documented in the patient record.

5. What are the areas defined in CPT guidelines that are considered counseling services?
    a. Diagnostic results, impressions, prognosis, risks and benefits, patient and family education
    b. Diagnostic results, impressions, medication list, problem list
    c. Instruction for treatment and follow-up, determination of diagnosis codes
    d. <u>Both a and c</u>

    Rationale: According to the CPT manual, the following elements are considered to be a part of counseling:
    •   Diagnostic results, impressions, and/or recommended diagnostic studies
    •   Prognosis
    •   Risks and benefits of management (treatment) options
    •   Instructions for management (treatment) and/or follow-up

- Importance of compliance with chosen management (treatment) options
- Risk factor reduction
- Patient and family education

6. Although it is not considered a key component, what role does the nature of presenting problem play in determining the level of E/M code?
   a. It determines the chief complaint
   b. <u>It helps the provider determine the amount of history, exam, and decision making required to treat the patient</u>
   c. It determines the diagnosis codes and decision making
   d. It does not factor into determining the level of E/M service

   Rationale: The nature of the presenting problem plays a critical role in determining the level of E/M code by providing documentation to support the medical necessity of the services provided.

7. Which is an example of additional information to determine ICD-10-CM code selection for the chief complaint of "my foot hurts?"
   a. What caused the pain?
   b. Do other body parts hurt?
   c. <u>Which foot?</u>
   d. Is the injury weather related?

   Rationale: In the ICD-10-CM coding system, laterality is required for proper code assignment, as shown below:
   - M79.67   Pain in foot and toes
   - M79.671   Pain in right foot
   - M79.672   Pain in left foot
   - M79.673   Pain in unspecified foot
   - M79.674   Pain in right toe(s)
   - M79.675   Pain in left toe(s)
   - M79.676   Pain in unspecified toe(s)

8. Of all the body areas/organ systems reviewed during an E/M encounter, which body system requires the greatest level of specificity in terms of documentation as it relates to ICD-10-CM?
   a. Neurological
   b. Respiratory
   c. Ears, nose, throat
   d. <u>Musculoskeletal</u>

   Rationale: The musculoskeletal system requires the most documentation in regard to specificity. The American Health Information Management Association (AHIMA) and other specialty societies note two factors that call for enhanced specificity when documenting conditions involving the musculoskeletal system. First, the musculoskeletal system contains a large number of codes because it includes both muscles and bones. Further, these codes are expanded in ICD-10-CM to accommodate laterality. The result is that the documentation for the musculoskeletal system requires significantly more specificity as compared to other body systems.

9. In the medical decision making (MDM) example seen on page 39, where a teenager with acne is also evaluated for a complaint of abdominal pain, why does the inclusion of clinical detail required for ICD-10-CM diagnosis assignment raise the MDM level potential from low to moderate?

    a. Acne is always a very serious medical condition

    b. Seeing the patient for acne and abdominal pain is very unusual

    c. Most E/M services require moderate decision making

    d. <u>The abdominal pain complaint required additional clinical detail</u>

    Rationale: Abdominal pain is the new problem while acne was the established problem. The new problem of abdominal pain gives the provider additional credit in medical decision making in addition to any further testing ordered to confirm the diagnosis. Future testing or additional prescriptions will also increase the medical decision making potential.

CHAPTER 3 QUESTIONS AND ANSWERS

1. Abbreviations can have multiple meanings and can confuse those who need to review the medical record documentation.

    a. <u>True</u>

    b. False

    Rationale: From a medico-legal standpoint, it is extremely important to have standardization in the use of abbreviations in medical records. Everyone who accesses the patient's record, from the clinicians to clinical staff, coders and even to auditors, must come to the same conclusion when reading an abbreviation to ensure that everyone infers the same meaning from the abbreviations used. Without consistency and uniformity, patient care and the meaning of what happened with the patient is compromised.

2. Why is legibility a key requirement of documentation?

    a. Patient care and treatment may be delayed and/or compromised

    b. <u>If the handwriting of the provider cannot be read, Medicare auditors, as well as other payers, consider the service as not billable or reimbursable</u>

    c. Legibility is not a key requirement of documentation at the present time

    d. None of the above

    Rationale: In a similar way to abbreviations, it is imperative for the provider's handwriting to be legible in order to correctly interpret the information in the patient's record. This is vitally important from a billing and reimbursement standpoint but also from a quality of care and continuity of care standpoint.

3. The benefits of the SOAP and SNOCAMP formats of documentation are that the SOAP format is a sequential record of how information is obtained, analyzed, and acted upon during the encounter and the "N" in the SNOCAMP format provides a place to document the nature of the presenting problem, which most often drives the depth of the components within the SOAP format.
   a. <u>True</u>
   b. False

   Rationale: See chapter 3 for more information on the benefits of these two formats.

4. Define over-coding and under-documenting.
   a. Over-coding is selecting the same code for every encounter and under-documenting is not completing a template
   b. Over-coding is selecting the highest code for every encounter and under-documenting is completing only the exam and decision making portions
   c. <u>Over-coding is reporting a higher level code than documented and under-documenting is having a lower level of history and exam than decision making</u>
   d. Over-coding is reporting a code based solely on the history and exam components and under-documenting is reporting a code based solely on the decision making

   Rationale: Government regulators define a service that is not supported by documentation as "over-coded." However, if the level of decision making generally points toward the correct code level and is supported in the medical record, then it is the history or exam or both that fail to support that level of service based on the code type. The encounter is more accurately described as "under-documented."

5. What is a common reason a provider might over-document an encounter?
   a. <u>Using a template as a documentation mandate and completing all fields regardless of the presenting problem and misinterpretation of the Table of Risk</u>
   b. Using a template as a prompter to record the history and exam completed
   c. Using nursing and ancillary staff as scribes
   d. Using the Table of Risk for the final level of E/M service

   Rationale: Providers that have not been properly trained in the use of EHR templates may consider the list of check boxes to be mandatory documentation requirements rather than prompts. Misinterpretation of the table of risk can also cause providers to unintentionally increase the level of medical decision making.

6. What is an advantage to using templates with an electronic health record?
   a. Templates are used to document all necessary elements for a specific level of E/M service
   b <u>Templates help provide consistent format and tools for electronic documentation</u>
   c. Templates allow other staff to fill in blank data
   d. Templates are mandated by the EHR legislation

   Rationale: Templates serve as documentation prompts and do not mandate specific elements of history, exam, or testing. Documentation should reflect the provider's history, exam, and decision making based on the patient's presenting problems. A template should never be used to direct a provider to a specific level of E/M.

7. Why should billing patterns be evaluated after implementing an EHR?
   a. To penalize providers not using an EHR
   b. <u>To verify any shift in coding patterns</u>
   c. To keep the coders busy
   d. Both a and b

   Rationale: One of the largest concerns when adopting an EHR system, especially one with an encoder, is that the level of services reported suddenly increases. This can be due to a misunderstanding of how to use a template and providers feeling that they need to complete every check box or blank on the template.

CHAPTER 4 QUESTIONS AND ANSWERS

1. Medical necessity is a critical element to medical record documentation because without it claims may be rejected or outright denied.
   a. <u>True</u>
   b. False

   Rationale: Section 1862(a)(1)(A) of the Social Security Act states that Medicare will not cover services that "are not reasonable and necessary for the diagnosis or treatment of illness or injury or to improve the functioning of a malformed body member."

   In addition, the CMS Pub. 100-04, *Medicare Claims Processing Manual* says that medical necessity is the "overarching criterion for payment in addition to the individual requirements of a CPT code. It would not be medically necessary or appropriate to bill a higher level of evaluation and management service when a lower level of service is warranted. The volume of documentation should not be the primary influence upon which a specific level of service is billed. Documentation should support the level of service reported."

   Simply put, medical necessity becomes the main factor considered during an audit or claim review, even over the history, examination, and medical decision making. Therefore, a claim determined to be lacking in medical necessity may end up rejected or denied and subsequently not paid.

2. What is the description of "incident-to" services?
    a. Services provided by auxiliary personnel of a facility for a physician
    b. Services provided by a nurse practitioner using their own provider identification number
    c. <u>Services provided by auxiliary personal under the supervision of and billed by the physician</u>
    d. Services provided directly by the physician for secondary conditions

    Rationale: Incident-to services and supplies are furnished as an integral, although incidental, part of the physician's personal professional services in the course of diagnosis or treatment of an illness or injury. Auxiliary personnel performing these services must be employed by the physician or clinic and services must be performed under the direct supervision of the physician and billed by the physician.

3. Where is the best place to find what set of documentation guidelines private payers are using?
    a. In the office or practice's policy and procedure manual.
    b. Within the contract itself.
    c. <u>In the provider's manual issued by your third-party payers.</u>
    d. None of the above

    Rationale: The provider manual may be a hard copy version or an online version. When this information is not readily available, the practice staff should request the payer to specify, in writing, which set of documentation guidelines are used for audits and reviews.

4. What are the advantages to learning only one set of documentation guidelines?
    a. The practice may not always know what coverage is in effect for a given service and who secondary payers might be
    b. It can be very difficult for providers to remember different sets of rules for different payers
    c. There really are no distinct advantages; it is better to learn both sets of guidelines thoroughly
    d. <u>Both a and b</u>

    Rationale: Focusing on learning one set of documentation guidelines ensures that the practice has consistency in the documentation process and permits staff and clinicians to learn, understand and apply the concepts from the single set of guidelines uniformly and regularly.

5. What are the disadvantages of using documentation templates?
    a. They can be abused by providing "stock" or comprehensive prerecorded, histories or exams
    b. No disadvantages; they are designed to replace provider work
    c. May not be used solely as a prompt to document elements performed
    d. <u>Both a and c</u>

    Rationale: See rationale for question 5 in chapter 18.

6. The teaching physician does not need to be present for the key portion of an encounter if the resident relays all pertinent information in chart notes.
   a. True
   b. <u>False</u>

   Rationale: Guidelines state that in order for teaching physicians to bill for services, they must be present during the key portion of the exam and document appropriately.

7. Which of the following is acceptable teaching physician documentation?
   a. Seen and agreed
   b. No changes
   c. <u>Patient evaluated, care plan reviewed with resident and agreed with findings, no additional changes</u>
   d. Signature and date

   Rationale: Teaching physician documentation does not need to restate the resident notes but it must demonstrate that the teaching physician has seen the patient, reviewed the care plan with the resident, including changes to treatment, testing, and medications, and agreed with the findings.

8. What is the responsibility of the teaching physician in a primary care exception program?
   a. Supervise residents in providing all E/M services
   b. <u>Supervise up to four residents providing primary responsibility for the patient's care and review each case with the resident during or immediately after the encounter</u>
   c. Have a full schedule of patients concurrent with the residents
   d. Cosign all resident notes

   Rationale: See complete guidelines under the subheading "Exception: E/M Services Furnished in Certain Primary Care Centers" in chapter 4.

9. What is conveyed with modifier GC?
   a. The teaching physician completed the service without resident participation
   b. <u>The teaching physician and the resident provided the service</u>
   c. The resident provided the service under the primary care exception
   d. The resident acted as scribe for the teaching physician

   Rationale: Modifier GC, (this service has been performed, in part, by a resident under the direction of a teaching physician), is to be reported with all services provided by a teaching physician except in circumstances where modifier GE, which certifies that the physician was present during the key portion of the service and was immediately available during the other parts of the services, is applicable.

10. What special criteria must a teaching physician utilize for psychiatric services?
    a. <u>The resident service is concurrently monitored using one-way mirrors or video equipment and audio transmission</u>
    b. The teaching physician records the audio transmission for review
    c. The teaching physician is not required to participate in the service due to patient privacy
    d. The teaching physician is only required to review medication changes

Rationale: For psychiatry services furnished under an approved GME program, the requirement that the teaching physician be present during the service may be met by concurrent observation of the service using one-way mirror or video equipment. Audio-only equipment does not suffice.

CHAPTER 5 QUESTIONS AND ANSWERS

1. History and physical examination elements are no longer used in selection of the level of office or other outpatient visit and therefore don't have to be documented in the medical record.
   a. True
   b. <u>False</u>

   Rationale: These elements must still be documented for continuity of patient care. The change based on the new guideline is that they will no longer be factors in code level selection for office or other outpatient E/M services. The nature and extent of history and physical examination is determined by the treating provider and per CMS must be "medically appropriate."

2. Total time on the date of the encounter includes non-face-to-face time. Which of the following activities personally performed by the treating provider may count toward the total time reported for purposes of code level selection? Select all that apply.
   a. <u>Reviewing tests or other records</u>
   b. <u>Documenting clinical information in the medical record</u>
   c. <u>Ordering tests/procedures or medications</u>
   d. <u>Counseling and educating the patient or caregiver</u>

   Rationale: Per the 2021 CPT guidelines, all of these count toward the total time personally spent by the provider on the date of the encounter. Refer to the General Guidelines sections in Chapter 5 for the complete list.

3. Based on the time documented at the end of the sample documentation for 99205 that starts on page 114, code 99205 could be reported based on time alone.
   a. <u>True</u>
   b. False

   Rationale: In the sample, a total of 70 minutes is documented. The new time range listed in the code descriptor for 99205 is 60–74 minutes.

4. A new patient presents to the office with two stable chronic illnesses. Limited data is reviewed, and changes are made to the patient's prescription drug regimen. Based on MDM elements, what level of service would be reported?

    a. 99203

    b. <u>99204</u>

    c. 99214

    d. 99205

    Rationale: Levels of MDM, based on the redefined table published by the AMA and adopted by CMS, are based on two out of three elements. In this example, there is moderate complexity of problems (two stable chronic illnesses), limited data reviewed, and moderate risk based on the prescription drug management. Two out of three elements of MDM are moderate, which equates to a moderate level of MDM or a level four.

CHAPTER 6 QUESTIONS AND ANSWERS

1. Based on the sample documentation for code 99219 on page 138, what is the chief complaint?

    a. <u>Left-sided renal colic</u>

    b. Hypercalcemic stone

    c. Hyperparathyroidism

    d. All of the above

    Rationale: The patient was admitted for sudden onset of left-sided renal colic. The documentation must always include a chief complaint (the symptoms or condition that precipitated the visit).

2. Based on the sample documentation for code 99219 on page 138, what level of MDM was documented?

    a. Minimal

    b. Low

    c. <u>Moderate</u>

    d. High

    Rationale: Patient has an acute illness with systemic symptoms, multiple labs and a KUB were ordered and reviewed, and the patient was given IV fluids with additives. All of these quantify the visit as moderate MDM.

3. What elements pertaining to the MDM in the sample documentation starting on page 148 qualify the visit as a 99226 or high MDM?

    a. Numerous diagnoses

    b. Extensive amount of data reviewed

    c. New problem—chest pain

    d. <u>All of the above</u>

    Rationale: All of the factors listed above give a clear picture of the patient's health and are vital in treating the patient. The management of several chronic conditions, the new onset of chest pain, and an extensive medical history collectively point to high complexity MDM.

4. Documentation for a level 2 initial hospital visit (99222) requires a complete ROS. How many systems must be reviewed?
   a. Eight or more
   b. <u>Ten or more</u>
   c. Depends on what physician is documenting the visit
   d. Four or more

   Rationale: See chapter 2 for more information on ROS requirements.

5. Based on the sample documentation for 99222 on page 155, what statement did the physician use to document that enough systems were reviewed to qualify as a complete ROS?

   <u>All systems reviewed and are otherwise within normal limits</u>

   Rationale: The 1995 and 1997 E/M guidelines state that "in the absence of a notation for each of ten systems, a notation of otherwise normal or negative is sufficient." Therefore, if all pertinent positive systems are specified and the other systems are reviewed a notation of 'all other ROS negative'."

6. Codes 99234–99236 are used to report E/M services provided to an observation patient or inpatient admitted and discharged on the same day.
   a. <u>True</u>
   b. False

   Rationale: See the general guidelines section in chapter 6 for "Subsequent Hospital Care and Hospital Discharge Services (99231–99239)" for more information on this code range.

7. Based on the first documentation sample for 99233 on page 167 and using the Table of Risk provided with the 1995 and 1997 E/M documentation guidelines in appendix C or D, what elements were documented that qualify this visit as high complexity MDM? (Select all that apply.)
   a. Moderate discomfort
   b. Pain does not change with position
   c. <u>New onset of chest pain with associated symptoms</u>
   d. <u>Starting a heparin drip</u>

   Rationale: Using the Table of Risk, new onset of chest pain after suffering a subendocardial MI four days earlier, qualifies as a high-risk presenting problem, acute illness that poses a threat to life or bodily function. The physician ordered a heparin drip, which qualifies as a high-risk management option, drug therapy requiring intensive monitoring for toxicity.

CHAPTER 7 QUESTIONS AND ANSWERS

1. Which of the following are appropriate places of service for use of office or other outpatient consultation codes (99241–99245)?
    a. <u>Physician office</u>
    b. <u>Patient's home</u>
    c. Hospital inpatient
    d. <u>Emergency department</u>

    Rationale: In addition to the above places of service, these may also be performed in outpatient or other ambulatory facilities, a hospital observation unit, rest home, or custodial care facility.

2. Codes 99241–99255 may be used to report consults initiated by a physician or the patient themselves.
    a. True
    b. <u>False</u>

    Rationale: Consults cannot be initiated by the patient, they must be requested by a physician who is seeking the opinion or advice of another physician regarding a specific problem.

3. Medicare no longer recognizes consultation codes but they are still used and reimbursable by some carriers.
    a. <u>True</u>
    b. False

    Rationale: Although Medicare no longer recognizes 99241–99255 as viable codes, other carriers may still reimburse for these codes. Check with the specific carrier to determine use.

4. Based on the documentation for code 99243 on page 184, which data element qualifies the PFSH as pertinent?
    a. Periodically evaluated for retinopathy
    b. <u>Diabetes was diagnosed at age 12</u>
    c. The patient is not hypertensive
    d. She has had no vision changes or problems

    Rationale: A pertinent PFSH requires only one element from past, family or social history to be reviewed and documented. The statement that the patient's diabetes was diagnosed at age 12 qualifies as past medical history and meets this requirement.

5. Select the HPI elements documented in the coding sample on page 196.
    a. <u>Duration</u>
    b. Severity
    c. <u>Modifying factors</u>
    d. Context

    Rationale: The consulting physician is only treating the anemia—not the fall. The applicable HPI in this case would be duration of three years, and modifying factors since the patient receives monthly B12 injections to control the anemia.

CHAPTER 8 QUESTIONS AND ANSWERS

1. To qualify as an emergency department service, the encounter must be performed in a hospital-based facility that is open 24 hours a day.
   a. <u>True</u>
   b. False

   Rationale: Per the guidelines, the service must be provided in a hospital-based facility open 24 hours a day and is reported regardless if the patient is new or established.

2. Both 99283 and 99284 require moderate MDM. From an MDM standpoint, what distinguishes these two codes from one another?
   a. Amount of history reviewed
   b. Number of diagnoses
   c. How long the person has had the problem
   d. <u>Problem severity or urgency</u>

   Rationale: Problem severity distinguishes these two codes. Code 99283 addresses problems of moderate severity or moderate risk of morbidity or mortality, while 99284 addresses problems of high severity or high risk of morbidity or mortality.

3. What code would be reported when a physician or other qualified health professional at the hospital is in two-way communication with rescue workers on site at a major traffic accident?
   a. This is not a billable service
   b. <u>99288</u>
   c. 99285
   d. 99291

   Rationale: Although 99288 is a valid code, typically these communications are bundled in to the emergency department physicians E/M service and are not separately reported.

4. The physician documented that 75 minutes was spent monitoring a critical patient who was given fluids and pressors after becoming hypoxic and hypotensive. What critical care code(s) would be reported?
   a. <u>99291 and 99292</u>
   b. 99291
   c. 99292
   d. 99291, 99292 x 2

   Rationale: Using the table for critical services provided in this chapter, the table indicates that 75 to 104 minutes of critical-care time would be reported with 99291x1 and 99292x1.

5. When additional procedures are performed by the same physician on the same date as critical care services, the time spent performing the additional procedures is counted toward the total critical-care time.
   a. True
   b. <u>False</u>

   Rationale: Per the *Medicare Claims Processing Manual*, Pub. 100-04, chapter 12, 30.6.12, time spent performing procedures not bundled in to the critical care service may not be factored into the total critical care time.

6. What code is assigned for 25 minutes of total critical-care time?
   a. 99291
   b. 99292
   c. Not reportable
   d. <u>Another appropriate level of E/M but not a critical-care code</u>

   Rationale: Guidelines in the *Medicare Claims Processing Manual*, Pub. 100-04, state that a minimum of 30 minutes must be spent providing critical care services in order to report a critical care code. If at least 15 minutes but less than 30 minutes of critical care services are provided, another appropriate level of E/M service may be reported. Critical care services of less than 15 minutes are not reported separately.

CHAPTER 9 QUESTIONS AND ANSWERS

1. What level of history and exam are required to report 99305 or 99306?
   a. Detailed
   b. Detailed or comprehensive
   c. <u>Comprehensive</u>
   d. Expanded problem focused

   Rationale: The differentiating factor between these two codes is the problem severity or level of MDM. Code 99305 requires moderate complexity MDM concerning a problem of moderate severity and 99306 requires high complexity MDM concerning a problem of high severity.

2. It is acceptable for a physician assistant to perform the initial nursing facility encounter as long as the physician reviews and signs the medical record.
   a. True
   b. <u>False</u>

   Rationale: Per the guidelines, the physician must perform the first assessment in the nursing facility.

3. Based on the sample documentation for a 99304 on page 234, which of the following organ systems was not examined by the physician?
   a. Genitourinary
   b. Eyes
   c. <u>Lymphatic</u>
   d. Cardiovascular

   Rationale: The organ systems examined include; constitutional, eyes, ENT, respiratory, cardiovascular, gastrointestinal, musculoskeletal, integumentary, neurological, and GU. Although the documentation states the GU exam was deferred, a rectal exam was performed, which qualifies as a GU exam.

4. What code would be assigned when the physician documents a subsequent nursing facility visit where the physician spent 25 minutes with the patient and 15 of those minutes was spent counseling the patient on a recent hip fracture and depressive symptoms as a result of being in a nursing home?
   a. <u>99309</u>
   b. 99304
   c. 99315
   d. 99308

   Rationale: Since time was documented and more than 50 percent of the encounter was spent in counseling the patient, this service was billed based on time. See chapter 2 for more information on using time to determine the level service.

5. Code 99318 is a subsequent care code. How many of the key components must be documented in order to bill 99318 for an annual nursing facility assessment?
   a. Two out of three
   b. None—this is a time-based code
   c. Only the physical exam
   d. <u>All three must be documented</u>

   Rationale: Subsequent care codes and established patient codes typically require only two out of three key components. However, 99318 is the exception to this and requires that all three key components be documented in order to determine correct code assignment.

6. What code is reported when a detailed history and exam with low complexity MDM are documented for a new patient in an assisted living facility?
   a. 99324
   b. <u>99325</u>
   c. 99326
   d. 99327

   Rationale: Code 99325 requires an expanded problem focused history and exam and low complexity MDM. Although the history and exam were detailed, medical decision making of low complexity kept this at a 99325. Moderate complexity MDM would have quantified this is a 99326.

7. Codes 99339 and 99340 are used to report care plan oversight services for patients using home health or in a nursing facility.
   a. True
   b. <u>False</u>

   Rationale: Care plan oversight for these places of service should be reported with codes 99374–99380.

CHAPTER 10 QUESTIONS AND ANSWERS

1. What codes are used to report new patient encounters in the patient's home?
   a. <u>99341–99345</u>
   b. 99241–99245
   c. 99347–99350
   d. 99202–99205

   Rationale: Codes 99341–993445 are used to report new patient encounters and codes 99347–99350 are used to report established patient encounters.

2. What home services code would be assigned for an established patient with a comprehensive history and exam and moderate MDM?
   a. 99349
   b. <u>99350</u>
   c. 99344
   d. None of the above

   Rationale: Code 99350 would also be reported if the above scenario involved high complexity MDM.

3. What modifier should be appended to codes 99341–99350 when services were mandated by a court order?
   a. 25
   b. 52
   c. 59
   d. <u>32</u>

   Rationale: Modifier 32 is appended to a service formally ordered by a court or other superior official.

4. Based on the 1995 E/M documentation guidelines, how many organ systems must be examined in order to bill a 99350?
   a. At least two
   b. <u>Eight or more</u>
   c. Ten or more
   d. Two to four

   Rationale: Code 99350 requires a comprehensive examination, based on the 1995 guidelines eight or more organ systems must be examined. See appendix C for more information on the 1995 E/M guidelines .

5. What home services code would be assigned for a new patient with moderate MDM, a comprehensive history, and a detailed physical examination?
   a. 99344
   b. <u>99343</u>
   c. 99349
   d. None of the above

Rationale: When assigning a new patient code all three key components must meet or exceed the level of service specified in the guidelines. See the Quick Comparison Table for Home Services–New Patient on page 255 for details. In this case, a comprehensive history was performed but only a detailed examination; therefore, the correct code is 99343. Since both 99343 and 99344 require moderate complexity MDM, if a comprehensive examination was warranted and documented, the service may have coded out to the higher level, 99344.

CHAPTER 11 QUESTIONS AND ANSWERS

1. When coding prolonged services, what major element out of the following is the determining factor for when to use 99354–99357 vs. 99358–99359?
   a. New vs. established
   b. Office or outpatient facility
   c. <u>With or without direct patient contact</u>
   d. All of the above

Rationale: A close look at these code ranges in this chapter and in the CPT book include "direct" or "without direct" patient contact in the description and should be the first consideration when assigning the correct code for these services.

2. Codes 99354, 99356, and 99358 may only be used once per date of service.
   a. <u>True</u>
   b. False

Rationale: These codes constitute the first 30 to 74 minutes of prolonged service time and may only be billed once for a given date of service. Codes 99355, 99357, and 99359 report each additional 30 minutes and may be billed as many times as necessary to report the total amount of time spent providing prolonged services. See the documentation requirements in this chapter for more detail on properly billing these codes.

3. Codes 99354, 99355, 99356, 99357, and 99359 are all add-on codes and can be billed alone with sufficient documentation.
   a. True
   b. <u>False</u>

Rationale: Add-on codes should never be billed as stand-alone codes. They are always billed with a primary code.

4. In order to bill prolonged services 99354–99357, the total time of the encounter must exceed the basic service by at least _____ minutes.
   a. 15
   b. <u>30</u>
   c. 45
   d. 60

   Rationale: Per the E/M guidelines, prolonged services of less than 30 minutes are not reported separately.

5. To report prolonged services provided by the clinical staff (99415–99416), direct supervision by a physician is required.
   a. <u>True</u>
   b. False

   Rationale: A physician or other qualified healthcare professional must be available to provide direct supervision to the clinical staff in order to report codes 99415 and 99416. See the general guidelines section under 99415–99416 for more information.

6. A clinician may not report standby services if the standby service period ends with the standby clinician performing a global surgery package procedure.
   a. <u>True</u>
   b. False

   Rationale: If the standby period ends with the standby clinician performing a procedure that is subject to the surgical package, this code is not reported separately.

CHAPTER 12 QUESTIONS AND ANSWERS

1. How many healthcare professionals of different specialties must participate in order to bill for a medical team conference (99366–99368)?
   a. Two or more
   b. Four or more
   c. More than 10
   d. <u>Three or more</u>

   Rationale: At least three healthcare professionals of different specialties who provide direct care to the patient must participate in order to report the team conference codes. Each provider must document his or her participation and care recommendations.

2. Which of the following activities would not count toward total time when billing for care plan oversight services?
   a. Adding new information to the treatment plan
   b. <u>Discussing treatment adjustments with the patient or a caregiver</u>
   c. Revisions to the plan of care
   d. Reviewing treatment plans and lab results

   Rationale: Besides the above activities, communication with other healthcare professionals involved in the care of the patient but not employed in the same practice, would also count towards total time for care plan oversight services.

3. What is the appropriate code for a well-visit/preventive service provided to a 20-year-old established patient?
   a. 99215
   b. 99385
   c. <u>99395</u>
   d. 99396

   Rationale: The preventive service codes are based on patient age and whether the patient is new or established. New patients are billed using codes 99381–99387 and established patients are billed using codes 99391–99397.

4. To bill telephone services (99441–99443,) the following guidelines must be met. (Select all that apply.)
   a. The service cannot be within the postoperative period of a previous procedure
   b. The service cannot result in the decision to see the patient within 24 hours or the next available appointment
   c. The service must be initiated by an established patient or his or her guardian
   d. <u>All of the above</u>

   Rationale: In addition to the above, these services cannot be reported if a related E/M service has been provided within the last seven days. Bill only for the time involved in the telephone discussion. These services are not reportable if performed concurrently with other billable services.

CHAPTER 13 QUESTIONS AND ANSWERS

1. Patients from birth to 28 days of age are considered newborns when assigning codes 99460–99486.
   a. <u>True</u>
   b. False

   Rationale: By definition, a patient is considered a newborn from birth to 28 days of age.

2. What codes would be used to report physician attendance of a critically ill infant less than 24 months of age being transported to the hospital?
   a. 99485–99486
   b. <u>99466–99467</u>
   c. 99291–99292
   d. None of the above

   Rationale: Codes 99466–99467 are time-based codes and are billed for services of at least 30 minutes. Critical care services of less than 30 minutes should be reported with the appropriate outpatient visit or subsequent hospital care code. Codes 99291–99292 are used to report transport of patients older than 24 months of age.

3. What codes are used to report inpatient critical care services of a 3-year-old patient?
   a. 99291 and 99292
   b. 99468 and 99469
   c. <u>99475 and 99476</u>
   d. 99471 and 99472

   Rationale: Neonatal and pediatric inpatient critical care codes are based on the patient's age and whether the encounter is an initial or subsequent service.

4. Subsequent *intensive* critical care codes, 99478–99480, are determined based on the patient's body weight.
   a. <u>True</u>
   b. False

   Rationale: Initial intensive critical care for a patient less than 28 days old is reported with code 99477. Codes 99478–99480 for subsequent intensive critical care are selected based on the patient's weight; 99478 for weight of less than 1500 grams, 99479 for weight of 1500 to 2500 grams, and 99480 for weight of 2501 to 5000 grams.

5. What code is reported when a newborn is admitted and discharged in the hospital or birthing center on the same date of service?
   a. 99460
   b. 99461
   c. 99462
   d. <u>99463</u>

   Rationale: The official code description for 99463 states, "Initial hospital or birthing center care, per day, for evaluation and management of normal newborn infant admitted and discharged on the same date."

6. Adult critical care codes are reported based on the amount of time spent with the patient. What factors determine which neonatal or pediatric critical care code is appropriate?
   a. Type of visit (initial or subsequent)
   b. Time
   c. Patient age
   d. <u>a and c</u>

Rationale: CPT guidelines state that neonatal and pediatric critical care services are reported per day—not on the amount of face-to-face time spent with the patient. Instead, proper code selection is based on the age of the patient, as well as whether the service is considered to be an initial or subsequent visit.

CHAPTER 14 QUESTIONS AND ANSWERS

1. A patient's chart indicates that 15 minutes of chronic care management services were provided for the month. What code would be reported for this service?
   a. 99490
   b. 99487
   c. 99489
   d. <u>The service is not reportable</u>

Rationale: Chronic care management services of less than 20 minutes are not separately reported.

2. Care management services include both face-to-face and non-face-to-face time spent by clinical staff with the patient, caregiver, or other professionals and agencies involved in the patient's care.
   a. <u>True</u>
   b. False

Rationale: See the general guidelines section in this chapter for more information on appropriate use of these codes.

3. Which of the following would be included in the care plan documentation?
   a. Expected outcomes
   b. Medication management
   c. Planned interventions
   d. <u>All of the above</u>

Rationale: In addition to the above, the care plan may also include a problem list, prognosis, treatment objectives, identification of providers providing each service ordered, periodic review, and revision of the care plan as necessary.

4. Care management services may only be provided by a physician or other qualified healthcare professional.
   a. True
   b. <u>False</u>

Rationale: These services may be performed in part by other clinical staff under direction of a physician or other qualified healthcare professional.

5. There are 10 required elements listed in the description for code 99483. For this patient only eight were performed. What code should be reported for the services provided?
   a. 99483-52
   b. 99483
   c. <u>An appropriate E/M code</u>
   d. None of the above

   Rationale: Guidance regarding 99483 from the AMA states that if all elements listed in the code description are not performed or are deemed unnecessary for the patient's condition, see the appropriate E/M code.

6. Behavioral health intervention codes 99484, 99492, and 99493, may only be reported once by the same provider in a calendar month.
   a. <u>True</u>
   b. False

   Rationale: These codes may only be reported once in a calendar month.

7. A patient's chart indicates that a total of 1 hour and 30 minutes of subsequent psychiatric collaborative care management services was provided for the calendar month. Which code(s) would be reported for these services?
   a. 99492 and 99494 x 1
   b. 99493
   c. 99492 and 99493
   d. <u>99493 and 99494 x 1</u>

   Rationale: Subsequent psychiatric care services of less than 31 minutes are not reported separately, 31–75 minutes are reported with 99493, and 76–105 minutes are reported with 99493 and add-on code 99494. Code 99494 is reported with 99492 (initial services) or 99493 (subsequent services) for each additional increment of 30 minutes above the base time.

8. Psychiatric collaborative care management services are provided by a care team that includes a treating provider, a behavioral healthcare manager, and a psychiatric consultant. Which care team member reports codes 99492, 99493, and 99494 for the services provided?
   a. Behavioral healthcare manager
   b. <u>Treating provider</u>
   c. Psychiatric consultant
   d. Each provider reports their own services

   Rationale: The treating provider reports these services on behalf of the care team. In some cases, all team members may be part of the same group practice. In most situations the psychiatric consultant will be contracted directly with the treating provider to provide consultation services.

9. General behavioral health integration management services of less than 20 minutes are not reportable.
   a. <u>True</u>
   b. False

   Rationale: General BHI services of less than 20 minutes are not reported separately.

CHAPTER 15 QUESTIONS AND ANSWERS

1. Transitional care services may only be reported when a face-to-face visit by a physician or other qualified healthcare professional has been performed.
   a. <u>True</u>
   b. False

   Rationale: These codes may only be reported if at least one face-to-face visit is provided by the physician or other qualified healthcare professional. These codes are based on level of MDM and how soon after discharge the face-to-face service is provided, within the first seven days or within eight to 14 days after discharge.

2. When does the 30-day transitional care management period begin?
   a. The day after the patient is discharged from the inpatient setting
   b. <u>The day the patient is discharged from the inpatient setting</u>
   c. The day the physician performs the face-to-face visit
   d. The first Monday following discharge

   Rationale: See the general guidelines section in this chapter for more guidance on appropriate use of these codes.

3. If the physician or other qualified healthcare professional provides more than one face-to-face visit in a month, these services are included in the transitional care codes and are not separately reportable.
   a. True
   b. <u>False</u>

   Rationale: If a physician or other qualified healthcare professional provides more than one face-to-face visit in a month, the additional visits should be reported with the appropriate E/M code.

4. Transitional care management services require interactive contact with the patient or caregiver within how many business days of discharge?
   a. Seven
   b. <u>Two</u>
   c. One
   d. Five

   Rationale: CPT guidelines state that transitional care management services require a:
   - Face-to-face visit
   - Initial patient contact, and
   - Medication reconciliation within a specified period of time

   In addition, the guidelines also require "an interactive contact with the patient or caregiver, as appropriate within two business days of discharge."

5. Which of the following are acceptable methods of communication for the required interactive contact? Select all that apply.
   a. <u>Telephone</u>
   b. Mail
   c. <u>Face to face</u>
   d. <u>E-mail</u>

   Rationale: Per CPT guidelines, the interactive contact may be rendered face to face, over the phone or by other electronic means such as the internet or email.

CHAPTER 16 QUESTIONS AND ANSWERS

1. Which range of E/M codes should not be reported with 99497–99498 on the same date of service?
   a. 99202–99215
   b. 99304–99310
   c. 99381–99397
   d. <u>99475–99480</u>

   Rationale: In addition to 99475–99480, codes 99291–99292, 99468–99469, and 99471–99472 should not be reported with the advance care planning codes.

2. The physician provides active management of the patient's problems as part of the advance care planning.
   a. True
   b. <u>False</u>

   Rationale: Advance care planning does not include any active management of the patient's problems. Time used to report these codes includes only the time spent in counseling and discussion of advance care directives.

CHAPTER 17 QUESTIONS AND ANSWERS

1. What code is reported for a Medicare patient who received 30 minutes of physician supervised care plan oversight services in the calendar month under a Medicare-approved hospice program?
    a. G0181
    b. <u>G0182</u>
    c. 99378
    d. The service is not reportable

    Rationale: Physician supervision of a patient receiving complex and multidisciplinary care under a Medicare approved hospice is reimbursable when 30 minutes or more are spent within a calendar month providing these services.

2. Code G0180 for physician certification for Medicare-covered, home health services can only be reported if the patient has not received any Medicare-covered, home health services for a period of at least 31 days.
    a. True
    b. <u>False</u>

    Rationale: Certification under a home health plan of care can only be reported when the patient has not received Medicare-covered, home health services for a period of at least 60 days.

3. Medicare does not cover preventive medicine services (99381–99429); however, the agency does cover a welcome to Medicare visit or initial preventive physical exam (IPPE). What code is used to report this visit?
    a. <u>G0402</u>
    b. 99387
    c. 99397
    d. G0438

    Rationale: HCPCS Level II code G0402 is used to report the IPPE for new Medicare beneficiaries, codes G0403–G0405 are used to report the global screening EKG if performed at the time of the IPPE.

4. How do providers reporting telehealth services to Medicare administrative contractors (MAC) indicate that the service was provided via telehealth real-time telecommunication systems?
    a. Report only the G code if the word telehealth is part of the code description
    b. Append modifier GT to the G code
    c. <u>Submit using place of service (POS) code 02</u>
    d. Both b and c

    Rationale: Beginning January 1, 2018, providers submitting for telehealth services to MAC's are not required to append modifier GT to the CPT or HCPCS code. The use of telehealth POS code 02 is sufficient to certify that the reported service meets the real-time telehealth requirements. For asynchronous telehealth services continue to append modifier GQ to the appropriate G code.

5. Which of the following are approved distant site telehealth practitioners?
    a. Nurse practitioner
    b. Clinical psychologist
    c. Nurse midwife
    d. <u>All of the above</u>

    Rationale: The following list identifies approved distant site practitioners:
    *   Physician
    *   Physician assistant (PA)
    *   Nurse practitioner (NP)
    *   Clinical nurse specialist (CNS)
    *   Nurse midwife
    *   Clinical psychologist
    *   Clinical social worker
    *   Registered dietitian or nutrition professional
    *   Certified registered nurse anesthetists

6. Codes G0425–G0427 and G0406–G0408 are only used to report telehealth consultations provided to Medicare beneficiaries.
    a. <u>True</u>
    b. False

    Rationale: G codes are only accepted by Medicare.

CHAPTER 18 QUESTIONS AND ANSWERS

1. Out of the following, which are considered part of a global surgery package?
    a. Postoperative visits
    b. Postsurgical pain management
    c. Preoperative visits
    d. All postoperative complications not requiring a return to the operating room
    e. <u>All of the above</u>

    Rationale: The CMS national definition of global surgery package includes all the items listed here as well as; intraoperative services, supplies, and miscellaneous services (i.e., dressing changes, removal of packing material, local incisional wound care, etc.). To review Medicare guidelines regarding payment for hospital observation services and observation or inpatient care services" see *Medicare Claims Processing Manual*, Pub. 100-04, chapter 12, section 30.6.8.

2. Where is Medicare's official list of postoperative days included in each surgical procedure found?
   a. *Medicare Claims Processing Manual*
   b. <u>Medicare Physician Fee Schedule Database</u>
   c. *Medicare Program Integrity Manual*
   d. National Correct Coding Initiative

   Rationale: The Medicare Physician Fee Schedule Database (MPFSDB) contains the number of days included in the postoperative period of each surgical procedure.

3. Preoperative visits for major procedures begin the day before a major procedure.
   a. <u>True</u>
   b. False

   Rationale: According to CMS guidelines preoperative visits occur after the decision for surgery has been made and begin on the day prior to a major procedure (90 global days) and begin the day of surgery for minor procedures (000 or 010 global days).

4. How many distinct components must be provided or referred to another physician, in order to bill for Medicare's initial preventive physician examination (IPPE)?
   a. Four
   b. <u>Seven</u>
   c. The number varies based on preventive services already provided to the patient
   d. 10

   Rationale: The IPPE face-to-face exam consists of the following seven distinct components:

   - Review of patient's medical and social history
   - Review the patient's potential risk factors for depression
   - Review the patient's functional ability and level of safety
   - Physical examination that includes height, weight, blood pressure, visual acuity, and BMI
   - End-of-life planning
   - Education, counseling, and referral based on the results of the review and evaluation services described above
   - Education, counseling, and referral, including a brief written plan or checklist, for obtaining the appropriate screening or other Part B preventive services

5. How should providers delivering critical care services to the same patient on the same date of service representing the same specialty and group practice report their services?

   a. <u>As a single provider</u>

   b. One provider would report 99291 and the other providers would report 99292 for each additional 30 minutes of critical care time provided

   c. Each provider reports services separately

   d. None of the above

   Rationale: Medicare policy states that physicians in the same practice in the same specialty must report these claims as though they were a single physician. To review Medicare's guidance on the use of critical care services see: *Medicare Claims Processing Manual*, Pub. 100-04, chapter 12, section 30.6.12.

6. When a patient is admitted under observation status but before the end of the day is subsequently admitted as an inpatient, what category of code(s) is used?

   a. Office/outpatient code

   b. <u>Inpatient code only</u>

   c. Observation code only

   d. Both an inpatient code and observation code

   Rationale: When the physician who admitted the patient to observation care services subsequently admits the patient to inpatient status prior to the end of the date on which the patient was assigned to observation status, report the appropriate initial inpatient hospital visit code. It is not appropriate to report observation care codes and initial inpatient hospital visit codes on the same date of service.

Glossary

1995 guidelines. Guidelines for determining level and type of evaluation and management services released by the Centers for Medicare and Medicaid Services (CMS) in 1995. These guidelines define levels of history, exam, and medical decision making, and the contributing nature of counseling, coordination of care, nature of presenting problem, as well as time.

1997 guidelines. Guidelines for determining level and type of evaluation and management services released by the Centers for Medicare and Medicaid Services (CMS) in 1997. These guidelines are a more defined measure using bullet points for determining the levels of history, exam, and medical decision making, and the contributing nature of counseling, coordination of care, nature of presenting problem, as well as time.

25. CPT modifier, for use with CPT evaluation and management (E/M) codes, that identifies when the patient's condition requires a significant, separately identifiable E/M service(s) above and beyond other services provided or above and beyond the usual preoperative and postoperative care associated with the procedure that was performed on the same date of service. Medical record documentation must clearly support all necessary criteria required for use of the E/M service being reported, including identifying signs or symptoms of the condition for which the service was rendered. Not all payers require a separate diagnosis when billing for a procedure and E/M service on the same date of service.

57. CPT modifier, for use with CPT evaluation and management (E/M) codes, that identifies an E/M service that resulted in the initial decision to perform surgery. This modifier should be used only with procedure codes considered major surgery (90-day global period).

abstractor. Person who selects and extracts specific data from the medical record and enters the information into computer files.

abuse. Medical reimbursement term that describes an incident that is inconsistent with accepted medical, business, or fiscal practices and directly or indirectly results in unnecessary costs to the Medicare program, improper reimbursement, or reimbursement for services that do not meet professionally recognized standards of care or which are medically unnecessary. Examples of abuse include excessive charges, improper billing practices, billing Medicare as primary instead of other third-party payers that are primary, and increasing charges for Medicare beneficiaries but not to other patients.

accountable care organization. Recognized legal entity under state law comprised of providers of services and suppliers with an established mechanism for shared governance who work together to coordinate care for Medicare fee-for-service beneficiaries. Section 3022 of the Affordable Care Act required CMS to develop a shared savings program to promote coordination and cooperation among providers for the purposes of improving the quality of care for Medicare fee-for-service beneficiaries and minimize costs.

Accredited Standards Committee. Organization accredited by the American National Standards Institute (ANSI) for the development of American national standards.

ACG. 1) Ambulatory care group. 2) American College of Gastroenterologists. Professional organization for gastroenterology medical specialty.

ACH. Automated clearinghouse. Entity that processes or facilitates the processing of information received from another entity in a nonstandard format or containing nonstandard data content into standard data elements or a standard transaction, or that receives a standard transaction from another entity and processes or facilitates the processing of that information into nonstandard format or nonstandard data content for a receiving entity.

activities of daily living. Self-care activities often used to determine a patient's level of function, such as bathing, dressing, using a toilet, transferring in and out of bed or a chair, continence, eating, and walking.

acute. Sudden, severe. Documentation and reporting of an acute condition is important to establishing medical necessity.

acute care facility. Health care institution primarily engaged in providing treatment to inpatients and diagnostic and therapeutic services for medical diagnosis, treatment, and care of injured, disabled, or sick persons who are in an acute phase of illness.

add-on code. CPT code representing a procedure performed in addition to the primary procedure and designated with a + symbol in the CPT book. Add-on codes are never reported for stand-alone services but are reported secondarily in addition to the primary procedure.

adjudication. Processing and review of a submitted claim resulting in payment, partial payment, or denial. In relationship to judicial hearings, it is the process of hearing and settling a case through an objective, judicial procedure.

admission. Formal acceptance of a patient by a health care facility.

admission date. Date the patient was admitted to the health care facility for inpatient care, outpatient service, or the start of care.

against medical advice. Discharge status of patients who leave the hospital after signing a form that releases the hospital from responsibility, or those who leave the hospital premises without notifying hospital personnel.

age restriction. In health care contracting, limitation of benefits when a patient reaches a certain age.

AHA. American Hospital Association. Health care industry association that represents the concerns of institutional providers. The AHA hosts the National Uniform Billing Committee (NUBC), which has a formal consultative role under HIPAA. The AHA also publishes <i>Coding Clinic</i> for ICD-10 and HCPCS.

AHIMA. American Health Information Management Association. Association of health information management professionals offering various certification examinations for physician- and facility-based coders, clinical documentation improvement practitioners, and other technology and health informatics specialists.

allowable charge. Fee schedule amount for a medical service as determined by the physician fee schedule methodology published annually by CMS.

altering patient records. Inappropriately changing or amending patient records, usually to obtain reimbursement or because of pending audits and legal review of records.

AMA. American Medical Association. Professional organization for physicians. The AMA is the secretariat of the National Uniform Claim Committee (NUCC), which has a formal consultative role under HIPAA. The AMA also maintains the Physicians' Current Procedural Terminology (CPT) coding system.

American Academy of Professional Coders. National organization for coders and billers offering certification examinations based on physician-, facility-, or payer-specific guidelines or coding documentation. Upon successful completion of the selected examination, the credential for that examination is obtained.

ancillary services. Services, other than routine room and board charges, that are incidental to the hospital stay. These services include operating room; anesthesia; blood administration; pharmacy; radiology; laboratory; medical, surgical, and central supplies; physical, occupational, speech pathology, and inhalation therapies; and other diagnostic services.

any willing provider. Provider who meets the network's usual selection criteria as defined in statutes requiring a provider network.

appeal. Specific request made to a payer for reconsideration of a denial or adverse coverage or payment decision and potential restriction of benefit reimbursement.

appeal process. Steps required for appealing negative decisions related to payer denials such as denied authorization for requested services or denied charges.

arbitration. Settling of a dispute through a designated individual, group, or committee that is assigned to hear both sides of the story and has the authority to make a binding decision.

ARRA. American recovery and reinvestment act of 2009.

assessment. Process of collecting and studying information and data, such as test values, signs, and symptoms.

audit. Examination or review that establishes the extent to which performance or a process conforms to predetermined standards or criteria. An audit may target utilization, quality of care, coding, or reimbursement.

auditing and monitoring. Regular review of an organization's claim development and submission process from the point where service for a patient is initiated to the submission of a claim for payment. Monitoring involves a system of checks of and controls over, as well as a method of reporting, all areas of compliance, including regulations and audits.

auditor. Professional who evaluates a provider's utilization, quality of care, or level of reimbursement.

authentication. Characteristic of electronic signature. Under HIPAA, authentication is the product of a technology that, when it affixes a signature to a document, also includes a means of establishing that the person or entity signing the document is who he or she claims to be.

authorization. Verbal or written agreement indicating that a third-party payer will pay for services rendered by the provider as set forth in the authorization.

auxiliary personnel. Individual acting under a physician's supervision. It may be an employee, leased employee, or independent contractor of the physician (or other practitioner) or of the same entity that employs or contracts with the physician (or other practitioner).

behavior management. Education and modification techniques or methodologies aimed at helping a patient change undesirable habits or behaviors.

bullet. Under the 1997 E/M guidelines, each physical examination element is commonly referred to as a bullet point or bullet.

care plan oversight services. Physician's ongoing review and revision of a patient's care plan involving complex or multidisciplinary care modalities.

charts. Compilation of documents maintained by the provider for each patient that includes treatment/progress notes, test orders and results, correspondence from other health care providers, and other documents pertinent to the patient's care.

chief complaint. Term used in evaluation and management documentation and coding that identifies the reason or presenting problem that necessitated the patient's encounter for treatment. Typically, this is documented in the medical record using the patient's own words; for example, "My head hurts."

chronic. Persistent, continuing, or recurring.

claim. Statement of services rendered requesting payment from an insurance company or a government entity.

claim manual. Administrative guidelines used by claims processors to adjudicate claims according to company policy and procedure.

clinic. Outpatient facility that provides scheduled diagnostic, curative, rehabilitative, and educational services for walk-in (ambulatory) patients.

clinical quality measure. Tools that assist in measuring and tracking the quality of health care services rendered by eligible clinicians, eligible hospitals, and critical access hospitals (CAH). Measures use data associated with clinicians' ability to deliver high-quality care or relate to long-term goals for quality health care.

coder. Professional who translates documented, written diagnoses and procedures into numeric and alphanumeric codes.

coding guidelines. Criteria that specifies how procedure, diagnosis, or supply codes are to be translated and used in various situations. Coding guidelines are issued by the AHA, AMA, CMS, NCHVS, and various other groups. Guidelines may vary by payer, type of coding system, and intended use.

coding rules. Official rules and coding conventions used for diagnosis and procedure coding.

coding specificity. Selection of classification codes (e.g., ICD-10-CM) that provides the highest degree of accuracy and completeness based on clinical documentation. For example, a six-character ICD-10-CM code cannot be reported when the specific code requires a 7th character.

comorbid condition. Condition present that is not the primary reason for treating the patient, but one that affects the patient's care.

comorbidity. Preexisting condition that causes an increase in length of stay by at least one day in approximately 75 percent of cases. Used in DRG reimbursement.

complete past, family, and social history. Comprehensive review of all elements of the patient's past, family, and social history. Two or three history areas are required depending on the category of E/M service.

complete system review. Narrative of organ systems reviewed including systems related to the problems identified in the chief complaint and/or history of presenting illness plus a review of all other systems.

compliance audit. Internal or external monitoring and review of activities to ensure compliance with all laws, regulations, and guidelines related to health care.

comprehensive physical examination. Under the 1995 guidelines, examination of at least eight organ systems or one comprehensive single-system examination. Under the 1997 guidelines, an examination of at least nine organ systems or body areas, which must include all bullet point elements within each of the nine systems/areas for the multisystem exam or examination of all bullet point elements from one of the 10 single organ system exams.

concurrent care. Medical care provided by two or more physicians on the same day. If care is medically necessary, payers usually pay both physicians. Generally, payers expect the physicians to be of different specialties and caring for different conditions or different aspects of the same condition or disease process.

constitutional. Component of evaluation and management documentation. History component review of systems used to denote general symptoms such as fever, malaise, weight change. Exam component noting vital signs and general appearance.

consultation. Advice or opinion regarding diagnosis and treatment or determination to accept transfer of care of a patient rendered by a medical professional at the request of the primary care provider.

contractor. Entity who enters into a contractual agreement with CMS to service a component of the Medicare program administration, for example, fiscal intermediaries, carriers, program safeguard coordinators.

conversion. In health care contracting, shifting a member under a group contract to an individual contract in accordance with contract terms and occurring with a change in employer benefits or when the covered person leaves the group.

conversion factor. 1) Dollar value for each relative value unit. When this dollar amount is multiplied by the total relative value units, it yields the reimbursement rate for the service. 2) National multiplier that converts the geographically adjusted relative value units into Medicare fee schedule dollar amounts that applies to all services paid under the MPFS.

coordinated care. In health care contracting, system of health care delivery that influences utilization, quality of care, and cost of services. Managed care integrates financing and management with an employed or contracted organized provider network that delivers services to an enrolled population.

coordination of benefits. Agreement that prevents double payment for services when the member is covered by two or more sources. The agreement dictates which organization is primarily and secondarily responsible for payment.

coordination of care. Care provided concurrently with counseling that includes treatment instructions to the patient or caregiver; special accommodations for home, work, school, vacation, or other locations; coordination with other providers and agencies; and living arrangements.

copayment. Cost-sharing arrangement in which a covered person pays a specified portion of allowed charges. In relation to Medicare, the copayment designates the specific dollar amount that the patient must pay and coinsurance designates the percentage of allowed charges.

coronary care unit. Facility or service area dedicated to patients suffering from heart attack, stroke, or other serious cardiopulmonary problems.

counseling. Discussion with a patient and/or family concerning one or more of the following areas: diagnostic results, impressions, and/or recommended diagnostic studies; prognosis; risks and benefits of management (treatment) options; instructions for management (treatment) and/or follow-up; importance of compliance with chosen management (treatment) options; risk factor reduction; and patient and family education.

CPT. Current Procedural Terminology. Definitive procedural coding system developed by the American Medical Association that lists descriptive terms and identifying codes to provide a uniform language that describes medical, surgical, and diagnostic services for nationwide communication among physicians, patients, and third parties, used to report professional and outpatient services.

CPT codes. Codes maintained and copyrighted by the AMA and selected for use under HIPAA for outpatient facility and nondental professional transactions.

CPT modifier. Two-character code used to indicate that a service was altered in some way from the stated CPT or HCPCS Level II description, but not enough to change the basic definition of the service.

CQM. Clinical quality measure. Tools that assist in measuring and tracking the quality of health care services rendered by eligible clinicians, eligible hospitals, and critical access hospitals (CAH). Measures use data associated with clinicians' ability to deliver high-quality care or relate to long-term goals for quality health care.

critical care. Treatment of critically ill patients in a variety of medical emergencies that requires the constant attendance of the physician (e.g., cardiac arrest, shock, bleeding, respiratory failure, postoperative complications, critically ill neonate).

Current Procedural Terminology. Definitive procedural coding system developed by the American Medical Association that lists descriptive terms and identifying codes to provide a uniform language that describes medical, surgical, and diagnostic services for nationwide communication among physicians, patients, and third parties.

customary, prevailing, and reasonable charge. Categories used as the basis for Medicare's reimbursement rates before the resource-based relative value scale (RBRVS) was implemented. These rates were based on the lowest charge of the three categories rather than the relative values of each service, which caused wide variations in Medicare payments among physicians and specialties. "Customary" described a clinician's historical charges, "prevailing" represented the charges of other providers in the same specialty type residing in the same general locality, and "reasonable" was the lowest charge of all three categories.

date of service. Day the encounter or procedure is performed or the day a supply is issued.

detailed physical examination. Under the 1995 guidelines, examination of two to seven organ systems, with at least one system documented in detail. Under the 1997 guidelines, an examination of at least six organ systems or body areas, including at least two bullet point elements for each system/area or at least 12 bullet point elements from at least two organ systems or body areas.

diagnosis. Determination or confirmation of a condition, disease, or syndrome and its implications.

diagnostic laboratory services. Laboratory services that are required to diagnose a disease or injury, regardless of where the services are rendered. These services include certain mechanical or machine tests such as EKGs and EEGs. For Medicare purposes, these services are paid under a fee schedule.

diagnostic procedures. Procedure performed on a patient to obtain information to assess the medical condition of the patient or to identify a disease and to determine the nature and severity of an illness or injury.

diagnostic services. Examination or procedure performed on a patient to obtain information to assess the medical condition of the patient or to identify a disease and to determine the nature and severity of an illness or injury.

diagnostic x-ray services. X-ray and other related services performed for diagnostic purposes, including portable x-ray services.

direct supervision. Situation in which the physician must be present in the office suite and immediately available to provide assistance and direction throughout a given procedure. The physician is not, however, required to be present in the room when the procedure is performed.

discharge. Situation in which the patient leaves an acute care (prospective payment) hospital after receiving complete acute care treatment.

discharge date. For medical facilities, the date the patient is formally released, expires, or is transferred. In other situations, the date that medical care or treatment ended.

discharge plan. Treatment plan by the provider for continued patient care after discharge that may include home care, the services of case managers or other health care providers, or transfer to another facility.

discharge status. Disposition of the patient at discharge (e.g., left against medical advice, discharged home, transferred to an acute care hospital, expired).

discharge transfer. Discharge of a patient from one facility to another.

documentation. Physician's written or transcribed notations about a patient encounter, including a detailed operative report or written notes about a routine encounter. Source documentation must be the treating provider's own account of the encounter and may be transcribed from dictation, dictated by the physician into voice recognition software, or be hand- or typewritten. A signature or authentication accompanies each entry.

e-prescribing. Transmission of prescription or prescription-related information between the prescriber and the medication dispenser. For Medicare purposes, e-prescribing includes but is not limited to two-way transmission between the point of care and the dispenser.

E/M. Evaluation and management services. Assessment, counseling, and other services provided to a patient and reported through CPT codes.

E/M codes. Evaluation and management service codes.

E/M service components. Key components in determining the correct level of E/M codes are history, examination, and medical decision-making.

EC. Eligible clinician. Term used in the Quality Payment Program (QPP) Merit-based Incentive Payment System (MIPS) track to describe medical professionals who are eligible to participate in the program.

electronic health record. Electronic version of individual patients' health-related information that has the interoperability to be created, managed, and consulted by more than one health care organization's authorized staff and clinicians and designed to streamline the clinicians' workflow processes. Information contained in an EHR includes, but is not limited to, patient demographics, process notes, problems, medications, vital signs, past medical history, immunizations, laboratory data, and radiology reports.

electronic medical record. Electronic version of individual patients' health-related information that can be created, managed, and consulted by single care organizations' authorized staff and clinicians.

eligible professional. Nonhospital based physician receiving Medicare and/or Medicaid reimbursement who is using a certified electronic health record.

emergency. Serious medical condition or symptom (including severe pain) resulting from injury, sickness, or mental illness that arises suddenly and requires immediate care and treatment, generally received within 24 hours of onset, to avoid jeopardy to the life, limb, or health of a covered person.

emergency admission. Admission in which the patient requires immediate medical or psychiatric attention because of life-threatening, severe, and potentially disabling conditions.

emergency department. Organized hospital-based facility for the provision of unscheduled episodic services to patients who present for immediate medical attention. The facility must be available 24 hours a day.

emergency outpatient. Patient admitted for diagnosis and treatment of a condition requiring immediate attention but who will not stay at that facility or be transferred to another.

emergent care. Treatment for a medical or mental health condition or symptom that arises suddenly and requires care and treatment immediately or as soon as possible.

EMR. Electronic medical record.

encoder. Computer application that assists in the assignment of a diagnosis or procedure code and may also assign reimbursement categories and values.

encounter. 1) Direct personal contact between a registered hospital outpatient (e.g., medical clinic or emergency department) and a physician (or other person authorized by state law and hospital bylaws to order or furnish services) for the diagnosis and treatment of an illness or injury. Visits with more than one health professional that take place during the same session and at a single location within the hospital are considered a single visit. 2) Quality reporting term used to describe meetings with patients during the performance period as represented by the following: CPT Category I or Category II service or procedure code or a HCPCS Level II code located in a quality measure's denominator. Reporting of these codes counts as eligibility to meet a measure's inclusion requirements when the service occurs during the specified performance period.

end-stage renal disease. Chronic, advanced kidney disease requiring renal dialysis or a kidney transplant to prevent imminent death.

EP. Eligible professional.

episode of care. One or more health care services received during a period of relatively continuous care by a hospital or health care provider.

established patient. 1) Patient who has received professional services in a face-to-face setting within the last three years from the same physician/qualified health care professional or another physician/qualified health care professional of the exact same specialty and subspecialty who belongs to the same group practice. 2) For OPPS hospitals, patient who has been registered as an inpatient or outpatient in a hospital's provider-based clinic or emergency department within the past three years.

estimated length of stay. Average number of days of hospitalization required for a given illness or procedure, based on prior histories of patients who have been hospitalized for the same illness or procedure.

evaluation and management. Assessment, counseling, and other services provided to a patient reported through CPT codes.

evaluation and management codes. Assessment and management of a patient's health care.

evaluation and management service components. Key components of history, examination, and medical decision making that are key to selecting the correct E/M codes. Other non-key components include counseling, coordination of care, nature of presenting problem, and time.

examination. Comprehensive visual and tactile screening and specific testing leading to diagnosis or, as appropriate, to a referral to another practitioner.

expanded problem focused physical examination. Under the 1995 guidelines, examination of two to seven organ systems. Under the 1997 guidelines, examination of at least six bullet point elements in one or more organ systems from the general multisystem examination OR examination of at least six of the bullet point elements from one of the 10 single organ system exams.

extended care facility. Institution that provides any type of long-term care. Usually refers to a skilled nursing facility, but may be used in reference to other types of long-term institutions.

extended history of present illness. Detailed narrative of the presenting illness, including at least four elements: location, quality, severity, duration, timing, context, modifying factors, or associated signs and symptoms.

extended system review. Narrative of two to nine organ systems reviewed directly related to the chief complaint or history of present illness plus a review of a limited number of additional, related systems.

face to face. Interaction between two parties, usually provider and patient, that occurs in the physical presence of each other.

facility. Place of patient care, including inpatient and outpatient, acute or long term.

family history. Record of the health of family members, including the health status or cause of death of parents, siblings, and children, and specific diseases related to the patient's chief complaint, history of present illness, and/or review of systems.

fellow. Physician who has completed a basic residency program and is now in a formally organized and approved subspecialty program that may or may not be recognized as an approved residency program under Medicare for received GME funding.

health care provider. Entity that administers diagnostic and therapeutic services.

health history form. Document completed by the patient that contains a number of questions regarding health history; typically completed at the first patient encounter. The patient may be asked to periodically review the document at subsequent visits or as needed to ensure health history information remains current and up to date. The form should include a place for the patient to list all current prescription and over-the-counter (OTC) medications and supplements, including dosages and frequency, as well as a personal, family, and social history. All 14 body systems (constitutional, eyes, ears, nose, throat, mouth [ENT, M], respiratory, cardiovascular, gastrointestinal, genitourinary, musculoskeletal, integumentary [skin/breast], neurological, psychiatric, endocrine, hematologic/lymphatic, and allergy/immunologic) should be listed. Space should be included for any applicable insurance information, the phone number to the patient's pharmacy, and a next of kin contact.

history of present illness. Chronological account of signs and symptoms of the present condition.

HIT. Health information technology.

HITECH. Health information technology for economic and clinical health. Act that was included as part of the American Recovery and Reinvestment Act of 2009 and signed into law on February 17, 2009 for the meaningful use of health information technology. Within the Act, privacy and security measures are addressed regarding the electronic transmission of protected health information with civil and criminal enforcement of HIPAA rules defined.

home health. Palliative and therapeutic care and assistance in the activities of daily life to home bound Medicare and private plan members.

hospice. Organization that furnishes inpatient, outpatient, and home health care for the terminally ill. Hospices emphasize support and counseling services for terminally ill people and their families, pain relief, and symptom management. When the Medicare beneficiary chooses hospice benefits, all other Medicare benefits are discontinued, except physician services and treatment of conditions not related to the terminal illness.

hospital admission plan. Used to facilitate admission to the hospital and to assure prompt payment to the hospital.

HPI. History of present illness.

ICD-10. International Classification of Diseases, 10th Revision. Classification of diseases by alphanumeric code, used by the World Health Organization.

ICD-10-CM. International Classification of Diseases, 10th Revision, Clinical Modification. Clinical modification of the alphanumeric classification of diseases used by the World Health Organization, already in use in much of the world, and used for mortality reporting in the United States.

ICD-10-PCS. International Classification of Diseases, 10th Revision, Procedure Coding System. Inpatient hospital services and surgical procedures must be coded using ICD-10-PCS codes.

incident to. Provision of a service concurrently with another service. For example, additional covered supplies and materials that are furnished after surgery typically are billed as "incident to" a physician's services and not as hospital services. This term is used specifically for revenue codes for pharmacy, supplies, and anesthesia furnished along with radiology and other diagnostic services.

inpatient hospitalization. Period in which a patient is housed in a single hospital usually without interruption.

intern. Medical school graduate who is in the first year of postgraduate training under the direction of a teaching physician and/or senior resident.

interpretation. Professional health care provider's review of data with a written or verbal opinion.

interval history. History documenting what has occurred in a given area since the last visit, usually associated with subsequent hospital, nursing home, rest home, and home visit services.

key components. Three components of history, examination, and medical decision making are considered the keys to selecting the correct level of E/M codes. In most cases, all three components must be addressed in the documentation. However, in established, subsequent, and follow-up categories, only two of the three must be met or exceeded for a given code.

key portion. Part (or parts) of a service determined by the teaching physician to be the critical or key portion.

leased employee. Legal employment relationship established by a contract where an employer hires the services of an employee through another employer.

long-term care facility. Nursing home or, more specifically, a facility offering extended, nonacute care to a resident patient whose illness does not require acute care.

meaningful use. 1) Sets of guidelines that must be followed as part of the HITECH Act. Three main components are specified in the Act: use of certified EHR in a meaningful manner (e.g., e-prescribing), electronic exchange of health information to improve the quality of healthcare, and submission of clinical quality and other measures. 2) Use of certified electronic health technology in measurable ways of both quality and quantity. The Medicare EHR Incentive Program, aka meaningful use, ended reporting on 12/31/2016; components from this program have been included in the Quality Payment Program (QPP) mandated under the MACRA legislation.

medical consultation. Advice or an opinion rendered by a physician at the request of the primary care provider.

medical decision making. Consideration of the differential diagnoses, the amount and/or complexity of data reviewed and considered (medical records, test results, correspondence from previous treating physicians, etc.), current diagnostic studies ordered, and treatment or management options and risk (complications of the patient's condition, the potential for complications, continued morbidity, risk of mortality, any comorbidities associated with the patient's disease process).

medical documentation. Patient care records, including operative notes; physical, occupational, and speech-language pathology notes; progress notes; physician certification and recertifications; and emergency room records; or the patient's medical record in its entirety. When Medicare coverage cannot be determined based on the information submitted on the claim, medical documentation may be requested. The Medicare Administrative Contractor (MAC) will deny a claim for lack of medical necessity if medical documentation is not received within the stated time frame defined by the MAC (usually within 35-45 days after the date of request).

medical necessity. Medically appropriate and necessary to meet basic health needs; consistent with the diagnosis or condition and national medical practice guidelines regarding type, frequency, and duration of treatment; rendered in a cost-effective manner.

Medicare. Federally funded program authorized as part of the Social Security Act that provides for health care services for people age 65 or older, people with disabilities, and people with end-stage renal disease (ESRD).

Medicare administrative contractor. Jurisdictional entity that contracts with CMS to adjudicate professional claims under Part A and Part B, responsible for daily claims processing, utilization review, record maintenance, dissemination of information based on CMS regulations, and whether services are covered and payments are appropriate.

Medicare carrier. Organization that contracts with CMS to adjudicate professional claims under Part B, the supplemental medical insurance program. Medicare carriers are responsible for daily claims processing, utilization review, record maintenance, dissemination of information based on CMS regulations, and determining whether services are covered and payments are appropriate. This

organization has been replaced by Medicare administrative contractors.

Medicare fee schedule. Fee schedule based upon physician work, expense, and malpractice designed to slow the rise in cost for services and standardize payment to physicians regardless of specialty or location of service with geographic adjustments.

Medicare Part B. Supplemental medical insurance that includes outpatient hospital care and physician and other qualified professional care. Claims from providers or suppliers other than a hospital are submitted to carriers for reimbursement. Hospital outpatient claims are submitted to their FI/MAC.

Merit-based Incentive Payment System. CMS Quality Payment Program (QPP) track that combines parts of three retired quality reporting programs—the Physician Quality Reporting System (PQRS), the Value Modifier (VM or Value-based Payment Modifier), and the Medicare EHR Incentive Program (EHR) and another CMS created performance category called Improvement Activities —into a single program. Eligible clinicians (EC) are measured on all four categories. The QPP became effective January 1, 2017.

minor procedure. Self-limited procedure, usually with an assignment of 0 or 10 follow-up days by payers. A minor procedure may be considered by many payers to be part of the global package for a primary surgical service and cannot be billed separately from the primary procedure.

MIPS. Merit-Based Incentive Payment System.

miscoding. Incorrect coding or using a code that does not apply to the procedure.

modifier. Two characters that can be appended to a HCPCS code as a means of identifying circumstances that alter or enhance the description of a service or supply.

morbidity. Diseased condition or state.

mortality. Condition of being mortal (subject to death).

new patient. Patient who is receiving face-to-face care from a provider/qualified health care professional or another physician/qualified health care professional of the exact same specialty and subspecialty who belongs to the same group practice for the first time in three years. For OPPS hospitals, a patient who has not been registered as an inpatient or outpatient, including off-campus provider based clinic or emergency department, within the past three years.

newborn admission. Infant born in the facility.

newborn intensive care unit. Special care unit for premature and seriously ill infants.

noninstitutional setting. All settings other than a hospital or skilled nursing facility.

observation patient. Patient who needs to be monitored and assessed for inpatient admission or referral to another site for care.

observation services. Services furnished on a hospital's premises, including use of a bed and periodic monitoring by a hospital's nursing or other staff, that are reasonable and necessary to evaluate an outpatient's condition or determine the need for a possible admission to the hospital as an inpatient. Such services are covered only when provided by the order of a physician or another individual authorized by state license laws and hospital staff bylaws to admit patients to the hospital or to order outpatient tests. Observation services normally do not extend beyond 23 hours.

on-call physician encounter. Physician/qualified health care professional who is on call or covering for another physician/qualified health care professional and classifies the patient's encounter as it would have been by the physician/qualified health care professional who is not available.

ONC. Office of the national coordinator for health information technology.

outpatient. Person who has not been admitted as an inpatient but who is registered on the hospital or CAH records as an outpatient and receives services (rather than supplies alone) directly from the hospital or CAH. (Code of Federal Regulations, section 410.2.)

outpatient services. Medical and other services, diagnostic or therapeutic, provided to a person who has not been admitted to the hospital as an inpatient but is registered on the hospital records as an outpatient. Outpatient services usually require a stay of less than 24 hours.

outpatient visit. Encounter in a recognized outpatient facility.

overutilization. Services rendered by providers more frequently than usual.

past history. Record of prior illnesses or conditions occurring in childhood and adulthood, such as infectious diseases, allergies, accidents, current medications, hospitalizations, and surgical/medical procedures.

patient problem. Disease, condition, illness, injury, symptom, sign, finding, complaint, or other reason for an encounter, with or without a diagnosis being established at the time of the encounter.

pediatric patient. Patient usually younger than 14 years of age.

pertinent past, family, and/or social history (PFSH). Brief narrative of the past, family, or social history elements directly related to the problems identified in the chief complaint, history of present illness, or the review of systems.

physically present. Teaching physicians must be in the same room, or a partitioned or curtained area, as the patient and resident and/or perform a face-to-face service.

physician. Legally authorized practitioners including a doctor of medicine or osteopathy, a doctor of dental surgery or of dental medicine, a doctor of podiatric medicine, a doctor of optometry, and a chiropractor only with respect to treatment by means of manual manipulation of the spine (to correct a subluxation).

physician services. Professional services performed by physicians, including surgery, consultations, and home, office, and institutional calls.

physician work. One of three components used to develop relative value units (RVU) under the resource-based relative value scale. Physician work represents the value of the skill and time required to perform a service.

physicians at teaching hospitals. Set up by the Office of Inspector General (OIG), initiative of the National Recovery Project targeting reimbursement practices at teaching hospitals, focusing on the use of residents and the services they perform under Medicare Part B that are paid as part of Medicare Part A.

Physicians' Current Procedural Terminology. Definitive procedural coding system developed and owned by the American Medical Association that is a listing of descriptive terms and identifying codes used for reporting medical services and procedures.

plan of treatment. Written documentation of the type of therapy services (e.g., physical, occupational, speech-language pathology, cardiac rehabilitation) to be provided to a patient and of the amount, frequency, and duration (in days, weeks, months) of the services to be provided. An active treatment plan must identify the diagnosis, the anticipated goals of the treatment, the date the plan was established, and the type of modality or procedure to be used.

practitioner. Physician or nonphysician practitioner authorized to receive payment for services or incident-to services rendered.

preexisting condition. Symptom that causes a person to seek diagnosis, care, or treatment for which medical advice or treatment was recommended or received by a physician within a certain time period before the effective date of medical insurance coverage. The preexisting condition waiting period is the time the beneficiary must wait after buying health insurance before coverage begins for a condition that existed before coverage was obtained.

present illness. Current problem, from the onset of symptoms to the time of the encounter.

presenting problem. Disease, condition, illness, injury, symptom, sign, finding, complaint, or other reason for the patient encounter.

preventive medicine service. Evaluation and management service provided as a periodic health screening and/or prophylactic service that does not typically include management of new or existing diagnoses or problems.

primary care. Basic or general health care, traditionally provided by family practice, pediatrics, and internal medicine practitioners.

primary care physician. Physician who makes an initial diagnosis and referral and retains control over the patient and utilization of services both in and outside of the plan.

primary diagnosis. Current, most significant reason for the services or procedures provided.

problem focused physical examination. Under the 1995 guidelines, an examination of one organ system or body area. Under the 1997 guidelines, examination of one to five bullet point elements in one or more organ system or body areas.

problem pertinent system review. Narrative of the organ systems reviewed related to the system identified in the chief complaint and/or history of present illness.

procedure. Diagnostic or therapeutic service provided for the care and treatment of a patient, usually conforming to a specific set of steps or instructions.

prognosis. Forecast of the probable outcome of a condition or disease and the prospects of recovery and disease residual, dependent on the nature of the disease and the patient's response to treatment.

prolonged physician services. Extended pre- or post-service care provided to a patient whose condition requires services beyond the usual.

psychiatric hospital. Specialized institution that provides, under the supervision of physicians, services for the diagnosis and treatment of mentally ill persons.

QPP. Quality Payment Program. Program that is part of the larger goal of the Centers for Medicare and Medicaid Services (CMS) to improve Medicare through a greater focus and emphasis on the quality of medical care provided to beneficiaries. The Medicare Access and CHIP Reauthorization Act of 2015 (MACRA) repealed the Sustainable Growth Rate (SGR) formula and consolidated multiple quality reporting programs into a single system called the Merit-based Incentive Payment System (MIPS), one of two tracks that makes up the Quality Payment Program. The QPP provides incentive payments to clinicians for participating in MIPS or through the second track, Advanced Alternative Payment Models (APM). The QPP's purpose is to give providers new tools and resources to help provide patients with the best possible care. Clinicians can choose how they wish to participate based on practice size, specialty, location, or patient population. Clinicians who opt to participate in an Advanced APM through Medicare Part B may earn an incentive payment for participating in an innovative payment model. However, if clinicians choose to participate in traditional Medicare Part B, they will participate in MIPS where they are eligible to earn a performance-based payment adjustment. The QPP became effective on January 1, 2017.

qualified health care professional. Educated, licensed or certified, and regulated professional operating under a specified scope of practice to provide patient services that are separate and distinct from other clinical staff. Services may be billed independently or under the facility's services.

referral. Approval from the primary care physician to see a specialist or receive certain services. May be required for coverage purposes before a patient receives care from anyone except the primary physician.

referred outpatient. Person sent to a special diagnostic facility or to a hospital service department for the diagnostic tests or procedures.

rehabilitation hospital. Institution that serves inpatients of whom the vast majority require intensive rehabilitative services for the treatment of certain conditions (e.g., stroke, amputation, brain or spinal cord injuries, and neurological disorders).

resident. Individual participating in an approved graduate medical education (GME) program or a physician who is not in an approved GME program but who is authorized to practice only in a hospital setting including interns and fellows but not medical students.

rural health clinic. Clinic in an area where there is a shortage of health services staffed by a nurse practitioner, physician assistant, or certified nurse midwife under physician direction that provides routine diagnostic services, including clinical laboratory services, drugs, and biologicals, and that has prompt access to additional diagnostic services from facilities meeting federal requirements.

second opinion. Medical opinion obtained from another health care professional, relevant to clinical evaluation, before the performance of a medical service or surgical procedure. Includes patient education regarding treatment alternatives and/or to determine medical necessity.

secondary care. Services provided by medical specialists, such as cardiologists, urologists, and dermatologists who generally do not have first contact with patients.

self-referral. Patient who was not referred by a physician or other health care practitioner, but who chose that facility or provider on his or her own.

severity of illness. Relative levels of loss of function and mortality that may be experienced by patients with a particular disease.

short-stay patients. Inpatients admitted for 48 hours or less, or outpatients who stay 24 hours or less.

signature. Physician's signature acknowledges that he/she has performed or supervised the service or procedure and that the transcription has been read and corrections made before signing. Signed or initialed laboratory and x-ray results show auditors that the physician has reviewed the information.

skilled nursing facility. Institution or a distinct part of an institution that is primarily engaged in providing skilled nursing care and related services for residents who require medical or nursing care; or rehabilitation services for the rehabilitation of injured, disabled, or sick persons.

SOAP. Subjective, objective, assessment, plan. When documenting patients' visits, the SOAP approach has been used historically as it standardizes physician documentation and easily adapts to history, exam, and medical decision-making. The steps are defined as follows: 1) Subjective: The information the patient tells the physician. 2) Objective: The physician's observed, objective overview, including the patient's vital signs and the findings of the physical exam and any diagnostic tests. 3) Assessment: A list the physician prepares in response to the patient's condition, including the problem, diagnoses, and reasons leading the physician to the diagnoses. 4) Plan: The physician's workup or treatment planned for each problem in the assessment.

social history. Review of pertinent past and current activities of the patient including marital status, employment or occupation, use of drugs, alcohol and tobacco, educational background, sexual history, and other related social factors such as travel, avocations, and hobbies.

swing bed. Bed used for acute or long-term care, depending on the patient's need and the hospital's level of occupancy. Swing beds typically are available in small and rural hospitals. A swing-bed patient may be admitted and discharged from acute care and readmitted to a swing bed to receive skilled or intermediate levels of care. At times, the patient may remain in the same bed while changes occur in his or her care, charges, and payment.

teaching physician. Physician, other than another resident, who involves residents in the care of his or her patients.

telehealth service. Care by a provider with the patient at a remote site, usually rural, utilizing electronic communication to evaluate, monitor, and treat a patient.

tertiary care facility. Hospital providing specialty care to patients referred from other hospitals because of the severity of their injuries or illnesses.

treatment plan. Plan of care established by the provider outlining specific deficits and planned treatment that may be submitted to the case manager when seeking certification for a plan member.

type A emergency department. Emergency department licensed and advertised to be available to provide emergent care 24 hours a day, seven days a week. Type A emergency departments must meet both the CPT book definition of an emergency department and the EMTALA definition of a dedicated emergency department.

type B emergency department. Emergency department licensed and advertised to provide emergent care less than 24 hours a day, seven days a week. Type B emergency departments must meet the EMTALA definition of a dedicated emergency department.

UCR. Usual, customary, and reasonable. Fees charged for medical services that are considered normal, common, and in line with the prevailing fees in a given geographical area. May also be referred to as "customary, prevailing, and reasonable" charges.

upcoding. Practice of billing a code that represents a higher reimbursement than the code for the procedure actually performed.

Appendix A: Physician E/M Code Self-Audit Forms

Note: For 2021, the forms contained in this appendix will also be available as a downloadable PDF. To access the forms, use the following URL and password:

www.optum360coding.com/2021EMCAForms
Password: o360emca21

EXAMPLE 1: 1997 GUIDELINES

Physician offices may want to adopt a checklist like the one below, for providers to use to correctly identify accurate E/M code levels or as a self-audit tool.

Patient name _____

Account number _____   Date of service _____

Providing physician or other qualified healthcare provider_____

Requesting provider's name and UPIN _____

Diagnoses:

1.   3.

2.   4.

Type of Patient:
- ❑ New
- ❑ Established

Type of History (check one only):
- ❑ **Problem focused** (chief complaint, brief history of present problem)
- ❑ **Expanded problem focused** (chief complaint, brief history and system review pertinent to problem)
- ❑ **Detailed** (chief complaint, extended history, extended system review and pertinent past, family and/or social history **or** minimum of three chronic/inactive conditions reviewed.)
- ❑ **Comprehensive** (chief complaint, extended history, complete system review and complete past, family and social history)

Type of Examination-Multisystem[1] (check one only):
- ❑ **Problem focused** (one to five elements, one or more systems/areas)
- ❑ **Expanded problem focused** (at least six elements, one or more systems/areas)
- ❑ **Detailed** (at least two elements in six systems/areas)
- ❑ **Comprehensive** (all elements in 9 systems/areas)

---

1   **Change as appropriate to use for single organ system physical examinations**

(EXAMPLE 1 CONTINUED)

Level of Medical Decision Making:

	Straightforward	Low Complexity	Moderate Complexity	High Complexity
Number of management options	❑ Minimal	❑ Limited	❑ Multiple	❑ Extensive
Amount/complexity of data to be reviewed	❑ Minimal	❑ Limited	❑ Moderate	❑ Extensive
Risk of complications and/or morbidity or mortality	❑ Minimal	❑ Low	❑ Moderate	❑ High

Select highest level for which two or more criteria are met or exceeded:

❑ High complexity
❑ Moderate complexity
❑ Low complexity
❑ Straightforward

Time:

Total face-to-face time with patient: _____

Total counseling time_____
(required if more than 50 percent of the face-to-face time was spent in counseling or coordination of care—documentation of the extent of counseling and coordination of care is required)

CPT® Code: _____

E/M DOCUMENTATION/SELF-AUDIT FORM—EXAMPLE 2: 1997 GUIDELINES

Name of Patient _____ Date _____

Provider _____ Type of visit _____

DOCUMENTED HISTORY

History of Present Illness (HPI):

_____ Location   _____ Severity   _____ Timing   _____ Associated signs/symptoms
_____ Quality   _____ Duration   _____ Context   _____ Modifying factors
_____ **Brief History:** 1–3 elements   _____ **Extended History:** 4 or more elements
                                                 OR 3 or more chronic/inactive conditions

Review of Systems (ROS):

_____ Constitutional   _____ Respiratory   _____ Integumentary
_____ Eyes   _____ Gastrointestinal   _____ Neurological
_____ Ears/Nose/Throat   _____ Genitourinary   _____ Psychiatric
_____ Cardiovascular   _____ Musculoskeletal   _____ Endocrine
_____ Hematologic/Lymphatic   _____ Allergic/Immunologic

ROS:

_____ None   _____ Problem-related   _____ Problem relating to the
                                                            HPI 10/more OR plus 2–9 systems

Past, Family, Social History (PFSH):

_____ None   _____ Pertinent (1 or 2)   _____ Complete (3 for new, 2 for est pt)

Documented History Summary:

HPI	Brief	Brief	Extended	Extended
ROS	None	Problem pertinent	Extended	Complete
PFSH	None	None	Pertinent	Complete
None	Problem focused	Expanded problem focused	Detailed	Comprehensive

Documented level of the history is:

_____

COMPLEXITY OF EXAMINATION

(See general multisystem exam in this example or specialty-specific exams in appendix C.)

COMPLEXITY OF MEDICAL DECISION MAKING:

Number of diagnoses/management options:

_____ New problem   _____ Established problem, improved
_____ Established problem stable   _____ Workup planned
_____ Established problem worsening _____ No workup planned

(EXAMPLE 2 CONTINUED)

System/Body Area	Elements of Examination
Constitutional	• Measurement of any three of the following seven vital signs: 1) sitting or standing blood pressure, 2) supine blood pressure, 3) pulse rate and regularity, 4) respiration, 5) temperature, 6) height, 7) weight (May be measured and recorded by ancillary staff). • General appearance of patient (e.g., development, nutrition, body habitus, deformities attention to grooming)
Eyes	• Inspection of conjunctivae and lids • Examination of pupils and irises (e.g., reaction to light and accommodation, size and symmetry) • Ophthalmoscopic examination of optic discs (e.g., size, C/D ratio, appearance) and posterior segments (e.g., vessel changes, exudates, hemorrhages)
Ears, Nose, Mouth and Throat	• External inspection of ears and nose (e.g., overall appearance, scars, lesions, masses) • Otoscopic examination of external auditory canals and tympanic membranes • Assessment of hearing (e.g., whispered voice, finger rub, tuning fork) • Inspection of nasal mucosa, septum and turbinates • Inspection of lips, teeth and gums • Examination of oropharynx: oral mucosa, salivary glands, hard and soft palates, tongue, tonsils and posterior pharynx
Neck	• Examination of neck (e.g., masses, overall appearance, symmetry, tracheal position, crepitus) • Examination of thyroid (e.g., enlargement, tenderness, mass)
Respiratory	• Assessment of respiratory effort (e.g., intercostal retractions, use of accessory muscles, diaphragmatic movement) • Percussion of chest (e.g., dullness, flatness, hyperresonance) • Palpation of chest (e.g., tactile fremitus) • Auscultation of lungs (e.g., breath sounds, adventitious sounds, rubs)
Cardiovascular	• Palpation of heart (e.g., location, size, thrills) • Auscultation of heart with notation of abnormal sounds and murmurs Examination of: • carotid arteries (e.g., pulse amplitude, bruits) • abdominal aorta (e.g., size, bruits) • femoral arteries (e.g., pulse amplitude, bruits) • pedal pulses (e.g., pulse amplitude) • extremities for edema and/or varicosities
Chest (Breasts)	• Inspection of breasts (e.g., symmetry, nipple discharge) • Palpation of breasts and axillae (e.g., masses or lumps, tenderness)
Gastrointestinal (Abdomen)	• Examination of abdomen with notation of presence of masses or tenderness • Examination of liver and spleen • Examination for presence or absence of hernia • Examination (when indicated) of anus, perineum and rectum, including sphincter tone, presence of hemorrhoids, rectal masses • Obtain stool sample for occult blood test when indicated
Genitourinary	**Male**: • Examination of the scrotal contents (e.g., hydrocele, spermatocele, tenderness of cord, testicular mass) • Examination of the penis • Digital rectal examination of prostate gland (e.g., size, symmetry, nodularity tenderness)

General Multisystem Examination

System/Body Area	Elements of Examination
Genitourinary (continued)	**Female**: Pelvic examination (with or without specimen collection for smears and cultures), including: • Examination of external genitalia (e.g., general appearance, hair distribution, lesions) and vagina (e.g., general appearance, estrogen effect, discharge, lesions, pelvic support, cystocele, rectocele) • Examination of urethra (e.g., masses, tenderness, scarring) • Examination of bladder (e.g., fullness, masses, tenderness) • Cervix (e.g., general appearance, lesions, discharge) • Uterus (e.g., size, contour, position, mobility, tenderness, consistency, descent or support) • Adnexa/parametria (e.g., masses, tenderness, organomegaly, nodularity)
Lymphatic	Palpation of lymph nodes in **two or more** areas: • Neck • Groin • Axillae • Other
Musculoskeletal	• Examination of gait and station • Inspection and/or palpation of digits and nails (e.g., clubbing, cyanosis, inflammatory conditions, petechiae, ischemia, infections, nodes) Examination of joints, bones and muscles of **one or more of the following six areas**: 1) head and neck; 2) spine, ribs and pelvis; 3) right upper extremity; 4) left upper extremity; 5) right lower extremity; and 6) left lower extremity. The examination of a given area includes: • Inspection and/or palpation with notation of presence of any misalignment, asymmetry, crepitation, defects, tenderness, masses, effusions • Assessment of range of motion with notation of any pain, crepitation or contracture • Assessment of stability with notation of any dislocation (luxation), subluxation or laxity • Assessment of muscle strength and tone (e.g., flaccid, cog wheel, spastic) with notation of any atrophy or abnormal movements
Skin	• Inspection of skin and subcutaneous tissue (e.g., rashes, lesions, ulcers) • Palpation of skin and subcutaneous tissue (e.g., induration, subcutaneous nodules, tightening)
Neurologic	• Test cranial nerves with notation of any deficits • Examination of deep tendon reflexes with notation of pathological reflexes (e.g., Babinski) • Examination of sensation (e.g., by touch, pin, vibration, proprioception)
Psychiatric	• Description of patient's judgment and insight Brief assessment of mental status, including: • orientation to time, place and person • recent and remote memory • mood and affect (e.g., depression, anxiety, agitation)

Content and Documentation Requirements

Level of Exam	Perform and Document
Problem focused	**One to five** elements identified by a bullet.
Expanded Problem focused	**At least six** elements identified by a bullet.
Detailed	**At least two** elements identified by a bullet **from each of six areas/systems or at least twelve elements** identified by a bullet in **two or more areas/systems.**
Comprehensive	Perform **all elements** identified by a bullet in **at least nine** organ systems or body areas and document **at least two** elements identified by a bullet **from each of nine areas/systems.**

Amount and complexity of data obtained/analyzed/reviewed:

_____ Review/order lab tests

_____ Review/order routine x-rays

_____ Review/order EKG, EEG, ECHO, cardiac cath, noninvasive vascular studies, PETS

_____ Discussion of test results with performing provider

_____ Decision to obtain old records

_____ Review and summarization of old records

Overall risk of complications/morbidity/mortality:

Assess risk based on number of conditions (presenting problem plus underlying/additional conditions) being managed, diagnostic procedures ordered, management options selected such as decision for surgical procedures, etc.

_____ Minimal

_____ Low

_____ Moderate

_____ High

DOCUMENTED COMPLEXITY OF MEDICAL DECISION MAKING:

Decision Making	Number of diagnoses/management options	Amount/complexity of data	Overall risks
_____ Straightforward/minimal	Minimal	Minimal or none	Minimal
_____ Low complexity	Limited	Limited	Low
_____ Moderate complexity	Multiple	Moderate	Moderate
_____ High complexity	Extensive	Extensive	High

Documented complexity of medical decision making is: _____

_____ YES   Does the chart documentation of history, physical examination and complexity of medical decision making for today's encounter clearly and

_____ NO   adequately support the E/M code AND the medical need for all diagnostic and therapeutic services provided or ordered?

E/M Code Documented_____ E/M Code Assigned_____

E/M DOCUMENTATION/SELF-AUDIT MATRIX—EXAMPLE 3: 1995 GUIDELINES

E/M Documentation Auditors' Instructions

1. History

Refer to data section (table below) in order to quantify. After referring to data, circle the entry farthest to the RIGHT in the table, which best describes the HPI, ROS and PFSH. If one column contains three circles, draw a line down that column to the bottom row to identify the type of history. If no column contains three circles, the column containing a circle farthest to the LEFT, identifies the type of history.

After completing this table which classifies the history, circle the type of history within the appropriate grid in Section 5.

HPI (history of present illness) elements:

☐ Location	☐ Severity	☐ Timing	☐ Modifying factors	Brief (1-3)	Brief (1-3)	Extended* (4 or more)	Extended* (4 or more)
☐ Quality	☐ Duration	☐ Context	☐ Associated signs and symptoms				

ROS (review of systems):

				None	Pertinent to problem (1 system)	Extended (2-9 systems)	Complete
☐ Constitutional (wt loss,etc.)	☐ GI	☐ Integumentary (skin, breast)	☐ Endo				
☐ Eyes	☐ GU	☐ Neuro	☐ Hem/lymph				
☐ Card/vasc	☐ Musculo	☐ Psych	☐ All/immuno				
☐ Resp	☐ Ears, nose, rnouth,throat		☐ All others negative				

10 or more systems, or some systems with statement all others negative

PFSH (past medical, family, social history) areas:

	None	None	Pertinent (1 history area)	Complete (2 or 3 history areas)
☐ Past history (the patient's past experiences with illnesses, operation, injuries and treatments) ☐ Family history (a review of medical events in the patient's family, including diseases which may be hereditary or place the patient at risk) ☐ Social history (an age appropriale review of past and current activities)				

Complete PFSH:
2 hx areas: a) Establish pts, office (outpt) care, b) Emergency dept, c) Subseq nursing facility care
3 hx areas: a) New pts, office (outpt) care, domiciliary care, b) Consultations, c) Initial hospital care, d) Hospital observation, e) Comprehensive nursing facility assessments.

Problem Focused	Exp. Prob Focused	Detailed	Comprehensive

*Status of 3 or more chronic/inactive conditions

2. Examination

Refer to data section (table below) in order to quantify. After referring to data, identify the type of examination. Circle the type of examination within the appropriate grid in Section 5.

Limited to affected body area or organ system (one body area or system related to problem)	Problem Focused Exam
Affected body area or organ system and other symptomatic or related organ system(s) (additional systems up to total of 7)	Expanded Problem Focused Exam
Extended exam of affected area(s) and other symptomatic or related organ system(s) (additional sysems up to total of 7 or more depth than above)	Detailed Exam
General multi-system exam (8 or more systems) or complete exam of a single organ system (complete single system exam not defined in these instructions)	Comprehensive Exam

Body areas:

			☐ 1 body area or system	☐ Up to 7 systems	☐ Up to 7 systems	☐ 8 or more systems
☐ Head, including face,	☐ Abdomen	☐ Genitilia, groin, buttocks				
☐ Chest, including each extremity	☐ Neck	☐ Back. including spine				
		☐ Breasts and axilla				

Organ Systems:

☐ Constitutional (e.g., vitals, gen app)	☐ Ears, nose, mouth, throat	☐ Musculo	☐ Psych				
☐ Cardiovascular	☐ Resp	☐ Skin	☐ Hem/lymph/imm				
	☐ GI	☐ Neuro	☐ Eyes				
		☐ GU					

Problem Focused	Exp. Prob. Focused	Detailed	Comprehensive

(Example 3 Continued)

3. Medical Decision Making

Number of Diagnoses or Treatment Options

Identify each problem or treatment option mentioned in the record. Enter the number in each of the categories in Column B in the table below. (There are maximum number in two categories.) Do not categorize the problem(s) if the encounter is dominated by counseling/coordinating of care, and duration of time is not specified. In that case, enter 3 in the total box.

Number of Diagnoses or Treatment Options			
A	B	x C =	D
Problem(s) Status	Number	Point	Result
Self-limited or minor (stable, improved or worsening)	Max =2	1	
Est. problem (to examiner); stable. improved		1	
Est. problem (to examiner); worsening		2	
New problem (to examiner); no additional workup planned	Max =1	3	
New prob. (to examiner); add. workup planned		4	
	TOTAL		

Multiply the number in columns B & C and put the product in column D. Enter a total for Column D. Bring total to line A in Final Result for Complexity (table below)

Amount and/or Complexity of Data Reviewed

For each category of reviewed data identified, circle the number points column. Total the points.

Amount and/or Complexity of Data Reviewed	
Reviewed Data	Points
Review and/or order of clinical lab test	1
Review and/or order of tests in the radiology section of CPT	1
Review and/or order of tests in the medicine section of CPT	1
Discussion of tests results with performing providers	1
Discussion to obtain old records and/or obtain history from someone other than patient	1
Review and summarization of old records and/or obtaining history from someone other than patient and /or discussion of case with another health care provider	2
Independent visualization of image, tracing or specimen itself (not simply review of report)	2
TOTAL	

Bring total to line C in Final Result for Complexity (table below)

Use the risk table below as a guide to assign risk factors. It is understood that the ta below does not contain all specific instances of medical care; the table is intended to used as a guide. Circle the most appropriate factor(s) in each category. The overall measure of risk is the highest level circled. Enter the level of risk identified in Final F for Complexity (table below)

	Risk of Complications and/or Morbidity or Mortality		
Level of Risk	Presenting Problem(s)	Diagnostic Procedure(s) Ordered	Management Options Selected
Minimal	● One self-limited or minor problem, e.g., cold, insect bite, tinea corporis	● Laboratory tests requiring venipuncture ● Chest x-rays ● EKG/EEG ● Urinalysis ● Ultrasound, e.g., echo ● KOH prep	● Rest ● Gargles ● Elastic bandages ● Superficial dressings
Low	● Two or more self-limited or minor problems ● One stable chronic illness, e.g., well controlled hypertension of non-insulin dependent diabetes, cataract, BPH ● Acute uncomplicated illness or injury e.g. cystitis, allergic rhinitis, simple sprain	● Physiologic tests not under stress, e.g., pulmonary function tests ● Non-cardiovascular imaging studies with contrast, e.g., barium enema ● Superficial needle biopsies ● Clinical laboratory tests requiring arterial puncture ● Skin biopsies	● Over-the-counter drugs ● Minor surgery with no identified risk factors ● Physical therapy ● Occupational therapy ● IV fluids without additives
Moderate	● One or more chronic illnesses with mild exacerbation, progression, or side effects of treatment ● Two or more stable chronic illnesses ● Undiagnosed new problem with uncertain prognosis, e.g., lump in breast ● Acute illness with systemic symptoms, e.g., pyelonephritis, pneumonitis, colitis ● Acute complicated injury, e.g., head injury with brief loss of consciousness	● Physiologic tests not under stress, e.g., cardiac stress tests, fetal contraction stress test ● Diagnostic endoscopies with no identified risk factors ● Deep needle or incisional biopsies ● Cardiovascular imaging studies with contrast and no identified risk factors, e.g., arteriogram cardiac cath ● Obtain fluid from body cavity, e.g., lumbar puncture, thoracentesis, culdocentesis	● Minor surgery with identified risk factors ● Elective major surgery (open, percutaneous or endoscopic) with no identified risk factors ● Prescription drug management ● Therapeutic nuclear medicine ● IV fluids with additives ● Closed treatment of fracture or dislocation without manipulation
High	● One or more chronic illnesses with severe exacerbation, progression or side effects of treatment ● Acute or chronic illnesses or injuries that may pose a threat to life or bodily function, e.g., multiple trauma, acute MI pulmonary embolus, severe respiratory distress, progressive severe rheumatoid arthritis, psychiatric illness with potential threat to self or others, peritonitis, acute renal failure ● An abrupt change in neurologic status, seizure, TIA, weakness or sensory loss	● Cardiovascular imaging studies with contrast with identified risk factors ● Cardiac electrophysiological tests ● Diagnostic endoscopies with identified risk factors ● Discography	● Elective major surgery (open, percutaneous or endoscopic with identified risk factors) ● Emergency major surgery (open, percutaneous or endoscopic) ● Parenteral controlled substances ● Drug therapy requiring intensive monitoring for toxicity ● Decision not to resuscitate or to de-escalate care because of poor prognosis

MEDICAL DECISION MAKING

(EXAMPLE 3 CONTINUED)

Final Result for Complexity
Draw a line down any column with 2 or 3 circles to identify the type of decision making in that column. Otherwise, draw a line down the column with the 2nd circle from the left. After completing this table, which classifies complexity, circle the type of decision making within the appropriate grid in Section 5.

	Final Result for Complexity				
A	Number of diagnoses or treatment options	≤1 Minimal	2 Limited	3 Multiple	≥4 Extensive
B	Highest Risk	Minimal	Low	Moderate	High
C	Amount and complexity of data	≤1 Minimal	2 Limited	3 Multiple	≥4 Extensive
	Type of decision making	STRAIGHT FORWARD	LOW COMPLEX.	MODERATE COMPLEX.	HIGH COMPLEX

4. Time

If the provider documents total time and suggests that counseling or coordinating care dominates (more than 50%) the encounter, time may determine level of service. Documentation may refer to: prognosis, differential diagnosis, risks, benefits of treatment, instructions, compliance, risk reduction or discussion with another health care provider.

Does documentation reveal total time? Time: Face-to-face in outpatient setting. Unit/floor in inpatient setting
☐ Yes ☐ No

Does documentation describe the content of counseling or coordinating care?
☐ Yes ☐ No

Does documentation reveal that more than half of the time was counseling or coordinating care?
☐ Yes ☐ No

If all answers are "yes", select level based on time.

5. Level of Service

Outpatient, Consults (OUTPATIENT, INPATIENT & CONFIRMATION) and ER

	Consults/ER Requires 3 components within shaded area				
History	PF	EPF	D ER: EPF	C ER: D	C
Examination	PF	EPF	D ER: EPF	C ER: D	C
Complexity of medical decision	SF	SF ER: L	L ER:M	M	H
Average time (minutes) (Confirmatory consults & ER have no average time)	15 Outpt cons (99241) 20 Inpt cons (99251) Conf. cons (99271) ER (99281)	30 Outpt cons (99242) 40 Inpt cons (99252) Conf. cons (99272) ER (99282)	40 Outpt cons (99243) 55 Inpt cons (99253) Conf. cons (99273) ER (99283)	60 Outpt cons (99244) 80 Inpt cons (99254) Conf. cons (99274) ER (99284)	80 Outpt cons (99245) 110 Inpt cons (99255) Conf. cons (99275) ER (99285)
Level	I	II	III	IV	V

INPATIENT

	Initial Hospital/Observation Requires 3 components within shaded area			Subsequent Inpatient/Observation/Follow-up Consult Requires 2 components within shaded area		
History	D or C	C	C	PF interval	EPF interval	D interval
Examination	D or C	C	C	PF	EPF	D
Complexity of medical decision	SF/L	M	H	SF/L	M	H
Average time (minutes) (Init observation care has no average time)	30 Init hosp (99221) Init observ care (99218)	50 Init hosp (99222) Init observ care (99219)	70 Init hosp (99223) Init observ care (99220)	10 Subsequent Inpt. (99231) 10 FU con (99261) 15 Subsequent Observ (99224)	25 Subsequent Inpt. (99232) 20 FU con (99262) 25 Subsequent Observ (99225)	35 Subsequent Inpt. (99233) 30 FU con (99263) 35 Subsequent Observ (99226)
Level	I	II	III	I	II	III

NURSING FACILITY

	Annual Assessment/Admission			Subsequent Nursing Facility		
	Old Plan Review	New Plan	Admission			
	Requires 3 components within shaded area			Requires 2 components within shaded area		
History	D interval	D interval	C	PF interval	EPF interval	D interval
Examination	D or C	C	C	PF	EPF	D
Complexity of medical decision	SF/L	M to H	M to H	SF/L	M	M to H
Average time (minutes) (Confirmatory consults and ER have no average time)	30 (99301)	40 (99302)	50 (99303)	15 (99311)	25 (99312)	35 (99313)
Level	I	II	III	I	II	III

DOMICILIARY (Rest Home, Custodial Care) and Home Care

	New Requires 3 components within shaded area			Established Requires 2 components within shaded area		
History	PF	EPF	D	PF interval	EPF interval	D interval
Examination	PF	EPF	D	PF	EPF	D
Complexity of medical decision	SF/L	M to H	M to H	SF/L	M	H
No average time established	Domiciliary (99321) Home Care (99341)	Domiciliary (99322) Home Care (99342)	Domiciliary (99323) Home Care (99343)	Domiciliary (99331) Home Care (99351)	Domiciliary (99332) Home Care (99352)	Domiciliary (99333) Home Care (99353)
Level	I	II	III	I	II	III

PF= Problem focused   EPF= Expanded problem focused   D = Detailed   C= Comprehensive   L = Low   M = Moderate   H = High

DOMICILIARY OR REST HOME SERVICES

	Established			
	Requires 2 components within shaded area			
History	PF (interval)	EPF (interval)	D	C
Examination	PF	EPF	D	C
Complexity of medical decision	SF	L	M	M/H
Average time (minutes)	15 (99334)	25 (99335)	40 (99336)	60 (99337)

HOME SERVICES

	New				
	Requires 3 components within shaded area				
History	PF (interval)	EPF (interval)	D	C	C
Examination	PF	EPF	D	C	C
Complexity of medical decision	SF	L	M	M	H
Average time (minutes)	20 (99341)	30 (99342)	45 (99343)	60 (99344)	75 (99345)

HOME SERVICES

	Established			
	Requires 2 components within shaded area			
History	PF (interval)	EPF (interval)	D	C
Examination	PF	EPF	D	C
Complexity of medical decision	SF	L	M	M/H
Average time (minutes)	15 (99347)	25 (99348)	40 (99349)	60 (99350)

PF= Problem focused   EPF= Expanded problem focused   D = Detailed   C= Comprehensive   L = Low   M = Moderate   H = High

E/M Documentation/Self-Audit Matrix—Example 4: 1995 Guidelines

E/M Documentation Auditor's Instructions

Refer to data section (table below) in order to quantify. After referring to data, circle the entry farthest to the *RIGHT* in the table, which best describes the HPI, ROS and PFSH. If one column contains three circles, draw a line down that column to the bottom row to identify the type of history. If no column contains three circles, the column containing a circle farthest to the *LEFT*, identifies the type of history.

After completing this table which classifies the history, circle the type of history within the appropriate grid in Section 5.

H I S T O R Y					
HPI: Status of chronic conditions: ❑ 1 condition ❑ 2 conditions ❑ 3 conditions **OR**				❑ Status of 1-2 chronic conditions	❑ Status of 3 chronic conditions
HPI (history of present illness) elements: ❑ Location ❑ Severity ❑ Timing ❑ Modifying factors ❑ Quality ❑ Duration ❑ Context ❑ Associated signs and symptoms				❑ Brief (1-3)	❑ Extended (4 or more)
ROS (review of systems): ❑ Constitutional ❑ Ears,nose, ❑ GI ❑ Integumentary ❑ Endo (wt loss, etc) mouth, throat ❑ GU (skin, breast) ❑ Hem/lymph ❑ Eyes ❑ Card/vasc ❑ Musculo ❑ Neuro ❑ All/immuno ❑ Resp ❑ Psych ❑ All others negative	❑ None	❑ Pertinent to problem (1 system)	❑ Extended (2-9 systems)		❑ *Complete
PFSH (past medical, family, social history) areas: ❑ Past history (the patient's past experiences with illnesses, operation, injuries and treatments) ❑ Family history (a review of medical events in the patient's family, including diseases which may be hereditary or place the patient at risk) ❑ Social history (an age appropriate review of past and current activities)		❑ None	❑ Pertinent (1 history area)		❑ **Complete (2 or 3 history areas)
	PROBLEM FOCUSED	**EXP.PROB. FOCUSED**	**DETAILED**		**COMPRE- HENSIVE**

*Complete ROS: 10 or more systems or the pertinent positives and/or negatives of some systems with a statement "all others negative".

**Complete PFSH: 2 history areas: a) Established Patients - Office (Outpatient) Care; b) Emergency Department.

3 history areas: a) New Patients - Office (Outpatient) Care, Domiciliary Care, Home Care; b) Initial Hospital Care; c) Initial Hospital Observation; d) Initial Nursing Facility Care.

NOTE: For certain categories of E/M services that include only an interval history, it is not necessary to record information about the PFSH. Please refer to procedure code descriptions.

2. Examination

Refer to data section (table below) in order to quantify. After referring to data, identify the type of examination. Circle the type of examination within the appropriate grid in Section 5.

Limited to affected body area or organ system (one body area or system related to problem)	**PROBLEM FOCUSED EXAM**
Affected body area or organ system and other symptomatic or related organ system(s) (additional systems up to total of 7)	**EXPANDED PROBLEM FOCUSED EXAM**
Extended exam of affected area(s) and other symptomatic or related organ system(s) (additional systems up to total of 7 or more depth than above)	**DETAILED EXAM**
General multi-system exam (8 or more systems) or complete exam of a single organ system (complete single exam not defined in these instructions)	**COMPREHENSIVE EXAM**

E X A M				
Body areas: ❑ Head, including face ❑ Chest, including breasts and axillae ❑ Abdomen ❑ Neck ❑ Back, including spine ❑ Genitalia, groin, buttocks ❑ Each extremity **Organ systems:** ❑ Constitutional ❑ Ears,nose, ❑ Resp ❑ Musculo ❑ Psych (e.g., vitals, gen app) mouth, throat ❑ GI ❑ Skin ❑ Hem/lymph/imm ❑ Eyes ❑ Cardiovascular ❑ GU ❑ Neuro	❑ 1 body area or system	❑ Up to 7 systems	❑ Up to 7 systems	❑ 8 or more systems
	PROBLEM FOCUSED	**EXP.PROB. FOCUSED**	**DETAILED**	**COMPRE- HENSIVE**

(EXAMPLE 4 CONTINUED)

3. Medical Decision Making

Number of Diagnoses or Treatment Options

Identify each problem or treatment option mentioned in the record. Enter the number in each of the categories in Column B in the table below. (There are maximum number in two categories.)

MEDICAL DECISION MAKING

Number of Diagnoses or Treatment Options			
A	**B** X	**C** =	**D**
Problem(s) Status	**Number**	**Points**	**Result**
Self-limited or minor (stable, improved or worsening)	Max = 2	1	
Est. problem (to examiner); stable, improved		1	
Est. problem (to examiner); worsening		2	
New problem (to examiner); no additional workup planned	Max = 1	3	
New prob. (to examiner); add. workup planned		4	
		TOTAL	

Multiply the number in columns B & C and put the product in column D. Enter a total for column D.

Bring total to **line A** in Final Result for Complexity (table below)

Amount and/or Complexity of Data Reviewed

For each category of reviewed data identified, circle the number in the points column. Total the points.

Amount and/or Complexity of Data Reviewed	
Reviewed Data	**Points**
Review and/or order of clinical lab tests	1
Review and/or order of tests in the radiology section of CPT	1
Review and/or order of tests in the medicine section of CPT	1
Discussion of test results with performing physician	1
Decision to obtain old records and/or obtain history from someone other than patient	1
Review and summarization of old records and/or obtaining history from someone other than patient and/or discussion of case with another health care provider	2
Independent visualization of image, tracing or specimen itself (not simply review of report)	2
TOTAL	

Bring total to **line C** in Final Result for Complexity (table below)

Use the risk table below as a guide to assign risk factors. It is understood that the table below does not contain all specific instances of medical care; the table is intended to be used as a guide. Circle the most appropriate factor(s) in each category. The overall measure of risk is the highest level circled. Enter the level of risk identified in Final Result for Complexity (table below).

Risk of Complications and/or Morbidity or Mortality

Level of Risk	Presenting Problem(s)	Diagnostic Procedure(s) Ordered	Management Options Selected
Minimal	• One self-limited or minor problem, e.g., cold, insect bite, tinea corporis	• Laboratory tests requiring venipuncture • Chest x-rays • EKG/EEG • Urinalysis • Ultrasound, e.g., echo • KOH prep	• Rest • Gargles • Elastic bandages • Superficial dressings
Low	• Two or more self-limited or minor problems • One stable chronic illness, e.g., well controlled hypertension or non-insulin dependent diabetes, cataract, BPH • Acute uncomplicated illness or injury, e.g., cystitis, allergic rhinitis, simple sprain	• Physiologic tests not under stress, e.g., pulmonary function tests • Non-cardiovascular imaging studies with contrast, e.g., barium enema • Superficial needle biopsies • Clinical laboratory tests requiring arterial puncture • Skin biopsies	• Over-the-counter drugs • Minor surgery with no identified risk factors • Physical therapy • Occupational therapy • IV fluids without additives
Moderate	• One or more chronic illnesses with mild exacerbation, progression, or side effects of treatment • Two or more stable chronic illnesses • Undiagnosed new problem with uncertain prognosis, e.g., lump in breast • Acute illness with systemic symptoms, e.g., pyelonephritis, pneumonitis, colitis • Acute complicated injury, e.g., head injury with brief loss of consciousness	• Physiologic tests under stress, e.g., cardiac stress test, fetal contraction stress test • Diagnostic endoscopies with no identified risk factors • Deep needle or incisional biopsy • Cardiovascular imaging studies with contrast and no identified risk factors, e.g., arteriogram cardiac cath • Obtain fluid from body cavity, e.g., lumbar puncture, thoracentesis, culdocentesis	• Minor surgery with identified risk factors • Elective major surgery (open, percutaneous or endoscopic) with no identified risk factors • Prescription drug management • Therapeutic nuclear medicine • IV fluids with additives • Closed treatment of fracture or dislocation without manipulation
High	• One or more chronic illnesses with severe exacerbation, progression, or side effects of treatment • Acute or chronic illnesses or injuries that may pose a threat to life or bodily function, e.g., multiple trauma, acute MI, pulmonary embolus, severe respiratory distress, progressive severe rheumatoid arthritis, psychiatric illness with potential threat to self or others, peritonitis, acute renal failure • An abrupt change in neurologic status, e.g., seizure, TIA, weakness or sensory loss	• Cardiovascular imaging studies with contrast with identified risk factors • Cardiac electrophysiological tests • Diagnostic endoscopies with identified risk factors • Discography	• Elective major surgery (open, percutaneous or endoscopic with identified risk factors) • Emergency major surgery (open, percutaneous or endoscopic) • Parenteral controlled substances • Drug therapy requiring intensive monitoring for toxicity • Decision not to resuscitate or to de-escalate care because of poor prognosis

Final Result for Complexity

Draw a line down any column with 2 or 3 circles to identify the type of decision making in that column. Otherwise, draw a line down the column with the 2nd circle from the left. After completing this table, which classifies complexity, circle the type of decision making within the appropriate grid in Section 5.

	Final Result for Complexity				
A	Number diagnoses or treatment options	≤ 1 Minimal	2 Limited	3 Multiple	≥ 4 Extensive
B	Highest Risk	Minimal	Low	Moderate	High
C	Amount and complexity of data	≤ 1 Minimal or low	2 Limited	3 Multiple	≥ 4 Extensive
	Type of decision making	STRAIGHT-FORWARD	LOW COMPLEX.	MODERATE COMPLEX.	HIGH COMPLEX.

4. Time

If the physician documents total time *and* suggests that counseling or coordinating care dominates (more than 50%) the encounter, time may determine level of service. Documentation may refer to: prognosis, differential diagnosis, risks, benefits of treatment, instructions, compliance, risk reduction or discussion with another health care provider.

Does documentation reveal total time? Time: Face to face in outpatient setting / Unit/floor in inpatient setting		Yes	No
Does documentation describe the content of counseling or coordinating care?		Yes	No
Does documentation reveal that more than half of the time was counseling or coordinating care?		Yes	No

If all answers are "yes", select level based on time.

(EXAMPLE 4 CONTINUED)

5. Level of Service

Emergency Room

	Outpatient / ER				
	Requires 3 components within shaded area				
History	PF **ER: PF**	EPF **ER: EPF**	D **ER: EPF**	C **ER: D**	C **ER: C**
Examination	PF **ER: PF**	EPF **ER: EPF**	D **ER: EPF**	C **ER: D**	C **ER: C**
Complexity of medical decision	SF **ER: SF**	SF **ER: L**	L **ER: M**	M **ER: M**	H **ER: H**
Average time (minutes) ER has no average time	ER (99281)	ER (99282)	ER (99283)	ER (99284)	ER (99285)
Level	I	II	III	IV	V

Hospital Care

	Initial Hospital/Observation			Subsequent Hospital/Observation		
	Requires 3 components within shaded area			**Requires 2 components within shaded area**		
History	D/C	C	C	PF interval	EPF interval	D interval
Examination	D/C	C	C	PF	EPF	D
Complexity of medical decision	SF/L	M	H	SF/L	M	H
Average time (minutes)	30 Init hosp (99221) 30 Init observ Care (99218)	50 Init hosp (99222) 50 Init observ Care (99219)	70 Init hosp (99223) 70 Init observ care (99220)	15 Sub hosp (99231) 15 Sub observ care (99224)	25 Sub hosp (99232) 25 Sub observ care (99225)	35 Sub hosp (99233) 35 Sub observ care (99226)
Level	I	II	III	I	II	III

Nursing Facility Care

	Initial Nursing Facility			Subsequent Nursing Facility				Other Nursing Facility (Annual Assessment)
	Requires 3 components within shaded area			**Requires 2 components within shaded area**				**Requires 3 components within shaded area**
History	D/C	C	C	PF interval	EPF interval	D interval	C interval	D interval
Examination	D/C	C	C	PF	EPF	D	C	C
Complexity of medical decision	SF/L	M	H	SF	L	M	H	L/M
Average time (minutes)	25 99304	35 99305	45 99306	10 99307	15 99308	25 99309	35 99310	30 99318
Level	I	II	III	I	II	III	IV	

Domiciliary, Rest Home (eg, Boarding Home), or Custodial Care Services and Home Care

	Requires 3 components within shaded area					**Requires 2 components within shaded area**			
History	PF	EPF	D	C	C	PF interval	EPF interval	D interval	C interval
Examination	PF	EPF	D	C	C	PF	EPF	D	C
Complexity of medical decision	SF	L	M	M	H	SF	L	M	M/H
Average time (minutes)	20 Domiciliary (99324) Home care (99341)	30 Domiciliary (99325) Home care (99342)	45 Domiciliary (99326) Home care (99343)	60 Domiciliary (99327) Home care (99344)	75 Domiciliary (99328) Home care (99345)	15 Domiciliary (99334) Home care (99347)	25 Domiciliary (99335) Home care (99348)	40 Domiciliary (99336) Home care (99349)	60 Domiciliary (99337) Home care (99350)
Level	I	II	III	IV	V	I	II	III	IV

PF = Problem focused   EPF = Expanded problem focused   D = Detailed   C = Comprehensive   SF = Straightforward   L = Low   M = Moderate   H = High

E/M Documentation/Self-Audit Matrix—Example 5: Multi-System Specialty Exam

HIC#

DATE OF SERVICE

SPECIALTY EXAM: GENERAL MULTI-SYSTEM

Refer to data section (table below) in order to quantify. After reviewing the medical record documentation, identify the level of examination. Circle the level of examination within the appropriate grid in Section 5 (Page 3).

Performed and Documented	Level of Exam
One to five bullets	Problem Focused
At least six bullets	Expanded Problem Focused
At least two bullets from **each of six** body systems/areas **OR** at least twelve bullets in any two or more body systems/areas.	Detailed
At least two bullets from **each** of nine body systems/areas	Comprehensive

(Circle the bullets that are documented.)

NOTE: For the descriptions of the elements of examination containing the words "and", "and/or", only one (1) of those elements must be documented.

System/Body Area	Elements of Examination
Constitutional	• Measurement of **any three of the following seven** vital signs: 1) sitting or standing blood pressure, 2) supine blood pressure, 3) pulse rate and regularity, 4) respiration, 5) temperature, 6) height, 7) weight (May be measured and recorded by ancillary staff) • General appearance of patient (e.g., development, nutrition, body habitus, deformities, attention to grooming)
Eyes	• Inspection of conjunctivae and lids • Examination of pupils and irises (e.g., reaction to light and accommodation, size and symmetry) • Ophthalmoscopic examination of optic discs (e.g., size, C/D ratio, appearance) and posterior segments (e.g., vessel changes, exudates, hemorrhages)
Ears, Nose, Mouth and Throat	• External inspection of ears and nose (e.g., overall appearance, scars, lesions, masses) • Otoscopic examination of external auditory canals and tympanic membranes • Assessment of hearing (e.g., whispered voice, finger rub, tuning fork) • Inspection of lips, teeth and gums • Examination of oropharynx: oral mucosa, salivary glands, hard and soft palates, tongue, tonsils and posterior pharynx • Inspection of nasal mucosa, septum and turbinates

1a

System/Body Area	Elements of Examination
Neck	• Examination of neck (e.g., masses, overall appearance, symmetry, tracheal position, crepitus) • Examination of thyroid (e.g., enlargement, tenderness, mass)
Respiratory	• Assessment of respiratory effort (e.g., intercostal retractions, use of accessory muscles, diaphragmatic movement) • Percussion of chest (e.g., dullness, flatness, hyperresonance) • Palpation of chest (e.g., tactile fremitus) • Auscultation of lungs (e.g., breath sounds, adventitious sounds, rubs)
Cardiovascular	• Palpation of heart (e.g., location, size, thrills) • Auscultation of heart with notation of abnormal sounds and murmurs Examination of: • Carotid arteries (e.g., pulse amplitude, bruits) • Abdominal aorta (e.g., size, bruits) • Femoral arteries (e.g., pulse amplitude, bruits) • Pedal pulses (e.g., pulse amplitude) • Extremities for edema and/or varicosities
Chest (Breasts)	• Inspection of breasts (e.g., symmetry, nipple discharge) • Palpation of breasts and axillae (e.g., masses or lumps, tenderness)
Gastrointestinal (Abdomen)	• Examination of abdomen with notation of presence of masses or tenderness • Examination of liver and spleen • Examination for presence or absence of hernia • Examination of anus, perineum and rectum, including sphincter tone, presence of hemorrhoids, rectal masses • Obtain stool sample for occult blood test when indicated

1b

10229-1 11/97

Appendix B: Crosswalk for 1995 and 1997 E/M Documentation Guidelines

E/M Guidelines Crosswalk		
CPT® Code	**1995 Guidelines**	**1997 Guidelines**
Initial Hospital Observation Services		
99218	**History:** CC; extended HPI; problem-pertinent ROS including review of limited number additional systems; pertinent PFSH directly related to problem(s) or CC; extended HPI; ROS directly related to problem(s) plus review of all additional systems; complete PFSH	**History:** Same. Document two–nine systems for ROS. PFSH should document one item from any history area or Same. Document at least four elements of HPI or document at least three chronic/inactive conditions. ROS should document at least 10 organ systems
	Exam: Extended exam of affected body area(s)/organ system(s) & other related/symptomatic system(s) or General multisystem exam or complete exam of a single-organ system, basing exam on the seven recognized body areas and/or the 11 recognized organ systems	**Exam:** Two bullet elements in at least six organ systems/body areas OR 12 bullet elements in two or more organ systems/body areas. Single System-Eye or Psychiatric Exams: nine bullet elements are required or All bullet elements in at least nine organ systems/body areas. Document no less than two bullet elements in each area/system reviewed. Single System Exams: Must document all bullet elements in shaded boxes and at least one bullet element in each unshaded box
	MDM: Dx/management options-minimal; amount/complexity dataminimal or none; risk-minimal or Dx/management options-limited; amount/complexity data-limited; risk-low	**MDM:** Same or Same
99219	**History:** CC; extended HPI; ROS directly related to problem(s) plus review of all additional systems; complete PFSH	**History:** Same. Document at least four elements of HPI or document at least three chronic/inactive conditions. ROS should document at least 10 organ systems
	Exam: General multisystem exam or complete exam of a single-organ system, basing exam on the seven recognized body areas and/or the 11 recognized organ systems	**Exam:** All bullet elements in at least nine organ systems/body areas. Document no less than two bullet elements in each area/system reviewed. Single System Exams: Must document all bullet elements in shaded boxes and at least one bullet element in each unshaded box
	MDM: Dx/management options-minimal; amount/complexity datamoderate; risk-moderate	**MDM:** Same
99220	**History:** CC; extended HPI; ROS directly related to problem(s) plus review of all additional systems; complete PFSH	**History:** Same. Document at least 4 elements of HPI or document at least three chronic/inactive conditions. ROS should document at least 10 organ systems.
	Exam: General multisystem exam or complete exam of a single-organ system, basing exam on the seven recognized body areas and/or the 11 recognized organ systems	**Exam:** All bullet elements in at least nine organ systems/body areas. Document no less than two bullet elements in each area/system reviewed. Single-System Exams: Must document all bullet elements in shaded boxes and at least one bullet element in each unshaded box
	MDM: Dx/management options extensive; amount/complexity data-extensive; risk high	**MDM:** Same

E/M Guidelines Crosswalk

CPT® Code	1995 Guidelines	1997 Guidelines
Subsequent Hospital Observation Services (Resequenced)		
99224	**History:** CC; brief HPI	**History:** Same
	Exam: Limited exam of affected body area/organ system	**Exam:** One to five bullet elements in one or more organ systems or body areas
	MDM: Dx/management options minimal; amount/complexity data minimal or none; risk-minimal or Dx/management options-limited; amount/complexity data-limited risk-low	**MDM:** Same or Same
99225	**History:** CC; brief HPI; problem pertinent ROS	**History:** Same
	Exam: Limited exam of affected body area/organ system & other related/symptomatic system(s)	**Exam:** Six bullet elements in one or more organ systems or body areas
	MDM: Dx/management options multiple; amount/complexity data- moderate; risk-moderate	**MDM:** Same
99226	**History:** CC; extended HPI; problem-pertinent ROS including review of limited number additional systems; pertinent PFSH directly related to problem(s)	**History:** Same. Document two–nine systems for ROS. PFSH should document one item from any history area
	Exam: Extended exam of affected body area(s)/organ system(s) & other related/symptomatic system(s)	**Exam:** Two bullet elements in at least six organ systems/body areas OR 12 bullet elements in two or more organ systems/body areas. Single-System-Eye or Psychiatric Exams: nine bullet elements are required
	MDM: Dx/management options extensive; amount/complexity data-extensive; risk-high	**MDM:** Same
99221	**History:** CC; extended HPI problem-pertinent ROS including review of limited number additional systems; pertinent PFSH directly related to problem(s) or CC; extended HPI; ROS directly related to problem(s) plus review of all additional systems; complete PFSH	**History:** Same. Document two–nine systems for ROS. PFSH should document one item from any history area or Same. Document at least four elements of HPI or document at least three chronic/inactive conditions. ROS should document at least 10 organ systems
	Exam: Extended exam of affected body area(s)/organ system(s) & other related/symptomatic system(s) or General multisystem exam or complete exam of a single-organ system, basing exam on the seven recognized body areas and/or the 11 recognized organ systems	**Exam:** Two bullet elements in at least six organ systems/body areas OR 12 bullet elements in two or more organ systems/body areas. Single-System-Eye or Psychiatric Exams: nine bullet elements are required All bullet elements in at least nine organ systems/body areas. Document no less than two bullet elements in each area/system reviewed. Single-System Exams: Must document all bullet elements in shaded boxes and at least one bullet element in each unshaded box
	MDM: Dx/management options minimal; amount/complexity data- minimal or none; risk-minimal or Dx/management options-limited; amount/complexity data-limited; risk-low	**MDM:** Same or Same

E/M Guidelines Crosswalk		
CPT® Code	**1995 Guidelines**	**1997 Guidelines**
99222	**History:** CC; extended HPI; ROS directly related to problem(s) plus review of all additional systems; complete PFSH	**History:** Same. Document at least four elements of HPI or document at least three chronic/inactive conditions. ROS should document at least 10 organ systems
	Exam: General multisystem exam or complete exam of a single-organ system, basing exam on the seven recognized body areas and/or the 11 recognized organ systems	**Exam:** All bullet elements in at least nine organ systems/body areas. Document no less than two bullet elements in each area/system reviewed. Single-System Exams: Must document all bullet elements in shaded boxes and at least one bullet element in each unshaded box
	MDM: Dx/management options multiple; amount/complexity data moderate; risk-moderate	**MDM:** Same
99223	**History:** CC; extended HPI; ROS directly related to problem(s) plus review of all additional systems; complete PFSH	**History:** Same. Document at least four elements of HPI or document at least three chronic/inactive conditions. ROS should document at least 10 organ systems
	Exam: General multisystem exam or complete exam of a single-organ system, basing exam on the seven recognized body areas and/or the 11 recognized organ systems	**Exam:** All bullet elements in at least nine organ systems/body areas. Document no less than two bullet elements in each area/system reviewed. Single-System Exams: Must document all bullet elements in shaded boxes and at least one bullet element in each unshaded box
	MDM: Dx/management options multiple; amount/complexity data moderate; risk-moderate	**MDM:** Same
Hospital Inpatient Services, Subsequent Hospital Care		
99231	**History:** CC; brief HPI	**History:** Same.
	Exam: Limited exam of affected body area/organ system	**Exam:** one to five bullet elements in one or more organ systems or body areas
	MDM: Dx/management options minimal; amount/complexity data minimal or none; risk-minimal or Dx/management options-limited; amount/complexity data-limited risk-low	**MDM:** Same or Same
99232	**History:** CC; brief HPI; problem pertinent ROS	**History:** Same.
	Exam: Limited exam of affected body area/organ system & other related/symptomatic system(s)	**Exam:** Six bullet elements in one or more organ systems or body areas
	MDM: Dx/management options multiple; amount/complexity data- moderate; risk-moderate	**MDM:** Same
99233	**History:** CC; extended HPI; problem-pertinent ROS including review of limited number additional systems; pertinent PFSH directly related to problem(s)	**History:** Same. Document two–nine systems for ROS. PFSH should document one item from any history area
	Exam: Extended exam of affected body area(s)/organ system(s) & other related/symptomatic system(s)	**Exam:** Two bullet elements in at least six organ systems/body areas OR 12 bullet elements in two or more organ systems/body areas. Single-System-Eye or Psychiatric Exams: nine bullet elements are required
	MDM: Dx/management options extensive; amount/complexity data-extensive; risk-high	**MDM:** Same

E/M Guidelines Crosswalk		
CPT® Code	**1995 Guidelines**	**1997 Guidelines**
Observation or Inpatient Care Services (Including Admission and Discharge Services)		
99234	**History:** CC; extended HPI; problem-pertinent ROS including review of limited number additional systems; pertinent PFSH directly related to problem(s) or CC; extended HPI; ROS directly related to problem(s) plus review of all additional systems; complete PFSH	**History:** Same. Document two–nine systems for ROS. PFSH should document one item from any history area or Same. Document at least four elements of HPI or document at least three chronic/inactive conditions. ROS should document at least 10 organ systems
	Exam: Extended exam of affected body area(s)/organ system(s) & other related/symptomatic system(s) or General multisystem exam or complete exam of a single-organ system, basing exam on the seven recognized body areas and/or the 11 recognized organ systems	**Exam:** Two bullet elements in at least six organ systems/body areas OR 12 bullet elements in two or more organ systems/body areas. Single System-Eye or Psychiatric Exams: nine bullet elements are required or All bullet elements in at least nine organ systems/body areas. Document no less than two bullet elements in each area/system reviewed. Single System Exams: Must document all bullet elements in shaded boxes and at least one bullet element in each unshaded box
	MDM: Dx/management options- minimal; amount/complexity dataminimal or none; risk-minimal or Dx/management options-limited; amount/complexity data-limited; risk-low	**MDM:** Same or Same
99235	**History:** CC; extended HPI; ROS directly related to problem(s) plus review of all additional systems; complete PFSH	**History:** Same. Document at least four elements of HPI or document at least three chronic/inactive conditions. ROS should document at least 10 organ systems
	Exam: General multisystem exam or complete exam of a single-organ system, basing exam on the seven recognized body areas and/or the 11 recognized organ systems	**Exam:** All bullet elements in at least nine organ systems/body areas. Document no less than two bullet elements in each area/system reviewed. Single System Exams: Must document all bullet elements in shaded boxes and at least one bullet element in each unshaded box
	MDM: Dx/management options-multiple; amount/complexity data-moderate; risk-moderate	**MDM:** Same
99236	**History:** CC; extended HPI; ROS directly related to problem(s) plus review of all additional systems; complete PFSH	**History:** Same. Document at least four elements of HPI or document at least three chronic/inactive conditions. ROS should document at least 10 organ systems
	Exam: General multisystem exam or complete exam of a single-organ system, basing exam on the seven recognized body areas and/or the 11 recognized organ systems	**Exam:** All bullet elements in at least nine organ systems/body areas. Document no less than two bullet elements in each area/system reviewed. Single System Exams: Must document all bullet elements in shaded boxes and at least one bullet element in each unshaded box
	MDM: Dx/management options-extensive; amount/complexity data-extensive; risk-high	**MDM:** Same
Office or Other Outpatient Consultations		
99241	**History:** CC; brief HPI	**History:** Same.
	Exam: Limited exam of affected body area/organ system	**Exam:** one–five bullet elements in one or more organ systems or body areas
	MDM: Dx/management options minimal; amount/complexity data- minimal or none; risk-minimal	**MDM:** Same

E/M Guidelines Crosswalk

CPT® Code	1995 Guidelines	1997 Guidelines
99242	**History:** CC; brief HPI; problem-pertinent ROS	**History:** Same.
	Exam: Limited exam of affected body area/organ system related /symptomatic system(s)	**Exam:** Six bullet elements in one or more organ systems or body areas
	MDM: Dx/management options minimal; amount/complexity data- minimal or none; risk-minimal	**MDM:** Same
99243	**History:** CC; extended HPI; problem-pertinent ROS including review of limited number additional systems; pertinent PFSH directly related to problem(s)	**History:** Same. Document two–nine systems for ROS. PFSH should document one item from any history area
	Exam: Extended exam of affected body area(s)/organ system(s) & other related/symptomatic system(s)	**Exam:** Two bullet elements in at least six organ systems/body areas OR 12 bullet elements in two or more organ systems/body areas. Single System-Eye or Psychiatric Exams: nine bullet elements are required
	MDM: Dx/management options minimal; amount/complexity data- minimal or none; risk-low	**MDM:** Same
99244	**History:** CC; extended HPI; ROS directly related to problem(s) plus review of all additional systems; complete PFSH	**History:** Same. Document at least four elements of HPI or document at least three chronic/inactive conditions. ROS should document at least 10 organ systems
	Exam: General multisystem exam or complete exam of a single-organ system, basing exam on the seven recognized body areas and/or the 11 recognized organ systems	**Exam:** All bullet elements in at least nine organ systems/body areas. Document no less than two bullet elements in each area/system reviewed. Single-System Exams: Must document all bullet elements in shaded boxes and at least one bullet element in each unshaded box
	MDM: Dx/management options multiple; amount/complexity data- moderate; risk-moderate	**MDM:** Same
99245	**History:** CC; extended HPI; ROS directly related to problem(s) plus review of all additional systems; complete PFSH	**History:** Same. Document at least four elements of HPI or document at least three chronic/inactive conditions. ROS should document at least 10 organ systems
	Exam: General multisystem exam or complete exam of a single-organ system, basing exam on the seven recognized body areas and/or the 11 recognized organ systems	**Exam:** All bullet elements in at least nine organ systems/body areas. Document no less than two bullet elements in each area/system reviewed. Single-System Exams: Must document all bullet elements in shaded boxes and at least one bullet element in each unshaded box
	MDM: Dx/management options extensive; amount/complexity data-extensive; risk-high	**MDM:** Same

Inpatient Consultations

CPT® Code	1995 Guidelines	1997 Guidelines
99251	**History:** CC; brief HPI	**History:** Same.
	Exam: Limited exam of affected body area/organ system	**Exam:** 1-5 bullet elements in one or more organ systems or body areas
	MDM: Dx/management options minimal; amount/complexity data-minimal or none; risk-minimal	**MDM:** Same
99252	**History:** CC; brief HPI; problem pertinent ROS	**History:** Same.
	Exam: Limited exam of affected body area/organ system & other related/symptomatic system(s).	**Exam:** Six bullet elements in one or more organ systems or body areas
	MDM: Dx/management options minimal; amount/complexity data-minimal or none; risk-minimal	**MDM:** Same

E/M Guidelines Crosswalk

CPT® Code	1995 Guidelines	1997 Guidelines
99253	**History:** CC; extended HPI; problem-pertinent ROS including review of limited number additional systems; pertinent PFSH directly related to problem(s)	**History:** Same. Document two–nine systems for ROS. PFSH should document one item from any history area
	Exam: Extended exam of affected body area(s)/organ system(s) & other related/symptomatic system(s) elements in two or more organ systems/body areas.	**Exam:** Two bullet elements in at least six organ systems/body areas OR 12 bullet Single System-Eye or Psychiatric Exams: 9 bullet elements are required
	MDM: Dx/management options limited; amount/complexity data- limited; risk-low	**MDM:** Same
99254	**History:** CC; extended HPI; ROS directly related to problem(s) plus review of all additional systems; complete PFSH	**History:** Same. Document at least four elements of HPI or document at least three chronic/inactive conditions. ROS should document at least 10 organ systems
	Exam: General multisystem exam or complete exam of a single-organ system, basing exam on the seven recognized body areas and/or the 11 recognized organ systems	**Exam:** All bullet elements in at least nine organ systems/body areas. Document no less than two bullet elements in each area/system reviewed. Single-System Exams: Must document all bullet elements in shaded boxes and at least one bullet element in each unshaded box
	MDM: Dx/management options multiple; amount/complexity data- moderate; risk-moderate	**MDM:** Same
99255	**History:** CC; extended HPI; ROS directly related to problem(s) plus review of all additional systems; complete PFSH	**History:** Same. Document at least four elements of HPI or document at least three chronic/inactive conditions. ROS should document at least 10 organ systems
	Exam: General multisystem exam or complete exam of a single-organ system, basing exam on the seven recognized body areas and/or the 11 recognized organ systems	**Exam:** All bullet elements in at least nine organ systems/body areas. Document no less than two bullet elements in each area/system reviewed. Single-System Exams: Must document all bullet elements in shaded boxes and at least one bullet element in each unshaded box
	MDM: Dx/management options extensive; amount/complexity data- extensive; risk-high	**MDM:** Same
Emergency Department Services		
99281	**History:** CC; brief HPI	**History:** Same.
	Exam: Limited exam of affected body area/organ system	**Exam:** one–five bullet elements in one or more organ systems or body areas
	MDM: Dx/management options minimal; amount/complexity data-minimal or none; risk-minimal	**MDM:** Same
99282	**History:** CC; brief HPI; problem-pertinent ROS	**History:** Same.
	Exam: Limited exam of affected body area/organ system & other related/symptomatic system(s)	**Exam:** Six bullet elements in one or more organ systems or body areas
	MDM: Dx/management options limited; amount/complexity data- limited; risk-low	**MDM:** Same
99283	**History:** CC; brief HPI; problem-pertinent ROS	**History:** Same.
	Exam: Limited exam of affected body area/organ system & other related/symptomatic system(s)	**Exam:** Six bullet elements in one or more organ systems or body areas
	MDM: Dx/management options multiple; amount/complexity data- multiple; risk-moderate	**MDM:** Same

E/M Guidelines Crosswalk		
CPT® Code	**1995 Guidelines**	**1997 Guidelines**
99284	**History:** CC; extended HPI; problem-pertinent ROS including review of limited number additional systems; pertinent PFSH directly related to problem(s)	**History:** Same. Document two–nine systems for ROS. PFSH should document one item from any history area
	Exam: Extended exam of affected body area(s)/organ system(s) & other related/symptomatic organ system(s) or body area(s)	**Exam:** Two bullet elements in at least six organ systems/body areas OR 12 bullet elements in two or more organ systems/body areas. Single System-Eye or Psychiatric Exams: 9 bullet elements are required
	MDM: Dx/management options multiple; amount/complexity data- moderate; risk-moderate	**MDM:** Same
99285	**History:** CC; extended HPI; ROS directly related to problem(s) plus review of all additional systems; complete PFSH	**History:** Same. Document at least 4 elements of HPI or document at least 3 chronic/inactive conditions. ROS should document at least 10 organ systems
	Exam: General multisystem exam or complete exam of a single-organ system, basing exam on the 7 recognized body areas and/or the 11 recognized organ systems	**Exam:** All bullet elements in at least 9 organ systems/body areas. Document no less than 2 bullet elements in each area/system reviewed. Single-System Exams: Must document all bullet elements in shaded boxes and at least one bullet element in each unshaded box
	MDM: Dx/management options extensive; amount/complexity data- extensive; risk-high	**MDM:** Same
Nursing Facility Assessments		
99304	**History:** CC; extended HPI; problem-pertinent ROS including review of limited number of additional systems; pertinent PFSH directly related to problem(s) or CC; extended HPI; ROS directly related to problem(s) plus review of all additional systems; complete PFSH	**History:** Same. Document two–nine systems for ROS. PFSH should document one item from any history area or Same. Document at least four elements of HPI or document at least three chronic/inactive conditions. ROS should document at least 10 organ systems
	Exam: Extended exam of affected body area(s)/organ system(s) and other related/symptomatic system(s) or General multisystem exam or complete exam of a single-organ system, basing exam on the seven recognized body areas and/or the 11 recognized organ systems	**Exam:** Two bullet elements in two or more organ systems/body areas OR 12 bullet elements in two or more organ systems/body areas. Single System–Eye or psychiatric exams; nine bullet elements are required or All bullet elements in at least nine organ systems/body areas. Document no less than two bullet elements in each area/system reviewed. Single-System Exams: Must document all bullet elements in shaded boxes and at least one bullet element in each unshaded box
	MDM: Dx/management options-minimal; amount/complexity data-minimal or non; risk-minimal or Dx/management options-limited; amount/complexity data-limited; risk-low	**MDM:** Same
99305	**History:** CC; extended HPI; ROS directly related to problem(s) plus review of all additional systems; complete PFSH	**History:** Same
	Exam: General multisystem exam or complete exam of a single-organ system, basing exam on the seven recognized body areas and/or the 11 recognized organ systems	**Exam:** All bullet elements in at least nine organ systems/body areas. Document no less than two bullet elements in each area/system reviewed. Single-System Exams: Must document all bullet elements in shaded boxes and at least one bullet element in each unshaded box
	MDM: Dx/management options-multiple; amount/complexity data-moderate; risk-moderate	**MDM:** Same

E/M Guidelines Crosswalk

CPT® Code	1995 Guidelines	1997 Guidelines
99306	**History:**CC; extended HPI; ROS directly related to problem(s) plus review of all additional systems; complete PFSH	**History**: Same
	Exam: General multisystem exam or complete exam of a single-organ system, basing exam on the seven recognized body areas and/or the 11 recognized organ systems	**Exam**: All bullet elements in at least nine organ systems/body areas. Document no less than two bullet elements in each area/system reviewed. Single-System Exams: Must document all bullet elements in shaded boxes and at least one bullet element in each unshaded box
	MDM: Dx/management options-extensive: amount/complexity data-extensive; risk-high	**MDM**: Same
99307	**History**: CC; brief HPI	**History**: Same
	Exam: Limited exam of affected body area/organ system	**Exam**:One–five bullet elements in one or more organ systems of body areas
	MDM: Dx/management options-minimal; amount/complexity data-minimal or non; risk-minimal	**MDM**: Same
99308	**History**: CC; brief HPI; problem pertinent ROS	**History**: Same
	Exam: Limited exam of affected body area/organ system and other related/symptomatic system(s)	**Exam**: Six bullet elements in one or more organ systems or body areas
	MDM: Dx/management options-limited; amount/complexity data-limited; risk-low	**MDM**: Same
99309	**History**: CC; extended HPI; problem-pertinent ROS including review of limited number of additional systems; pertinent PFSH directly related to problem(s)	**History**: Same. Document two-nine systems for ROS. PFSH should document one item from any history area
	Exam: Extended exam of affected body area(s)/organ system(s) and other related/symptomatic system(s)	**Exam**: Two bullet elements in six organ systems/body areas OR 12 bullet elements in two or more organ systems/body areas. Single System–Eye or psychiatric exams; nine bullet elements are required
	MDM: Dx/management options-multiple; amount/complexity data-moderate; risk-moderate	**MDM**: Same
99310	**History:**CC; extended HPI; ROS directly related to problem(s) plus review of all additional systems; complete PFSH	**History**: Same. Document at least four elements of HPI or document at least three chronic/inactive conditions. ROS should document at least 10 organ systems
	Exam: General multisystem exam or complete exam of a single-organ system, basing exam on the seven recognized body areas and/or the 11 recognized organ systems	**Exam**: All bullet elements in at least nine organ systems/body areas. Document no less than two bullet elements in each area/system reviewed. Single-System Exams: Must document all bullet elements in shaded boxes and at least one bullet element in each unshaded box
	MDM: Dx/management options-extensive: amount/complexity data-extensive; risk-high	**MDM**: Same
99318	**History**: CC; extended HPI; problem-pertinent ROS including review of limited number of additional systems; pertinent PFSH directly related to problem(s)	**History**: Same. Document two-nine systems for ROS. PFSH should document one item from any history area
	Exam: General multisystem exam or complete exam of a single-organ system, basing exam on the seven recognized body areas and/or the 11 recognized organ systems	**Exam**: All bullet elements in at least nine organ systems/body areas. Document no less than two bullet elements in each area/system reviewed. Single-System Exams: Must document all bullet elements in shaded boxes and at least one bullet element in each unshaded box

E/M Guidelines Crosswalk		
CPT® Code	**1995 Guidelines**	**1997 Guidelines**
	MDM: Dx/management options-limited; amount/complexity data-limited; risk-low or Dx/management options-multiple; amount/complexity data-moderate; risk-moderate	**MDM**: Same

Domiciliary, Rest Home (e.g., Boarding Home), or Custodial Care Services

CPT® Code	1995 Guidelines	1997 Guidelines
99324	**History**: CC; brief HPI	**History**: Same
	Exam: Limited exam of affected body area/organ system	**Exam**:One-five bullet elements in one or more organ systems of body areas
	MDM: Dx/management options-minimal; amount/complexity data-minimal or non; risk-minimal	**MDM**: Same
99325	**History**: CC; brief HPI; problem pertinent ROS	**History**: Same
	Exam: Limited exam of affected body area/organ system and other related/symptomatic system(s)	**Exam**: Six bullet elements in one or more organ systems or body areas
	MDM: Dx/management options-limited; amount/complexity data-limited; risk-low	**MDM**: Same
99326	**History**: CC; extended HPI; problem-pertinent ROS including review of limited number of additional systems; pertinent PFSH directly related to problem(s)	**History**: Same. Document two-nine systems for ROS. PFSH should document one item from any history area
	Exam: Extended exam of affected body area(s)/organ system(s) and other related/symptomatic system(s)	**Exam**: Two bullet elements in six organ systems/body areas OR 12 bullet elements in two or more organ systems/body areas. Single System–Eye or psychiatric exams; nine bullet elements are required
	MDM: Dx/management options-multiple; amount/complexity data-moderate; risk-moderate	**MDM**: Same
99327	**History**: CC; extended HPI; ROS directly related to problem(s) plus review of all additional systems; complete PFSH	**History**: Same. Document at least four elements of HPI or document at least three chronic/inactive conditions. ROS should document at least 10 organ systems
	Exam: General multisystem exam or complete exam of a single-organ system, basing exam on the seven recognized body areas and/or the 11 recognized organ systems	**Exam**: All bullet elements in at least nine organ systems/body areas. Document no less than two bullet elements in each area/system reviewed. Single-System Exams: Must document all bullet elements in shaded boxes and at least one bullet element in each unshaded box
	MDM: Dx/management options-multiple; amount/complexity data-moderate; risk-moderate	**MDM**: Same
99328	**History**: CC; extended HPI; ROS directly related to problem(s) plus review of all additional systems; complete PFSH	**History**: Same. Document at least four elements of HPI or document at least three chronic/inactive conditions. ROS should document at least 10 organ systems
	Exam: General multisystem exam or complete exam of a single-organ system, basing exam on the seven recognized body areas and/or the 11 recognized organ systems	**Exam**: All bullet elements in at least nine organ systems/body areas. Document no less than two bullet elements in each area/system reviewed. Single-System Exams: Must document all bullet elements in shaded boxes and at least one bullet element in each unshaded box
	MDM: Dx/management options-extensive: amount/complexity data-extensive; risk-high	**MDM**: Same

E/M Guidelines Crosswalk		
CPT® Code	**1995 Guidelines**	**1997 Guidelines**
99334	**History**: CC; brief HPI	**History**: Same
	Exam: Limited exam of affected body area/organ system	**Exam**: One–five bullet elements in one or more organ systems of body areas
	MDM: Dx/management options-minimal; amount/complexity data-minimal or non; risk-minimal	**MDM**: Same
99335	**History**: CC; brief HPI; problem pertinent ROS	**History**: Same
	Exam: Limited exam of affected body area/organ system and other related/symptomatic system(s)	**Exam**: Six bullet elements in one or more organ systems or body areas
	MDM: Dx/management options-limited; amount/complexity data-limited; risk-low	**MDM**: Same
99336	**History**: CC; extended HPI; problem-pertinent ROS including review of limited number of additional systems; pertinent PFSH directly related to problem(s)	**History**: Same. Document two-nine systems for ROS. PFSH should document one item from any history area
	Exam: Extended exam of affected body area(s)/organ system(s) and other related/symptomatic system(s)	**Exam**: Two bullet elements in six organ systems/body areas OR 12 bullet elements in two or more organ systems/body areas. Single System–Eye or psychiatric exams; nine bullet elements are required
	MDM: Dx/management options-multiple; amount/complexity data-moderate; risk-moderate	**MDM**: Same
99337	**History**: CC; extended HPI; ROS directly related to problem(s) plus review of all additional systems; complete PFSH	**History**: Same. Document at least four elements of HPI or document at least three chronic/inactive conditions. ROS should document at least 10 organ systems
	Exam: General multisystem exam or complete exam of a single-organ system, basing exam on the seven recognized body areas and/or the 11 recognized organ systems	**Exam**: All bullet elements in at least nine organ systems/body areas. Document no less than two bullet elements in each area/system reviewed. Single-System Exams: Must document all bullet elements in shaded boxes and at least one bullet element in each unshaded box
	MDM: Dx/management options-extensive: amount/complexity data-extensive; risk-high	**MDM**: Same
Home Service, New Patient		
99341	**History:** CC; brief HPI	**History:** Same.
	Exam: Limited exam of affected body area/organ system	**Exam:** one–five bullet elements in one or more organ systems or body areas
	MDM: Dx/management options minimal; amount/complexity data-minimal or none; risk-minimal	**MDM:** Same
99342	**History:** CC; brief HPI; problem-pertinent ROS	**History:** Same.
	Exam: Limited exam of affected body area/organ system & other related/symptomatic system(s)	**Exam:** Six bullet elements in one or more organ systems or body areas
	MDM: Dx/management options multiple; amount/complexity data- moderate; moderate	**MDM:** Same

E/M Guidelines Crosswalk		
CPT® Code	**1995 Guidelines**	**1997 Guidelines**
99343	**History:** CC; extended HPI; problem-pertinent ROS including review of limited number additional systems; pertinent PFSH directly related to problem(s)	**History:** Same. Document two–nine systems for ROS. PFSH should document one item from any history area
	Exam: Extended exam of affected body area(s)/organ system(s) & other related/symptomatic system(s)	**Exam:** Two bullet elements in at least six organ systems/body areas OR 12 bullet elements in two or more organ systems/body areas. Single System-Eye or Psychiatric Exams: 9 bullet elements are required
	MDM: Dx/management options multiple; amount/complexity data-moderate; risk-moderate	**MDM:** Same
99344	**History:** CC; extended HPI; ROS directly related to problem(s) plus review of all additional systems; complete PFSH	**History:** Same. Document at least four elements of HPI or document at least three chronic/inactive conditions. ROS should document at least 10 organ systems
	Exam: General multisystem exam or complete exam of a single-organ system, basing exam on the seven recognized body areas and/or the 11 recognized organ systems	**Exam:** All bullet elements in at least nine organ systems/body areas. Document no less than two bullet elements in each area/system reviewed. Single-System Exams: Must document all bullet elements in shaded boxes and at least one bullet element in each unshaded box
	MDM: Dx/management options multiple; amount/complexity data-moderate or none; risk-moderate	**MDM:** Same
99345	**History:** CC; extended HPI; ROS directly related to problem(s) plus review of all additional systems; complete PFSH	**History:** Same. Document at least four elements of HPI or document at least three chronic/inactive conditions. ROS should document at least 10 organ systems
	Exam: General multisystem exam or complete exam of a single-organ system, basing exam on the seven recognized body areas and/or the 11 recognized organ systems	**Exam:** All bullet elements in at least nine organ systems/body areas. Document no less than two bullet elements in each area/system reviewed. Single-System Exams: Must document all bullet elements in shaded boxes and at least one bullet element in each unshaded box
	MDM: Dx/management options extensive; amount/complexity data-extensive; risk-high	**MDM:** Same
Home Services, Established Patient		
99347	**History:** CC; brief HPI	**History:** Same.
	Exam: Limited exam of affected body area/organ system	**Exam:** one–five bullet elements in one or more organ systems or body areas
	MDM: Dx/management options minimal; amount/complexity data- minimal or none; risk-minimal	**MDM:** Same
99348	**History:** CC; brief HPI; problem-pertinent ROS	**History:** Same.
	Exam: Limited exam of affected body area/organ system & other related/symptomatic system(s)	**Exam:** Six bullet elements in one or more organ systems or body areas
	MDM: Dx/management options limited; amount/complexity data- limited; risk-low	**MDM:** Same

E/M Guidelines Crosswalk

CPT® Code	1995 Guidelines	1997 Guidelines
99349	**History:** CC; extended HPI; problem-pertinent ROS including review of limited number additional systems; pertinent PFSH directly related to problem(s)	**History:** Same. Document two–nine systems for ROS. PFSH should document one item from any history area
	Exam: Extended exam of affected body area(s)/organ system(s) & other related/symptomatic system(s)	**Exam:** Two bullet elements in at least six organ systems/body areas OR 12 bullet elements in two or more organ systems/body areas. Single System-Eye or Psychiatric Exams: 9 bullet elements are required
	MDM: Dx/management options multiple; amount/complexity data-moderate; risk-moderate	**MDM:** Same
99350	**History:** CC; extended HPI; ROS directly related to problem(s) plus review of all additional systems; complete PFSH	**History:** Same. Document at least four elements of HPI or document at least three chronic/inactive conditions. ROS should document at least 10 organ systems
	Exam: General multisystem exam or complete exam of a single-organ system, basing exam on the seven recognized body areas and/or the 11 recognized organ systems	**Exam:** All bullet elements in at least nine organ systems/body areas. Document no less than two bullet elements in each area/system reviewed. Single-System Exams: Must document all bullet elements in shaded boxes and at least one bullet element in each unshaded box
	MDM: Dx/management options multiple; amount/complexity data-moderate; risk-moderate or Dx/management options extensive; amount/complexity data-extensive; risk-high	**MDM:** Same or Same

*For billing Medicare, a provider may choose either version of the documentation guidelines, not a combination of the two, to document a patient encounter. However, beginning for services performed on or after September 10, 2013 physicians may use the 1997 documentation guidelines for an extended history of present illness along with other elements from the 1995 guidelines to document an evaluation and management service.

Appendix C: 1995 Evaluation and Management Documentation Guidelines

1995 DOCUMENTATION GUIDELINES FOR EVALUATION AND MANAGEMENT

I. INTRODUCTION

WHAT IS DOCUMENTATION AND WHY IS IT IMPORTANT?

Medical record documentation is required to record pertinent facts, findings, and observations about an individual's health history including past and present illnesses, examinations, tests, treatments, and outcomes. The medical record chronologically documents the care of the patient and is an important element contributing to high quality care. The medical record facilitates:

- The ability of the physician and other healthcare professionals to evaluate and plan the patient's immediate treatment, and to monitor his/her healthcare over time
- Communication and continuity of care among physicians and other healthcare professionals involved in the patient's care
- Accurate and timely claims review and payment
- Appropriate utilization review and quality of care evaluations
- Collection of data that may be useful for research and education

An appropriately documented medical record can reduce many of the "hassles" associated with claims processing and may serve as a legal document to verify the care provided, if necessary.

WHAT DO PAYERS WANT AND WHY?

Because payers have a contractual obligation to enrollees, they may require reasonable documentation that services are consistent with the insurance coverage provided. They may request information to validate:

- The site of service
- The medical necessity and appropriateness of the diagnostic and/or therapeutic services provided and/or
- That services provided have been accurately reported

II. GENERAL PRINCIPLES OF MEDICAL RECORD DOCUMENTATION

The principles of documentation listed below are applicable to all types of medical and surgical services in all settings. For Evaluation and Management (E/M) services, the nature and amount of physician work and documentation varies by type of service, place of service and the patient's status. The general principles listed below may be modified to account for these variable circumstances in providing E/M services.

1. The medical record should be complete and legible.

2. The documentation of each patient encounter should include:
   - reason for the encounter and relevant history, physical examination findings and prior diagnostic test results
   - assessment, clinical impression or diagnosis plan for care, and
   - date and legible identity of the observer.

3. If not documented, the rationale for ordering diagnostic and other ancillary services should be easily inferred

4. Past and present diagnoses should be accessible to the treating and/or consulting physician

5. Appropriate health risk factors should be identified

6. The patient's progress, response to and changes in treatment, and revision of diagnosis should be documented

7. The CPT® and ICD-10-CM codes reported on the health insurance claim form or billing statement should be supported by the documentation in the medical record

III. DOCUMENTATION OF E/M SERVICES

This publication provides definitions and documentation guidelines for the three key components of E/M services and for visits which consist predominately of counseling or coordination of care. The three key components--history, examination, and medical decision making--appear in the descriptors for office and other outpatient services, hospital observation services, hospital inpatient services, consultations, emergency department services, nursing facility services, domiciliary care services, and home services. While some of the text of CPT has been repeated in this publication, the reader should refer to CPT for the complete descriptors for E/M services and instructions for selecting a level of service. Documentation guidelines are identified by the symbol ●DG.

The descriptors for the levels of E/M services recognize seven components which are used in defining the levels of E/M services. These components are:

- History
- Examination
- Medical decision making
- Counseling
- Coordination of care
- Nature of presenting problem; and
- Time

The first three of these components (i.e., history, examination and medical decision making) are the key components in selecting the level of E/M services. An exception to this rule is the case of visits which consist predominantly of counseling or coordination of care; for these services time is the key or controlling factor to qualify for a particular level of E/M service.

For certain groups of patients, the recorded information may vary slightly from that described here. Specifically, the medical records of infants, children, adolescents and pregnant women may have additional or modified information recorded in each history and examination area. As an example, newborn records may include under history of the present illness (HPI) the details of mother's pregnancy and the infant's status at birth; social history will focus on family structure; family history will focus on congenital anomalies and hereditary disorders in the family. In addition, information on growth and development and/or nutrition will be recorded. Although not specifically defined in these documentation guidelines, these patient group variations on history and examination are appropriate.

A. DOCUMENTATION OF HISTORY

The levels of E/M services are based on four types of history (Problem Focused, Expanded Problem Focused, Detailed, and Comprehensive.) Each type of history includes some or all of the following elements:

- Chief complaint (CC)
- History of present illness (HPI)
- Review of systems (ROS) and
- Past, family and/or social history (PFSH)

The extent of history of present illness, review of systems and past, family and/or social history that is obtained and documented is dependent upon clinical judgment and the nature of the presenting problem(s).

The chart below shows the progression of the elements required for each type of history. To qualify for a given type of history, **all three elements in the table must be met.** (A chief complaint is indicated at all levels.)

History of Present Illness	Review of Systems (ROS)	Past, Family, and/or (HPI) Social History (PFSH)	Type of History Brief
Brief	N/A	N/A	Problem Focused
Brief	Problem Pertinent	N/A	Expanded Problem Focused
Extended	Extended	Pertinent	Detailed
Extended	Complete	Complete	Comprehensive

- *DG: The CC, ROS and PFSH may be listed as separate elements of history, or they may be included in the description of the history of the present illness.*
- *DG: A ROS and/or a PFSH obtained during an earlier encounter does not need to be re-recorded if there is evidence that the physician reviewed and updated the previous information. This may occur when a physician updates his or her own record or in an institutional setting or group practice where many physicians use a common record. The review and update may be documented by:*
  - *describing any new ROS and/or PFSH information or noting there has been no change in the information*
  - *noting the date and location of the earlier ROS and/or PFSH.*
- *DG: The ROS and/or PFSH may be recorded by ancillary staff or on a form completed by the patient. To document that the physician reviewed the information, there must be a notation supplementing or confirming the information recorded by others.*
- *DG: If the physician is unable to obtain a history from the patient or other source, the record should describe the patient's condition or other circumstance which precludes obtaining a history.*

Definitions and specific documentation guidelines for each of the elements of history are listed below.

CHIEF COMPLAINT (CC)

The CC is a concise statement describing the symptom, problem, condition, diagnosis, physician recommended return, or other factor that is the reason for the encounter.

- *DG: The medical record should clearly reflect the chief complaint.*

HISTORY OF PRESENT ILLNESS (HPI)

The HPI is a chronological description of the development of the patient's present illness from the first sign and/or symptom or from the previous encounter to the present. It includes the following elements:

- Location
- Quality
- Severity
- Duration
- Timing
- Context
- Modifying factors and
- Associated signs and symptoms

Brief and extended HPIs are distinguished by the amount of detail needed to accurately characterize the clinical problem(s).

A brief HPI consists of one to three elements of the HPI.

- *DG: The medical record should describe one to three elements of the present illness (HPI).*

An extended HPI consists of four or more elements of the HPI.

- *DG: The medical record should describe four or more elements of the present illness (HPI) or associated comorbidities.*

REVIEW OF SYSTEMS (ROS)

A ROS is an inventory of body systems obtained through a series of questions seeking to identify signs and/or symptoms which the patient may be experiencing or has experienced. For purposes of ROS, the following systems are recognized:

- Constitutional symptoms (e.g., fever, weight loss)
- Eyes
- Ears, nose, mouth, throat
- Cardiovascular
- Respiratory
- Gastrointestinal
- Genitourinary
- Musculoskeletal
- Integumentary (skin and/or breast)
- Neurological
- Psychiatric
- Endocrine

- Hematologic/lymphatic
- Allergic/immunologic

A problem pertinent ROS inquires about the system directly related to the problem(s) identified in the HPI.

- *DG: The patient's positive responses and pertinent negatives for the system related to the problem should be documented.*

An extended ROS inquires about the system directly related to the problem(s) identified in the HPI and a limited number of additional systems.

- *DG: The patient's positive responses and pertinent negatives for two to nine systems should be documented.*

A complete ROS inquires about the system(s) directly related to the problem(s) identified in the HPI plus all additional body systems.

- *DG: At least ten organ systems must be reviewed. Those systems with positive or pertinent negative responses must be individually documented. For the remaining systems, a notation indicating all other systems are negative is permissible. In the absence of such a notation, at least ten systems must be individually documented.*

PAST, FAMILY AND/OR SOCIAL HISTORY (PFSH)

The PFSH consists of a review of three areas:

- Past history (the patient's past experiences with illnesses, operations, injuries and treatments);
- Family history (a review of medical events in the patient's family, including diseases which may be hereditary or place the patient at risk) and
- Social history (an age appropriate review of past and current activities).

For the categories of subsequent hospital care, follow-up inpatient consultations and subsequent nursing facility care, CPT requires only an "interval" history. It is not necessary to record information about the PFSH.

A pertinent PFSH is a review of the history area(s) directly related to the problem(s) identified in the HPI.

- *DG: At least one specific item from any of the three history areas must be documented for a pertinent PFSH.*

A complete PFSH is of a review of two or all three of the PFSH history areas, depending on the category of the E/M service. A review of all three history areas is required for services that by their nature include a comprehensive assessment or reassessment of the patient. A review of two of the three history areas is sufficient for other services.

- *DG: At least one specific item from two of the three history areas must be documented for a complete PFSH for the following categories of E/M services: office or other outpatient services, established patient; emergency department; subsequent nursing facility care; domiciliary care, established patient; and home care, established patient.*

- *DG: At least one specific item from each of the three history areas must be documented for a complete PFSH for the following categories of E/M services: office or other outpatient services, new patient; hospital observation services; hospital inpatient services, initial care; consultations; comprehensive nursing facility assessments; domiciliary care, new patient; and home care, new patient.*

B. DOCUMENTATION OF EXAMINATION

The levels of E/M services are based on four types of examination that are defined as follows:

- Problem focused: A limited examination of the affected body area or organ system.
- Expanded problem focused: A limited examination of the affected body area or organ system and other symptomatic or related organ system(s).
- Detailed: An extended examination of the affected body area(s) and other symptomatic or related organ system(s).
- Comprehensive: A general multi-system examination or complete examination of a single organ system.

For purposes of examination, the following body areas are recognized:

- Head, including the face
- Neck
- Chest, including breasts and axillae
- Abdomen
- Genitalia, groin, buttocks
- Back, including spine
- Each extremity

For purposes of examination, the following organ systems are recognized:

- Constitutional (e.g., vital signs, general appearance)
- Eyes
- Ears, nose, mouth and throat
- Cardiovascular
- Respiratory
- Gastrointestinal
- Genitourinary
- Musculoskeletal
- Skin
- Neurologic
- Psychiatric
- Hematologic/lymphatic/immunologic

The extent of examinations performed and documented is dependent upon clinical judgment and the nature of the presenting problem(s). They range from limited examinations of single body areas to general multi-system or complete single organ system examinations.

- *DG: Specific abnormal and relevant negative findings of the examination of the affected or symptomatic body area(s) or organ system(s) should be documented. A notation of "abnormal" without elaboration is insufficient.*

- *DG: Abnormal or unexpected findings of the examination of the unaffected or asymptomatic body area(s) or organ system(s) should be described.*
- *DG: A brief statement or notation indicating "negative" or "normal" is sufficient to document normal findings related to unaffected area(s) or asymptomatic organ system(s).*
- *DG: The medical record for a general multi-system examination should include findings about 8 or more of the 12 organ systems.*

C. DOCUMENTATION OF THE COMPLEXITY OF MEDICAL DECISION MAKING

The levels of E/M services recognize four types of medical decision making (straight-forward, low complexity, moderate complexity and high complexity). Medical decision making refers to the complexity of establishing a diagnosis and/or selecting a management option as measured by:

- The number of possible diagnoses and/or the number of management options that must be considered;
- The amount and/or complexity of medical records, diagnostic tests, and/or other information that must be obtained, reviewed and analyzed, and
- The risk of significant complications, morbidity and/or mortality, as well as comorbidities, associated with the patient's presenting problem(s), the diagnostic procedure(s) and/or the possible management options

The chart below shows the progression of the elements required for each level of medical decision making. To qualify for a given type of decision making, two of the three elements in the table must be either met or exceeded.

Number of diagnoses or management options	Amount and/or complexity of data to be reviewed	Risk of complications and/or morbidity or mortality	Type of decision making
Minimal	Minimal or None	Minimal	*Straightforward*
Limited	Limited	Low	*Low Complexity*
Multiple	Moderate	Moderate	*Moderate Complexity*
Extensive	Extensive	High	*High Complexity*

Each of the elements of medical decision making is described below.

NUMBER OF DIAGNOSES OR MANAGEMENT OPTIONS

The number of possible diagnoses and/or the number of management options that must be considered is based on the number and types of problems addressed during the encounter, the complexity of establishing a diagnosis and the management decisions that are made by the physician.

Generally, decision making with respect to a diagnosed problem is easier than that for an identified but undiagnosed problem. The number and type of diagnostic tests employed may be an indicator of the number of possible diagnoses. Problems which are improving or resolving are less complex than those which are worsening or failing to change as expected. The need to seek advice from others is another indicator of complexity of diagnostic or management problems.

- *DG: For each encounter, an assessment, clinical impression, or diagnosis should be documented. It may be explicitly stated or implied in documented decisions regarding management plans and/or further evaluation.*

— *For a presenting problem with an established diagnosis the record should reflect whether the problem is: a) improved, well controlled, resolving or resolved; or, b) inadequately controlled, worsening, or failing to change as expected.*

— *For a presenting problem without an established diagnosis, the assessment or clinical impression may be stated in the form of a differential diagnoses or as "possible," "probable," or "rule out" (R/O) diagnoses.*

- *DG: The initiation of, or changes in, treatment should be documented. Treatment includes a wide range of management options including patient instructions, nursing instructions, therapies, and medications.*
- *DG: If referrals are made, consultations requested or advice sought, the record should indicate to whom or where the referral or consultation is made or from whom the advice is requested.*

AMOUNT AND/OR COMPLEXITY OF DATA TO BE REVIEWED

The amount and complexity of data to be reviewed is based on the types of diagnostic testing ordered or reviewed. A decision to obtain and review old medical records and/or obtain history from sources other than the patient increases the amount and complexity of data to be reviewed. Discussion of contradictory or unexpected test results with the physician who performed or interpreted the test is an indication of the complexity of data being reviewed. On occasion the physician who ordered a test may personally review the image, tracing or specimen to supplement information from the physician who prepared the test report or interpretation; this is another indication of the complexity of data being reviewed.

- *DG: If a diagnostic service (test or procedure) is ordered, planned, scheduled, or performed at the time of the E/M encounter, the type of service, e.g., lab or x-ray, should be documented.*
- *DG: The review of lab, radiology and/or other diagnostic tests should be documented. An entry in a progress note such as "WBC elevated" or "chest x-ray unremarkable" is acceptable. Alternatively, the review may be documented by initialing and dating the report containing the test results.*
- *DG: A decision to obtain old records or decision to obtain additional history from the family, caretaker or other source to supplement that obtained from the patient should be documented.*
- *DG: Relevant findings from the review of old records, and/or the receipt of additional history from the family, caretaker or other source should be documented. If there is no relevant information beyond that already obtained, that fact should be documented. A notation of "Old records reviewed" or "additional history obtained from family" without elaboration is insufficient.*
- *DG: The results of discussion of laboratory, radiology or other diagnostic tests with the physician who performed or interpreted the study should be documented.*
- *DG: The direct visualization and independent interpretation of an image, tracing or specimen previously or subsequently interpreted by another physician should be documented.*

RISK OF SIGNIFICANT COMPLICATIONS, MORBIDITY, AND/OR MORTALITY

The risk of significant complications, morbidity, and/or mortality is based on the risks associated with the presenting problem(s), the diagnostic procedure(s), and the possible management options.

- *DG: Comorbidities/underlying diseases or other factors that increase the complexity of medical decision making by increasing the risk of complications, morbidity, and/or mortality should be documented.*
- *DG: If a surgical or invasive diagnostic procedure is ordered, planned or scheduled at the time of the E/M encounter, the type of procedure, e.g., laparoscopy, should be documented.*
- *DG: If a surgical or invasive diagnostic procedure is performed at the time of the E/M encounter, the specific procedure should be documented.*
- *DG: The referral for or decision to perform a surgical or invasive diagnostic procedure on an urgent basis should be documented or implied.*

The following table may be used to help determine whether the risk of significant complications, morbidity, and/or mortality is minimal, low, moderate, or high. Because the determination of risk is complex and not readily quantifiable, the table includes common clinical examples rather than absolute measures of risk. The assessment of risk of the presenting problem(s) is based on the risk related to the disease process anticipated between the present encounter and the next one.

The assessment of risk of selecting diagnostic procedures and management options is based on the risk during and immediately following any procedures or treatment. The highest level of risk in any one category (presenting problem(s), diagnostic procedure(s), or management options) determines the overall risk.

	Presenting Problem(s)	Diagnostic Procedure(s) Ordered	Management Options Selected
MINIMAL	• One self-limited or minor problem; e.g., cold, insect bite, tinea corporis	• Laboratory tests requiring venipuncture • Chest x-rays • EKG/EEG • Urinalysis • Ultrasound; e.g., echo • KOH prep	• Rest • Gargles • Elastic bandages • Superficial dressings
LOW	• Two or more self-limited or minor problems • One stable chronic illness; e.g., well controlled hypertension or non-insulin dependent diabetes, cataract, BPH • Acute uncomplicated illness or injury; e.g., cystitis, allergic rhinitis, simple sprain	• Physiological tests not under stress; e.g., pulmonary function tests • Non-cardiovascular imaging studies with contrast; e.g., barium enema • Superficial needle biopsies • Clinical laboratory tests requiring arterial puncture • Skin biopsies	• Over-the-counter drugs • Minor surgery with no identified risk factors • Physical therapy • Occupational therapy • IV fluids without additives
MODERATE	• One or more chronic illnesses with mild exacerbation, progression, or side effects of treatment • Two or more stable chronic illnesses • Undiagnosed new problem with uncertain prognosis; e.g., lump in breast • Acute illness with systemic symptoms; e.g., pyelonephritis, pneumonitis, colitis • Acute complicated injury; e.g., head injury with brief loss of consciousness	• Physiologic tests under stress; e.g., cardiac stress test, fetal contraction stress test • Diagnostic endoscopies with no identified risk factors • Deep needle or incisional biopsy • Cardiovascular imaging studies w/ contrast and no identified risk factors; e.g., arteriogram, cardiac catheterization • Obtain fluid from body cavity; e.g., lumbar puncture, thoracentesis, culdocentesis	• Minor surgery w/ identified risk factors • Elective major surgery (Open, percutaneous or endoscopic) w/ no identified risk factors • Prescription drug management • Therapeutic nuclear medicine • IV fluids with additives • Closed treatment of fracture or dislocation w/o manipulation
HIGH	• One or more chronic illnesses with severe exacerbation, progression, or side effects of treatment • Acute or chronic illnesses or injuries that pose a threat to life or bodily function; e.g., multiple trauma, acute MI, pulmonary embolus, severe respiratory distress, progressive severe rheumatoid arthritis, psychiatric illness with potential threat to self or others, peritonitis, ARF • An abrupt change in neurologic status; e.g., seizure, TIA, weakness or sensory loss	• Cardiovascular imaging studies with contrast with identified risk factors • Cardiac electrophysiological tests • Diagnostic endoscopies w/identified risk factors • Discography	• Elective major surgery (open, percutaneous or endoscopic) w/ identified risk factors • Emergency major surgery (open, percutaneous, endoscopic) • Parenteral controlled substances • Drug therapy requiring intensive monitoring for toxicity • Decision not to resuscitate or to de-escalate care because of poor prognosis

D. DOCUMENTATION OF AN ENCOUNTER DOMINATED BY COUNSELING OR COORDINATION OF CARE

In the case where counseling and/or coordination of care dominates (more than 50%) of the physician/patient and/or family encounter (face-to-face time in the office or other outpatient setting or floor/unit time in the hospital or nursing facility), time is considered the key or controlling factor to qualify for a particular level of E/M services.

- *DG: If the physician elects to report the level of service based on counseling and/or coordination of care, the total length of time of the encounter (face-to-face or floor time, as appropriate) should be documented and the record should describe the counseling and/or activities to coordinate care.*

Appendix D:
1997 Evaluation and Management Documentation Guidelines

1997 DOCUMENTATION GUIDELINES FOR EVALUATION AND MANAGEMENT SERVICES

I. INTRODUCTION

WHAT IS DOCUMENTATION AND WHY IS IT IMPORTANT?

Medical record documentation is required to record pertinent facts, findings, and observations about an individual's health history including past and present illnesses, examinations, tests, treatments, and outcomes. The medical recordchronologically documents the care of the patient and is an important element contributing to high quality care. The medical record facilitates:

- The ability of the physician and other healthcare professionals to evaluate and plan the patient's immediate treatment, and to monitor his/her healthcare over time
- Communication and continuity of care among physicians and other healthcare professionals involved in the patient's care
- Accurate and timely claims review and payment
- Appropriate utilization review and quality of care evaluations
- Collection of data that may be useful for research and education

An appropriately documented medical record can reduce many of the "hassles" associated with claims processing and may serve as a legal document to verify the care provided, if necessary.

WHAT DO PAYERS WANT AND WHY?

Because payers have a contractual obligation to enrollees, they may require reasonable documentation that services are consistent with the insurance coverage provided. They may request information to validate:

- The site of service
- The medical necessity and appropriateness of the diagnostic and/or therapeutic services provided
- That services provided have been accurately reported

II. GENERAL PRINCIPLES OF MEDICAL RECORD DOCUMENTATION

The principles of documentation listed below are applicable to all types of medical and surgical services in all settings. For Evaluation and Management (E/M) services, the nature and amount of physician work and documentation varies by type of service, place of service and the patient's status. The general principles listed below may be modified to account for these variable circumstances in providing E/M services.

1. The medical record should be complete and legible.

2. The documentation of each patient encounter should include:
    - reason for the encounter and relevant history, physical examination findings and prior diagnostic test results;
    - assessment, clinical impression or diagnosis;
    - plan for care; and
    - date and legible identity of the observer.

3. If not documented, the rationale for ordering diagnostic and other ancillary services should be easily inferred.

4. Past and present diagnoses should be accessible to the treating and/or consulting physician.

5. Appropriate health risk factors should be identified.

6. The patient's progress, response to and changes in treatment, and revision of diagnosis should be documented.

7. The CPT® and ICD-9-CM codes reported on the health insurance claim form or billing statement should be supported by the documentation in the medical record.

III. DOCUMENTATION OF E/M SERVICES

This publication provides definitions and documentation guidelines for the three key components of E/M services and for visits which consist predominately of counseling or coordination of care. The three key components--history, examination, and medical decision making–appear in the descriptors for office and other outpatient services, hospital observation services, hospital inpatient services, consultations, emergency department services, nursing facility services, domiciliary care services, and home services. While some of the text of CPT has been repeated in this publication, the reader should refer to CPT for the complete descriptors for E/M services and instructions for selecting a level of service. Documentation guidelines are identified by the symbol •DG.

The descriptors for the levels of E/M services recognize seven components which are used in defining the levels of E/M services. These components are:

- History
- Examination
- Medical decision making
- Counseling
- Coordination of care
- Nature of presenting problem
- Time

The first three of these components (i.e., history, examination and medical decision making) are the key components in selecting the level of E/M services. In the case of visits which consist *predominantly* of counseling or coordination of care, time is the key or controlling factor to qualify for a particular level of E/M service.

Because the level of E/M service is dependent on two or three key components, performance and documentation of one component (eg, examination) at the highest level does not necessarily mean that the encounter in its entirety qualifies for the highest level of E/M service.

These Documentation Guidelines for E/M services reflect the needs of the typical adult population. For certain groups of patients, the recorded information may vary slightly from that described here. Specifically, the medical records of infants, children, adolescents and pregnant women may have additional or modified information recorded in each history and examination area.

As an example, newborn records may include under history of the present illness (HPI) the details of mother's pregnancy and the infant's status at birth; social history will focus on family structure; family history will focus on congenital anomalies and hereditary disorders in the family. In addition, the content of a pediatric examination will vary with the age and development of the child. Although not specifically defined in these documentation guidelines, these patient group variations on history and examination are appropriate.

A. DOCUMENTATION OF HISTORY

The levels of E/M services are based on four types of history (Problem Focused, Expanded Problem Focused, Detailed, and Comprehensive). Each type of history includes some or all of the following elements:

- Chief complaint (CC)
- History of present illness (HPI)
- Review of systems (ROS)
- Past, family and/or social history (PFSH)

The extent of history of present illness, review of systems and past, family and/or social history that is obtained and documented is dependent upon clinical judgement and the nature of the presenting problem(s). The chart below shows the progression of the elements required for each type of history. To qualify for a given type of history all three elements in the table must be met. (A chief complaint is indicated at all levels.)

History of Present Illness (HPI)	Review of Systems Past (ROS)	Past Family, and/or Social History (PFSH)	Type of History
Brief	N/A	N/A	*Problem Focused*
Brief	Problem Pertinent	N/A	*Expanded Problem Focused*
Extended	Extended	Pertinent	*Detailed*
Extended	Complete	Complete	*Comprehensive*

- *DG: The CC, ROS and PFSH may be listed as separate elements of history, or they may be included in the description of the history of the present illness.*
- *DG: A ROS and/or a PFSH obtained during an earlier encounter does not need to be re-recorded if there is evidence that the physician reviewed and updated the previous information. This may occur when a physician updates his or her own record or in an institutional setting or group practice where many physicians use a common record. The review and update may be documented by:*
  - *describing any new ROS and/or PFSH information or noting there has been no change in the information; and*
  - *noting the date and location of the earlier ROS and/or PFSH.*

- *DG: The ROS and/or PFSH may be recorded by ancillary staff or on a form completed by the patient. To document that the physician reviewed the information, there must be a notation supplementing or confirming the information recorded by others.*
- *DG: If the physician is unable to obtain a history from the patient or other source, the record should describe the patient's condition or other circumstance which precludes obtaining a history.*

Definitions and specific documentation guidelines for each of the elements of history are listed below.

CHIEF COMPLAINT (CC)
The CC is a concise statement describing the symptom, problem, condition, diagnosis, physician recommended return, or other factor that is the reason for the encounter, usually stated in the patient's words.

- *DG: The medical record should clearly reflect the chief complaint.*

HISTORY OF PRESENT ILLNESS (HPI)
The HPI is a chronological description of the development of the patient's present illness from the first sign and/or symptom or from the previous encounter to the present. It includes the following elements:

- Location
- Quality
- Severity
- Duration
- Timing
- Context
- Modifying factors
- Associated signs and symptoms

Brief and *extended* HPIs are distinguished by the amount of detail needed to accurately characterize the clinical problem(s).

A *brief* HPI consists of one to three elements of the HPI.

- *DG: The medical record should describe one to three elements of the present illness (HPI).*

An *extended* HPI consists of at least four elements of the HPI or the status of at least three chronic or inactive conditions.

- *DG: The medical record should describe at least four elements of the present illness (HPI), or the status of at least three chronic or inactive conditions.*

REVIEW OF SYSTEMS (ROS)
A ROS is an inventory of body systems obtained through a series of questions seeking to identify signs and/or symptoms which the patient may be experiencing or has experienced. For purposes of ROS, the following systems are recognized:

- Constitutional symptoms (e.g., fever, weight loss)
- Eyes
- Ears, Nose, Mouth, Throat
- Cardiovascular
- Respiratory

- Gastrointestinal
- Genitourinary
- Musculoskeletal
- Integumentary (skin and/or breast)
- Neurological
- Psychiatric
- Endocrine
- Hematologic/Lymphatic
- Allergic/Immunologic

A *problem pertinent* ROS inquires about the system directly related to the problem(s) identified in the HPI.

- *DG: The patient's positive responses and pertinent negatives for the system related to the problem should be documented.*

An *extended* ROS inquires about the system directly related to the problem(s) identified in the HPI and a limited number of additional systems.

- *DG: The patient's positive responses and pertinent negatives for two to nine systems should be documented.*

A *complete* ROS inquires about the system(s) directly related to the problem(s) identified in the HPI plus all additional body systems.

- *DG: At least ten organ systems must be reviewed. Those systems with positive or pertinent negative responses must be individually documented. For the remaining systems, a notation indicating all other systems are negative is permissible. In the absence of such a notation, at least ten systems must be individually documented.*

PAST, FAMILY AND/OR SOCIAL HISTORY (PFSH)
The PFSH consists of a review of three areas:

- Past history (the patient's past experiences with illnesses, operations, injuries and treatments)
- Family history (a review of medical events in the patient's family, including diseases which may be hereditary or place the patient at risk)
- Social history (an age appropriate review of past and current activities)

For certain categories of E/M services that include only an interval history, it is not necessary to record information about the PFSH. Those categories are subsequent hospital care, follow-up inpatient consultations and subsequent nursing facility care.

A *pertinent* PFSH is a review of the history area(s) directly related to the problem(s) identified in the HPI.

- *DG: At least one specific item from any of the three history areas must be documented for a pertinent PFSH.*

A *complete* PFSH is of a review of two or all three of the PFSH history areas, depending on the category of the E/M service. A review of all three history areas is required for services that by their nature include a comprehensive

---

assessment or reassessment of the patient. A review of two of the three history areas is sufficient for other services.

- *DG: At least one specific item from two of the three history areas must be documented for a complete PFSH for the following categories of E/M services: office or other outpatient services, established patient; emergency department; domiciliary care, established patient; and home care, established patient.*
- *DG: At least one specific item from each of the three history areas must be documented for a complete PFSH for the following categories of E/M services: office or other outpatient services, new patient; hospital observation services; hospital inpatient services, initial care; consultations; comprehensive nursing facility assessments; domiciliary care, new patient; and home care, new patient.*

B. DOCUMENTATION OF EXAMINATION

The levels of E/M services are based on four types of examination:

- Problem Focused—a limited examination of the affected body area or organ system.
- Expanded Problem Focused—a limited examination of the affected body area or organ system and any other symptomatic or related body area(s) or organ system(s).
- Detailed—an extended examination of the affected body area(s) or organ system(s) and any other symptomatic or related body area(s) or organ system(s).
- Comprehensive—a general multi-system examination, or complete examination of a single organ system and other symptomatic or related body area(s) or organ system(s).

These types of examinations have been defined for general multi-system and the following single organ systems:

- Cardiovascular
- Ears, Nose, Mouth and Throat
- Eyes
- Genitourinary (Female)
- Genitourinary (Male)
- Hematologic/Lymphatic/Immunologic
- Musculoskeletal
- Neurological
- Psychiatric
- Respiratory
- Skin

A general multi-system examination or a single organ system examination may be performed by any physician regardless of specialty. The type (general multi-system or single organ system) and content of examination are selected by the examining physician and are based upon clinical judgement, the patient's history, and the nature of the presenting problem(s).

The content and documentation requirements for each type and level of examination are summarized below and described in detail in tables beginning on page 13. In the tables, organ systems and body areas recognized by CPT for purposes of describing examinations are shown in the left column. The content, or individual elements, of the examination pertaining to that body area or organ system are identified by bullets (•) in the right column.

Parenthetical examples, "(eg, ...)", have been used for clarification and to provide guidance regarding documentation. Documentation for each element must satisfy any numeric requirements (such as "Measurement of *any three of the following seven...*") included in the description of the element. Elements with multiple components but with no specific numeric requirement (such as "Examination of liver and spleen") require documentation of at least one component. It is possible for a given examination to be expanded beyond what is defined here. When that occurs, findings related to the additional systems and/or areas should be documented.

- *DG: Specific abnormal and relevant negative findings of the examination of the affected or symptomatic body area(s) or organ system(s) should be documented. A notation of "abnormal" without elaboration is insufficient.*
- *DG: Abnormal or unexpected findings of the examination of any asymptomatic body area(s) or organ system(s) should be described.*
- *DG: A brief statement or notation indicating "negative" or "normal" is sufficient to document normal findings related to unaffected area(s) or asymptomatic organ system(s).*

GENERAL MULTI-SYSTEM EXAMINATIONS

General multi-system examinations are described in detail beginning on page 13. To qualify for a given level of multi-system examination, the following content and documentation requirements should be met:

- Problem Focused Examination–should include performance and documentation of one to five elements identified by a bullet (•) in one or more organ system(s) or body area(s).
- Expanded Problem Focused Examination–should include performance and documentation of at least six elements identified by a bullet (•) in one or more organ system(s) or body area(s).
- Detailed Examination–should include at least six organ systems or body areas. For each system/area selected, performance and documentation of at least two elements identified by a bullet (•) is expected. Alternatively, a detailed examination may include performance and documentation of at least twelve elements identified by a bullet (•) in two or more organ systems or body areas.
- Comprehensive Examination–should include at least nine organ systems or body areas. For each system/area selected, all elements of the examination identified by a bullet (•) should be performed, unless specific directions limit the content of the examination. For each area/system, documentation of at least two elements identified by a bullet is expected.

SINGLE ORGAN SYSTEM EXAMINATIONS

The single organ system examinations recognized by CPT are described in detail beginning on page 18. Variations among these examinations in the organ systems and body areas identified in the left columns and in the elements of the examinations described in the right columns reflect differing emphases among specialties. To qualify for a given level of single organ system examination, the following content and documentation requirements should be met:

- Problem Focused Examination–should include performance and documentation of one to five elements identified by a bullet (•), whether in a box with a shaded or unshaded border.
- Expanded Problem Focused Examination–should include performance and documentation of at least six elements identified by a bullet (•), whether in a box with a shaded or unshaded border.
- Detailed Examination–examinations other than the eye and psychiatric examinations should include performance and documentation of at least twelve elements identified by a bullet (•), whether in box with a shaded or unshaded border.

Eye and psychiatric examinations should include the performance and documentation of at least nine elements identified by a bullet (•), whether in a box with a shaded or unshaded border.

- Comprehensive Examination–should include performance of all elements identified by a bullet (•), whether in a shaded or unshaded box. Documentation of every element in each box with a shaded border and at least one element in each box with an unshaded border is expected.

General Multisystem Examination

System/Body Area	Elements of Examination
Constitutional	• Measurement of **any three of the following seven** vital signs: 1) sitting or standing blood pressure, 2) supine blood pressure, 3) pulse rate and regularity, 4) respiration, 5) temperature, 6) height, 7) weight (May be measured and recorded by ancillary staff). • General appearance of patient (e.g., development, nutrition, body habitus, deformities attention to grooming)
Eyes	• Inspection of conjunctivae and lids • Examination of pupils and irises (e.g., reaction to light and accommodation, size and symmetry) • Ophthalmoscopic examination of optic discs (e.g., size, C/D ratio, appearance) and posterior segments (e.g., vessel changes, exudates, hemorrhages)
Ears, Nose, Mouth and Throat	• External inspection of ears and nose (e.g., overall appearance, scars, lesions, masses) • Otoscopic examination of external auditory canals and tympanic membranes • Assessment of hearing (e.g., whispered voice, finger rub, tuning fork) • Inspection of nasal mucosa, septum and turbinates • Inspection of lips, teeth and gums • Examination of oropharynx: oral mucosa, salivary glands, hard and soft palates, tongue, tonsils and posterior pharynx
Neck	• Examination of neck (e.g., masses, overall appearance, symmetry, tracheal position, crepitus) • Examination of thyroid (e.g., enlargement, tenderness, mass)
Respiratory	• Assessment of respiratory effort (e.g., intercostal retractions, use of accessory muscles, diaphragmatic movement) • Percussion of chest (e.g., dullness, flatness, hyperresonance) • Palpation of chest (e.g., tactile fremitus) • Auscultation of lungs (e.g., breath sounds, adventitious sounds, rubs)

Cardiovascular	• Palpation of heart (e.g., location, size, thrills)
	• Auscultation of heart with notation of abnormal sounds and murmurs
	• Examination of:
	  – carotid arteries (e.g., pulse amplitude, bruits)
	  – abdominal aorta (e.g., size, bruits)
	  – femoral arteries (e.g., pulse amplitude, bruits)
	  – pedal pulses (e.g., pulse amplitude)
	  – extremities for edema and/or varicosities

Chest (Breasts)	• Inspection of breasts (e.g., symmetry, nipple discharge) • Palpation of breasts and axillae (e.g., masses or lumps, tenderness)
Gastrointestinal (Abdomen)	• Examination of abdomen with notation of presence of masses or tenderness • Examination of liver and spleen • Examination for presence or absence of hernia • Examination (when indicated) of anus, perineum and rectum, including sphincter tone, presence of hemorrhoids, rectal masses • Obtain stool sample for occult blood test when indicated
Genitourinary	**Male**: • Examination of the scrotal contents (e.g., hydrocele, spermatocele, tenderness of cord, testicular mass) • Examination of the penis • Digital rectal examination of prostate gland (e.g., size, symmetry, nodularity tenderness)

General Multisystem Examination

System/Body Area	Elements of Examination
Genitourinary (continued)	**Female:** Pelvic examination (with or without specimen collection for smears and cultures), including: • Examination of external genitalia (e.g., general appearance, hair distribution, lesions) and vagina (e.g., general appearance, estrogen effect, discharge, lesions, pelvic support, cystocele, rectocele) • Examination of urethra (e.g., masses, tenderness, scarring) • Examination of bladder (e.g., fullness, masses, tenderness) • Cervix (e.g., general appearance, lesions, discharge) • Uterus (e.g., size, contour, position, mobility, tenderness, consistency, descent or support) • Adnexa/parametria (e.g., masses, tenderness, organomegaly, nodularity)

Lymphatic	• Palpation of lymph nodes in **two or more** areas:
	  – Neck
	  – Groin
	  – Axillae
	  – Other

Musculoskeletal	• Examination of gait and station
	• Inspection and/or palpation of digits and nails (e.g., clubbing, cyanosis, inflammatory conditions, petechiae, ischemia, infections, nodes)
	• Examination of joints, bones and muscles of **one or more of the following six** areas: 1) head and neck; 2) spine, ribs and pelvis; 3) right upper extremity; 4) left upper extremity; 5) right lower extremity; and 6) left lower extremity. The examination of a given area includes:
	  – Inspection and/or palpation with notation of presence of any misalignment, asymmetry, crepitation, defects, tenderness, masses, effusions
	  – Assessment of range of motion with notation of any pain, crepitation or contracture
	  – Assessment of stability with notation of any dislocation (luxation), subluxation or laxity
	  – Assessment of muscle strength and tone (e.g., flaccid, cog wheel, spastic) with notation of any atrophy or abnormal movements

Skin	• Inspection of skin and subcutaneous tissue (e.g., rashes, lesions, ulcers) • Palpation of skin and subcutaneous tissue (e.g., induration, subcutaneous nodules, tightening)
Neurologic	• Test cranial nerves with notation of any deficits • Examination of deep tendon reflexes with notation of pathological reflexes (e.g., Babinski) • Examination of sensation (e.g., by touch, pin, vibration, proprioception)

Psychiatric	• Description of patient's judgment and insight
	• Brief assessment of mental status, including:
	  – orientation to time, place and person
	  – recent and remote memory
	  – mood and affect (e.g., depression, anxiety, agitation)

Content and Documentation Requirements

Level of Exam	Perform and Document
Problem focused	**One to five** elements identified by a bullet.
Expanded Problem focused	**At least six** elements identified by a bullet.
Detailed	**At least two** elements identified by a bullet **from each of six areas/systems or at least twelve elements** identified by a bullet in **two or more areas/systems.**
Comprehensive	Perform **all elements** identified by a bullet in **at least nine** organ systems or body areas and document **at least two** elements identified by a bullet **from each of nine areas/systems.**

Cardiovascular Examination

System/Body Area	Elements of Examination
Constitutional	• Measurement of **any three of the following seven** vital signs: 1) sitting or standing blood pressure, 2) supine blood pressure, 3) pulse rate and regularity, 4) respiration, 5) temperature, 6) height, 7) weight (May be measured and recorded by ancillary staff). • General appearance of patient (e.g., development, nutrition, body habitus, deformities, attention to grooming)
Head and Face	
Eyes	• Inspection of conjunctivae and lids (e.g., xanthelasma)
Ears, Nose, Mouth and Throat	• Inspection of teeth, gums and palate • Examination of oral mucosa with notation of presence of pallor or cyanosis
Neck	• Examination of jugular veins (e.g., distension: a, v, or cannon waves) • Examination of thyroid (e.g., enlargement, tenderness, mass)
Respiratory	• Assessment of respiratory effort (e.g., intercostal retractions, use of accessory muscles, diaphragmatic movements) • Auscultation of lungs (e.g., breath sounds, adventitious sounds, rubs)

Cardiovascular	• Palpation of heart (e.g., location, size and forcefulness of the point of maximal impact; thrills; lifts; palpable S3 or S4)
	• Auscultation of heart including sounds, abnormal sounds and murmurs
	• Measurement of blood pressure in two or more extremities when indicated (e.g., aortic dissection, coarctation)
	• Examination of:
	  – carotid arteries (e.g., waveform, pulse amplitude, bruits, apical-carotid delay)
	  – abdominal aorta (e.g., size, bruits)
	  – femoral arteries (e.g., pulse amplitude, bruits)
	  – pedal pulses (e.g., pulse amplitude)
	  – extremities for peripheral edema and/or varicosities

Chest (Breasts)	
Gastrointestinal (Abdomen)	• Examination of abdomen with notation of presence of masses or tenderness • Examination of liver and spleen • Obtain stool sample for occult blood from patients who are being considered for thrombolytic or anticoagulant therapy
Genitourinary	
Lymphatic	
Musculoskeletal	• Examination of the back with notation of kyphosis or scoliosis • Examination of gait with notation of ability to undergo exercise testing and/or participation in exercise programs • Assessment of muscle strength and tone (e.g., flaccid, cog wheel, spastic) with notation of any atrophy or abnormal movements
Extremities	• Inspection and palpation of digits and nails (e.g., clubbing, cyanosis, inflammation, petechiae, ischemia, infections, Osler's nodes)
Skin	• Inspection and/or palpation of skin and subcutaneous tissue (e.g., stasis dermatitis, ulcers, scars, xanthomas) • Palpation of skin and subcutaneous tissue (e.g., induration, subcutaneous nodules, tightening)

Neurological/ Psychiatric	• Brief assessment of mental status including:
	  – orientation to time, place and person
	  – mood and affect (e.g., depression, anxiety, agitation)

Content and Documentation Requirements

Level of Exam	Perform and Document
Problem focused	**One to five** elements identified by a bullet.
Expanded Problem focused	**At least six** elements identified by a bullet.
Detailed	**At least twelve** elements identified by a bullet.
Comprehensive	Perform **all** elements identified by a bullet; document every element in each shaded box and at least one element in each unshaded box.

Ear, Nose and Throat Examination

System/Body Area	Elements of Examination
Constitutional	• Measurement of **any three of the following seven** vital signs: 1) sitting or standing blood pressure, 2) supine blood pressure, 3) pulse rate and regularity, 4) respiration, 5) temperature, 6) height, 7) weight (May be measured and recorded by ancillary staff). • General appearance of patient (e.g., development, nutrition, body habitus, deformities, attention to grooming) • Assessment of ability to communicate (e.g., use of sign language or other communication aids) and quality of voice
Head and Face	• Inspection of head and face (e.g., overall appearance, scars, lesions and masses) • Palpation and/or percussion of face with notation of presence or absence of sinus tenderness • Examination of salivary glands • Assessment of facial strength
Eyes	• Test ocular motility including primary gaze alignment
Ears, Nose, Mouth and Throat	• Otoscopic examination of external auditory canals and tympanic membranes including pneumootoscopy with notation of mobility of membranes • Assessment of hearing with tuning forks and clinical speech reception thresholds (e.g., whispered voice, finger rub) • External inspection of ears and nose (e.g., overall appearance, scars, lesions, masses) • Inspection of nasal mucosa, septum and turbinates • Inspection of lips, teeth and gums • Examination of oropharynx: oral mucosa, hard and soft palates, tongue, tonsils and posterior pharynx (e.g., asymmetry, lesions, hydration of mucosal surfaces) • Inspection of pharyngeal walls and pyriform sinuses (e.g., pooling of saliva, asymmetry, lesions) • Examination by mirror of larynx including the condition of the epiglottis, false vocal cords, true vocal cords and mobility of larynx (use of mirror not required in children) • Examination by mirror of nasopharynx including appearance of the mucosa, adenoids, posterior choanae and eustachian tubes (use of mirror not required in children)
Neck	• Examination of neck (e.g., masses, overall appearance, symmetry, tracheal position, crepitus) • Examination of thyroid (e.g., enlargement, tenderness, mass)
Respiratory	• Inspection of chest including symmetry, expansion and/or assessment of respiratory effort (e.g., intercostal retractions, use of accessory muscles, diaphragmatic movement) • Auscultation of lungs (e.g., breath sounds, adventitious sounds, rubs)
Cardiovascular	• Auscultation of heart with notation of abnormal sounds and murmurs • Examination of peripheral vascular system by observation (e.g., swelling, varicosities) and palpation (e.g., pulses, temperature, edema, tenderness)
Chest (Breasts)	
Gastrointestinal (Abdomen)	
Genitourinary	
Lymphatic	• Palpation of lymph nodes in neck, axillae, groin and/or other location
Musculoskeletal	

Ear, Nose and Throat Examination

System/Body Area	Elements of Examination
Extremities	
Skin	
Neurological/Psychiatric	• Test cranial nerves with notation of any deficits • Brief assessment of mental status including: – orientation to time, place and person – mood and affect (e.g., depression, anxiety, agitation)

Content and Documentation Requirements

Level of Exam	Perform and Document
Problem focused	**One to five** elements identified by a bullet.
Expanded Problem focused	**At least six** elements identified by a bullet.
Detailed	**At least twelve** elements identified by a bullet.
Comprehensive	Perform **all** elements identified by a bullet; document every element in each shaded box and at least one element in each unshaded box.

Eye Examination

System/Body Area	Elements of Examination
Constitutional	
Head and Face	
Eyes	• Test visual acuity (does not include determination of refractive error) • Gross visual field testing by confrontation • Test ocular motility including primary gaze alignment • Inspection of bulbar and palpebral conjunctivae • Examination of ocular adnexae including lids (e.g., ptosis or lagophthalmos), lacrimal glands, lacrimal drainage, orbits and preauricular lymph nodes • Examination of pupils and irises including shape, direct and consensual reaction (afferent pupil), size (e.g., anisocoria) and morphology • Slit lamp examination of the corneas including epithelium, stroma, endothelium, and tear film • Slit lamp examination of the anterior chambers including depth, cells, and flare • Slit lamp examination of the lenses including clarity, anterior and posterior capsule, cortex, and nucleus • Measurement of intraocular pressures (except in children and patients with trauma or infectious disease • Ophthalmoscopic examination through dilated pupils (unless contraindicated) of – optic discs including size, C/D ratio, appearance (e.g., atrophy, cupping, tumor elevation) and nerve fiber layer – posterior segments including retina and vessels (e.g., exudates and hemorrhages)
Ears, Nose, Mouth and Throat	
Neck	
Respiratory	
Cardiovascular	
Chest (Breasts)	
Gastrointestinal (Abdomen)	
Genitourinary	

Eye Examination

System/Body Area	Elements of Examination
Lymphatic	
Musculoskeletal	
Extremities	
Skin	

Neurological/ Psychiatric	• Brief assessment of mental status including:
	  – orientation to time, place and person
	  – mood and affect (e.g., depression, anxiety, agitation)

Content and Documentation Requirements

Level of Exam	Perform and Document
Problem focused	**One to five** elements identified by a bullet.
Expanded Problem focused	**At least six** elements identified by a bullet.
Detailed	**At least twelve** elements identified by a bullet.
Comprehensive	Perform **all** elements identified by a bullet; document every element in each shaded box and at least one element in each unshaded box.

Genitourinary Examination

System/Body Area	Elements of Examination
Constitutional	• Measurement of **any three of the following seven** vital signs: 1) sitting or standing blood pressure, 2) supine blood pressure, 3) pulse rate and regularity, 4) respiration, 5) temperature, 6) height, 7) weight (May be measured and recorded by ancillary staff). • General appearance of patient (e.g., development, nutrition, body habitus, deformities, attention to grooming)
Head and Face	
Eyes	
Ears, Nose, Mouth and Throat	
Neck	• Examination of neck (e.g., masses, overall appearance, symmetry, tracheal position, crepitus) • Examination of thyroid (e.g., enlargement, tenderness, mass)
Respiratory	• Assessment of respiratory effort (e.g., intercostal retractions, use of accessory muscles, diaphragmatic movements) • Auscultation of lungs (e.g., breath sounds, adventitious sounds, rubs)
Cardiovascular	• Auscultation of heart with notation of abnormal sounds and murmurs • Examination of peripheral vascular system by observation (e.g., swelling, varicosities and palpation (e.g., pulses, temperature, edema, tenderness)
Chest (Breasts)	[See Genitourinary (female)]
Gastrointestinal (Abdomen)	• Examination of abdomen with notation of presence of masses or tenderness • Examination for presence or absence of hernia • Examination of liver and spleen • Obtain stool sample for occult blood test when indicated

Genitourinary Examination

System/Body Area	Elements of Examination

Genitourinary	**Male:**
	• Inspection of anus and perineum
	• Examination (with or without specimen collection for smears and cultures) of genitalia including:
	  – scrotum (e.g., lesions, cysts, rashes)
	  – epididymides (e.g., size, symmetry, masses)
	  – testes (e.g., size, symmetry, masses)
	  – urethral meatus (e.g., size, location, lesions, discharge)
	  – penis (e.g., lesions, presence or absence of foreskin, foreskin retractability, plaque, masses, scarring deformities)
	• Digital rectal examination including:
	  – prostate gland (e.g., size, symmetry, nodularity, tenderness)
	  – seminal vesicles (e.g., symmetry, tenderness, masses, enlargement
	  – sphincter tone, presence of hemorrhoids, rectal masses
	Female:
	• Includes **at least seven of the following eleven** elements identified by bullets:
	  – Inspection and palpation of breasts (e.g., masses or lumps, tenderness, symmetry, nipple discharge)
	  – Digital rectal examination including sphincter tone, presence of hemorrhoids, rectal masses
	• Pelvic examination (with or without specimen collection for smears and cultures), including
	  – external genitalia (e.g., general appearance, hair distribution, lesions)
	  – urethral meatus (e.g., size, location, lesions, prolapse)
	  – urethra (e.g., masses, tenderness, scarring)
	  – bladder (e.g., fullness, masses, tenderness)
	  – vagina (e.g., general appearance, estrogen effect, discharge, lesions, pelvic support, cystocele, rectocele)
	  – cervix (e.g., general appearance, lesions, discharge)
	  – uterus (e.g., size, contour, position, mobility, tenderness, consistency, descent or support)
	  – adnexa/parametria (e.g., masses, tenderness, organomegaly, nodularity)
	  – anus and perineum

Lymphatic	• Palpation of lymph nodes in neck, axillae, groin and/or other location
Musculoskeletal	
Extremities	
Skin	• Inspection and/or palpation of skin and subcutaneous tissue (e.g., rashes, lesions, ulcers)

Neurological/ Psychiatric	• Brief assessment of mental status including:
	  – orientation to time, place and person and
	  – mood and affect (e.g., depression, anxiety, agitation)

Content and Documentation Requirements

Level of Exam	Perform and Document
Problem focused	**One to five** elements identified by a bullet.
Expanded Problem focused	**At least six** elements identified by a bullet.
Detailed	**At least twelve** elements identified by a bullet.
Comprehensive	Perform **all** elements identified by a bullet; document every element in each shaded box and at least one element in each unshaded box.

Hematologic/Lymphatic/Immunologic Examination

System/Body Area	Elements of Examination
Constitutional	• Measurement of **any three of the following seven** vital signs: 1) sitting or standing blood pressure, 2) supine blood pressure, 3) pulse rate and regularity, 4) respiration, 5) temperature, 6) height, 7) weight (May be measured and recorded by ancillary staff). • General appearance of patient (e.g., development, nutrition, body habitus, deformities, attention to grooming)
Head and Face	• Palpation and/or percussion of face with notation of presence or absence of sinus tenderness
Eyes	• Inspection of conjunctivae and lids
Ears, Nose, Mouth and Throat	• Otoscopic examination of external auditory canals and tympanic membranes • Inspection of nasal mucosa, septum and turbinates • Inspection of teeth and gums • Examination of oropharynx (e.g., oral mucosa, hard and soft palates, tongue, tonsils and posterior pharynx)
Neck	• Examination of neck (e.g., masses, overall appearance, symmetry, tracheal position, crepitus) • Examination of thyroid (e.g., enlargement, tenderness, mass)
Respiratory	• Assessment of respiratory effort (e.g., intercostal retractions, use of accessory muscles, diaphragmatic movements) • Auscultation of lungs (e.g., breath sounds, adventitious sounds, rubs)
Cardiovascular	• Auscultation of heart with notation of abnormal sounds and murmurs • Examination of peripheral vascular system by observation (e.g., swelling, varicosities) and palpation (e.g., pulses, temperature, edema, tenderness)
Chest (Breasts)	
Gastrointestinal (Abdomen)	• Examination of abdomen with notation of presence of masses or tenderness • Examination of liver and spleen
Genitourinary	
Lymphatic	• Palpation of lymph nodes in neck, axillae, groin, and/or other location
Musculoskeletal	
Extremities	• Inspection and palpation of digits and nails (e.g., clubbing, cyanosis, inflammation, petechiae, ischemia, infections, nodes)
Skin	• Inspection and/or palpation of skin and subcutaneous tissue (e.g., rashes, lesions, ulcers, ecchymoses, bruises)

Neurological/ Psychiatric	• Brief assessment of mental status including:
	  – orientation to time, place and person
	  – mood and affect (e.g., depression, anxiety, agitation)

Content and Documentation Requirements

Level of Exam	Perform and Document
Problem focused	**One to five** elements identified by a bullet.
Expanded Problem focused	**At least six** elements identified by a bullet.
Detailed	**At least twelve** elements identified by a bullet.
Comprehensive	Perform **all** elements identified by a bullet; document every element in each shaded box and at least one element in each unshaded box.

Musculoskeletal Examination

System/Body Area	Elements of Examination
Constitutional	• Measurement of **any three of the following seven** vital signs: 1) sitting or standing blood pressure, 2) supine blood pressure, 3) pulse rate and regularity, 4) respiration, 5) temperature, 6) height, 7) weight (May be measured and recorded by ancillary staff). • General appearance of patient (e.g., development, nutrition, body habitus, deformities, attention to grooming)
Head and Face	
Eyes	
Ears, Nose, Mouth and Throat	
Neck	
Respiratory	
Cardiovascular	• Examination of peripheral vascular system by observation (e.g., swelling, varicosities) and palpation (e.g., pulses, temperature, edema, tenderness)
Chest (Breasts)	
Gastrointestinal (Abdomen)	
Genitourinary	
Lymphatic	• Palpation of lymph nodes in neck, axillae, groin, and/or other location

Musculoskeletal	• Examination of gait and station
	• Examination of joint(s), bone(s) and muscle(s) tendon(s) of **four of the following six areas**: 1) head and neck; 2) spine, ribs and pelvis; 3) right upper extremity; 4) left upper extremity; 5) right lower extremity; and 6) left lower extremity. The examination of a given area includes:
	  – Inspection, percussion and/or palpation with notation of any misalignment, asymmetry, crepitation, defects, tenderness, masses or effusions
	  – Assessment of range of motion with notation of any pain (e.g., straight leg raising), crepitation or contrature
	  – Assessment of stability with notation of any dislocation (luxation), subluxation or laxity
	  – Assessment of muscle strength and tone (e.g., flaccid, cog wheel, spastic) with notation of any atrophy or abnormal movements
	Note: For the comprehensive level of examination, all four of the elements identified by a bullet must be performed and documented for each of four anatomic areas. For the three lower levels of examination, each element is counted separately for each body area. For example, assessing range of motion in two extremities constitutes two elements.

Extremities	[See Musculoskeletal and Skin]
Skin	• Inspection and/or palpation of skin and subcutaneous tissue (e.g., scars, rashes, lesions, cafe-au-lait spots, ulcers) in **four of the following six** areas: 1) head and neck; 2) trunk; 3) right upper extremity; 4) left upper extremity; 5) right lower extremity; and 6) left lower extremity. **Note:** For the comprehensive level, the examination of all four anatomic areas must be performed and documented. For the three lower levels of examination, each body area is counted separately. For example, inspection and/or palpation of the skin and subcutaneous tissue of two extremities constitutes two elements.

Neurological/Psychiatric	• Test coordination (e.g., finger/nose, heel/knee/shin, rapid alternating movements in the upper and lower extremities, evaluation of fine motor coordination in young children)
	• Examination of deep tendon reflexes and/or nerve stretch test with notation of pathological reflexes (e.g., Babinski)
	• Examination of sensation (e.g., by touch, pin, vibration, proprioception)
	• Brief assessment of mental status including:
	  – orientation to time, place and person
	  – mood and affect (e.g., depression, anxiety, agitation)

Content and Documentation Requirements

Level of Exam	Perform and Document
Problem focused	**One to five** elements identified by a bullet.
Expanded Problem focused	**At least six** elements identified by a bullet.
Detailed	**At least twelve** elements identified by a bullet.
Comprehensive	Perform **all** elements identified by a bullet; document every element in each shaded box **and** at least one element in each unshaded box.

Neurological Examination

System/Body Area	Elements of Examination
Constitutional	• Measurement of **any three of the following seven** vital signs: 1) sitting or standing blood pressure, 2) supine blood pressure, 3) pulse rate and regularity, 4) respiration, 5) temperature, 6) height, 7) weight (May be measured and recorded by ancillary staff). • General appearance of patient (e.g., development, nutrition, body habitus, deformities, attention to grooming)
Head and Face	
Eyes	• Ophthalmoscopic examination of optic discs (e.g., size, C/D ratio, appearance) and posterior segments (e.g., vessel changes, exudates, hemorrhages)
Ears, Nose, Mouth and Throat	
Neck	
Respiratory	
Cardiovascular	• Examination of carotid arteries (e.g., pulse amplitude, bruits) • Auscultation of heart with notation of abnormal sounds and murmurs • Examination of peripheral vascular system by observation (e.g., swelling, varicosities) and palpation (e.g., pulses, temperature, edema, tenderness)
Chest (Breasts)	
Gastrointestinal (Abdomen)	
Genitourinary	
Lymphatic	
Musculoskeletal	• Examination of gait and station • Assessment of motor function including: – muscle strength in upper and lower extremities – muscle tone in upper and lower extremities (e.g., flaccid, cog wheel, spastic) with notation of any atrophy or abnormal movements (e.g., fasciculation, tardive dyskinesia)
Extremities	[See Musculoskeletal]
Skin	

Neurological Examination

System/Body Area	Elements of Examination

Neurological	• Evaluation of higher integrative functions, including:
	  – orientation to time, place and person
	  – recent and remote memory
	  – attention span and concentration
	  – language (e.g., naming objects, repeating phrases, spontaneous speech)
	  – fund of knowledge (e.g., awareness of current events, past history, vocabulary)
	• Test the following cranial nerves:
	  – 2nd cranial nerve (e.g., visual acuity, visual fields, fundi)
	  – 3rd, 4th and 6th cranial nerves (e.g., pupils, eye movements)
	  – 5th cranial nerve (e.g., facial sensation, corneal reflexes)
	  – 7th cranial nerve (e.g., facial symmetry, strength)
	  – 8th cranial nerve (e.g., hearing with tuning fork, whispered voice and/or finger rub)
	  – 9th cranial nerve (e.g., spontaneous or reflex palate movement)
	  – 11th cranial nerve (e.g., shoulder shrug strength)
	  – 12th cranial nerve (e.g., tongue protrusion)
	• Examination of sensation (e.g., by touch, pin, vibration, proprioception)
	• Examination of deep tendon reflexes with notation of pathological reflexes (e.g., Babinski)
	• Test coordination (e.g., finger/nose, heel/knee/shin, rapid alternating movements in the upper and lower extremities, evaluation of fine motor coordination in young children)

Psychiatric	

Content and Documentation Requirements

Level of Exam	Perform and Document
Problem focused	**One to five** elements identified by a bullet.
Expanded Problem focused	**At least six** elements identified by a bullet.
Detailed	**At least twelve** elements identified by a bullet.
Comprehensive	Perform **all** elements identified by a bullet; document every element in each shaded box and at least one element in each unshaded box.

Psychiatric Examination

System/Body Area	Elements of Examination
Constitutional	• Measurement of **any three of the following seven** vital signs: 1) sitting or standing blood pressure, 2) supine blood pressure, 3) pulse rate and regularity, 4) respiration, 5) temperature, 6) height, 7) weight (May be measured and recorded by ancillary staff). • General appearance of patient (e.g., development, nutrition, body habitus, deformities, attention to grooming)
Head and Face	
Eyes	
Ears, Nose, Mouth and Throat	
Neck	
Respiratory	
Cardiovascular	
Chest (Breasts)	
Gastrointestinal (Abdomen)	
Genitourinary	
Lymphatic	
Musculoskeletal	• Assessment of muscle strength and tone (e.g., flaccid, cog wheel, spastic) with notation of any atrophy or abnormal movements • Examination of gait and station
Extremities	
Skin	
Neurological	

Psychiatric	• Description of speech including: volume; articulation; coherence; and spontaneity with notation of abnormalities (e.g., perseveration, paucity of language)
	• Description of thought processes including: rate of thoughts; content of thoughts (e.g., logical vs. illogical, tangential); abstract reasoning; and computation
	• Description of associations (e.g., loose, tangential, circumstantial, intact)
	• Description of abnormal or psychotic thoughts including: hallucinations; delusions; preoccupation with violence; homicidal or suicidal ideation; and obsessions
	• Description of the patient's judgment (e.g., concerning everyday activities and social situations) and insight (e.g., concerning psychiatric condition)
	• Complete mental status examination including:
	  – orientation to time, place and person
	  – recent and remote memory
	  – language (e.g., naming objects, repeating phrases)
	  – fund of knowledge (e.g., awareness of current events, past history, vocabulary)
	  – mood and affect (e.g., depression, anxiety, agitation, hypomania, lability)

Content and Documentation Requirements

Level of Exam	Perform and Document
Problem focused	**One to five** elements identified by a bullet.
Expanded Problem focused	**At least six** elements identified by a bullet.
Detailed	**At least nine** elements identified by a bullet.
Comprehensive	Perform **all** elements identified by a bullet; document every element in each shaded box and at least one element in each unshaded box.

Respiratory Examination

System/Body Area	Elements of Examination
Constitutional	• Measurement of **any three of the following seven** vital signs: 1) sitting or standing blood pressure, 2) supine blood pressure, 3) pulse rate and regularity, 4) respiration, 5) temperature, 6) height, 7) weight (May be measured and recorded by ancillary staff). • General appearance of patient (e.g., development, nutrition, body habitus, deformities, attention to grooming)
Head and Face	
Eyes	
Ears, Nose, Mouth and Throat	• Inspection of nasal mucosa, septum and turbinates • Inspection of teeth and gums • Examination of oropharynx (e.g., oral mucosa, hard and soft palates, tongue, tonsils and posterior pharynx)
Neck	• Examination of neck (e.g., masses, overall appearance, symmetry, tracheal position, crepitus) • Examination of thyroid (e.g., enlargement, tenderness, mass) • Examination of jugular veins (e.g., dissension; a, v or cannon a waves)
Respiratory	• Inspection of chest with notation of symmetry and expansion • Assessment of respiratory effort (e.g., intercostal retractions, use of accessory muscles, diaphragmatic movement) • Percussion of chest (e.g., dullness, flatness, hyperresonance) • Palpation of chest (e.g., tactile fremitus) • Auscultation of lungs (e.g., breath sounds, adventitious sounds, rubs)
Cardiovascular	• Auscultation of heart with notation of abnormal sounds and murmurs • Examination of peripheral vascular system by observation (e.g., swelling, varicosities) and palpation (e.g., pulses, temperature, edema, tenderness)
Chest (Breasts)	
Gastrointestinal (Abdomen)	• Examination of abdomen with notation of presence of masses or tenderness • Examination of liver and spleen
Genitourinary	
Lymphatic	• Palpation of lymph nodes in neck, axillae, groin and/or other location.
Musculoskeletal	• Assessment of muscle strength and tone (e.g., flaccid, cog wheel, spastic) with notation of any atrophy or abnormal movements • Examination of gait and station
Extremities	• Inspection and palpation of digits and nails (e.g., clubbing, cyanosis, inflammation, petechiae, ischemia, infections, nodes)
Skin	• Inspection and/or palpation of skin and subcutaneous tissue (e.g., rashes, lesions, ulcers)

Neurological/ Psychiatric	• Brief assessment of mental status including:
	  – orientation to time, place and person
	  – mood and affect (e.g., depression, anxiety, agitation)

Content and Documentation Requirements

Level of Exam	Perform and Document
Problem focused	**One to five** elements identified by a bullet.
Expanded Problem focused	**At least six** elements identified by a bullet.
Detailed	**At least twelve** elements identified by a bullet.
Comprehensive	Perform **all** elements identified by a bullet; document every element in each shaded box and at least one element in each unshaded box.

Skin Examination

System/Body Area	Elements of Examination
Constitutional	• Measurement of any **three of the following seven** vital signs: 1) sitting or standing blood pressure, 2) supine blood pressure, 3) pulse rate and regularity, 4) respiration, 5) temperature, 6) height, 7) weight (May be measured and recorded by ancillary staff). • General appearance of patient (e.g., development, nutrition, body habitus, deformities, attention to grooming)
Head and Face	
Eyes	• Inspection of conjunctivae and lids
Ears, Nose, Mouth and Throat	• Inspection of lips, teeth and gums • Examination of oropharynx (e.g., oral mucosa, hard and soft palates, tongue, tonsils and posterior pharynx)
Neck	• Examination of thyroid (e.g., enlargement, tenderness, mass)
Respiratory	
Cardiovascular	• Examination of peripheral vascular system by observation (e.g., swelling, varicosities) and palpation (e.g., pulses, temperature, edema, tenderness)
Chest (Breasts)	
Gastrointestinal (Abdomen)	• Examination of liver and spleen • Examination of anus for condyloma and other lesions
Genitourinary	
Lymphatic	• Palpation of lymph nodes in neck, axillae, groin and/or other location
Musculoskeletal	
Extremities	• Inspection and palpation of digits and nails (e.g., clubbing, cyanosis, inflammation, petechiae, ischemia, infections, nodes)
Skin	• Palpation of scalp and inspection of hair of scalp, eyebrows, face, chest, pubic area (when indicated) and extremities • Inspection and/or palpation of skin and subcutaneous tissue (e.g., rashes, lesions, ulcers, susceptibility to and presence of photo damage) in **eight of the following ten areas**: • Head, including the face • Neck • Chest, including breasts and axillae • Abdomen • Genitalia, groin, buttocks • Back • Right upper extremity • Left upper extremity • Right lower extremity • Left lower extremity **Note:** For the comprehensive level, the examination of at least eight anatomic areas must be performed and documented. For the three lower levels of examination, each body area is counted separately. For example, inspection and/or palpation of the skin and subcutaneous tissue of the right upper extremity and the left upper extremity constitutes two elements. • Inspection of eccrine and apocrine glands of skin and subcutaneous tissue with identification and location of any hyperhidrosis, chromhidroses or bromhidrosis

Neurological/Psychiatric	• Brief assessment of mental status including:
	  – orientation to time, place and person
	  – mood and affect (e.g., depression, anxiety, agitation)

Content and Documentation Requirements

Level of Exam	Perform and Document
Problem focused	**One to five** elements identified by a bullet.
Expanded Problem focused	**At least six** elements identified by a bullet.
Detailed	**At least twelve** elements identified by a bullet.
Comprehensive	Perform **all** elements identified by a bullet; document every element in each shaded box and at least one element in each unshaded box.

C. DOCUMENTATION OF THE COMPLEXITY OF MEDICAL DECISION MAKING

The levels of E/M services recognize four types of medical decision making (straightforward, low complexity, moderate complexity and high complexity). Medical decision making refers to the complexity of establishing a diagnosis and/or selecting a management option as measured by:

- The number of possible diagnoses and/or the number of management options that must be considered;
- The amount and/or complexity of medical records, diagnostic tests, and/or other information that must be obtained, reviewed and analyzed, and
- The risk of significant complications, morbidity and/or mortality, as well as comorbidities, associated with the patient's presenting problem(s), the diagnostic procedure(s) and/or the possible management options

The chart below shows the progression of the elements required for each level of medical decision making. To qualify for a given type of decision making, **two of the three elements in the table must be either met or exceeded.**

Number of diagnoses or management options	Amount and/or complexity of data to be reviewed	Risk of complications and/or morbidity or mortality	Type of decision making
Minimal	Minimal or None	Minimal	**Straightforward**
Limited	Limited	Low	**Low Complexity**
Multiple	Moderate	Moderate	**Moderate Complexity**
Extensive	Extensive	High	**High Complexity**

Each of the elements of medical decision making is described below.

NUMBER OF DIAGNOSES OR MANAGEMENT OPTIONS

The number of possible diagnoses and/or the number of management options that must be considered is based on the number and types of problems addressed during the encounter, the complexity of establishing a diagnosis and the management decisions that are made by the physician.

Generally, decision making with respect to a diagnosed problem is easier than that for an identified but undiagnosed problem. The number and type of diagnostic tests employed may be an indicator of the number of possible diagnoses. Problems which are improving or resolving are less complex than those which are worsening or failing to change as expected. The need to seek advice from others is another indicator of complexity of diagnostic or management problems.

- *DG: For each encounter, an assessment, clinical impression, or diagnosis should be documented. It may be explicitly stated or implied in documented decisions regarding management plans and/or further evaluation.*
  - *for a presenting problem with an established diagnosis the record should reflect whether the problem is: a) improved, well controlled, resolving or resolved; or, b) inadequately controlled, worsening, or failing to change as expected.*
  - *for a presenting problem without an established diagnosis, the assessment or clinical impression may be stated in the form of a differential diagnoses or as "possible", "probable", or "rule out" (R/O) diagnoses.*
- *DG: The initiation of, or changes in, treatment should be documented. Treatment includes a wide range of management options including patient instructions, nursing instructions, therapies, and medications.*
- *DG: If referrals are made, consultations requested or advice sought, the record should indicate to whom or where the referral or consultation is made or from whom the advice is requested.*

AMOUNT AND/OR COMPLEXITY OF DATA TO BE REVIEWED

The amount and complexity of data to be reviewed is based on the types of diagnostic testing ordered or reviewed. A decision to obtain and review old medical records and/or obtain history from sources other than the patient increases the amount and complexity of data to be reviewed. Discussion of contradictory or unexpected test results with the physician who performed or interpreted the test is an indication of the complexity of data being reviewed. On occasion the physician who ordered a test may personally review the image, tracing or specimen to supplement information from the physician who prepared the test report or interpretation; this is another indication of the complexity of data being reviewed.

- *DG: If a diagnostic service (test or procedure) is ordered, planned, scheduled, or performed at the time of the E/M encounter, the type of service, e.g., lab or x-ray, should be documented.*
- *DG: The review of lab, radiology and/or other diagnostic tests should be documented. An entry in a progress note such as "WBC elevated" or "chest x-ray unremarkable" is acceptable. Alternatively, the review may be documented by initialing and dating the report containing the test results.*
- *DG: A decision to obtain old records or decision to obtain additional history from the family, caretaker or other source to supplement that obtained from the patient should be documented.*
- *DG: Relevant findings from the review of old records, and/or the receipt of additional history from the family, caretaker or other source to supplement that obtained from the patient should be documented. If there is no relevant information beyond that already obtained, that fact should be documented. A notation of "Old records reviewed" or "additional history obtained from family" without elaboration is insufficient.*
- *DG: The results of discussion of laboratory, radiology or other diagnostic tests with the physician who performed or interpreted the study should be documented.*
- *DG: The direct visualization and independent interpretation of an image, tracing or specimen previously or subsequently interpreted by another physician should be documented.*

RISK OF SIGNIFICANT COMPLICATIONS, MORBIDITY, AND/OR MORTALITY

The risk of significant complications, morbidity, and/or mortality is based on the risks associated with the presenting problem(s), the diagnostic procedure(s), and the possible management options.

- *DG: Comorbidities/underlying diseases or other factors that increase the complexity of medical decision making by increasing the risk of complications, morbidity, and/or mortality should be documented.*
- *DG: If a surgical or invasive diagnostic procedure is ordered, planned or scheduled at the time of the E/M encounter, the type of procedure, e.g., laparoscopy, should be documented.*
- *DG: If a surgical or invasive diagnostic procedure is performed at the time of the E/M encounter, the specific procedure should be documented.*
- *DG: The referral for or decision to perform a surgical or invasive diagnostic procedure on an urgent basis should be documented or implied.*

The following table may be used to help determine whether the risk of significant complications, morbidity, and/or mortality is minimal, low, moderate, or high. Because the determination of risk is complex and not readily quantifiable, the table includes common clinical examples rather than absolute measures of risk. The assessment of risk of the presenting problem(s) is based on the risk related to the disease process anticipated between the present encounter and the next one.

The assessment of risk of selecting diagnostic procedures and management options is based on the risk during and immediately following any procedures or treatment. **The highest level of risk in any one category (presenting problem(s), diagnostic procedure(s), or management options) determines the overall risk.**

TABLE OF RISK

	Presenting Problem(s)	Diagnostic Procedure(s) Ordered	Management Options Selected
MINIMAL	• One self-limited or minor problem; e.g., cold, insect bite, tinea corporis	• Laboratory tests requiring venipuncture • Chest x-rays • EKG/EEG • Urinalysis • Ultrasound; e.g., echo • KOH prep	• Rest • Gargles • Elastic bandages • Superficial dressings
LOW	• Two or more self-limited or minor problems • One stable chronic illness; e.g., well controlled hypertension or non-insulin dependent diabetes, cataract, BPH • Acute uncomplicated illness or injury; e.g., cystitis, allergic rhinitis, simple sprain	• Physiological tests not under stress; e.g., pulmonary function tests • Non-cardiovascular imaging studies with contrast; e.g., barium enema • Superficial needle biopsies • Clinical laboratory tests requiring arterial puncture • Skin biopsies	• Over-the-counter drugs • Minor surgery with no identified risk factors • Physical therapy • Occupational therapy • IV fluids without additives
MODERATE	• One or more chronic illnesses with mild exacerbation, progression, or side effects of treatment • Two or more stable chronic illnesses • Undiagnosed new problem with uncertain prognosis; e.g., lump in breast • Acute illness with systemic symptoms; e.g., pyelonephritis, pneumonitis, colitis • Acute complicated injury; e.g., head injury with brief loss of consciousness	• Physiologic tests under stress; e.g., cardiac stress test, fetal contraction stress test • Diagnostic endoscopies with no identified risk factors • Deep needle or incisional biopsy • Cardiovascular imaging studies w/ contrast and no identified risk factors; e.g., arteriogram, cardiac catheterization • Obtain fluid from body cavity; e.g., lumbar puncture, thoracentesis, culdocentesis	• Minor surgery w/ identified risk factors • Elective major surgery (Open, percutaneous or endoscopic) w/ no identified risk factors • Prescription drug management • Therapeutic nuclear medicine • IV fluids with additives • Closed treatment of fracture or dislocation w/o manipulation
HIGH	• One or more chronic illnesses with severe exacerbation, progression, or side effects of treatment • Acute or chronic illnesses or injuries that pose a threat to life or bodily function; e.g., multiple trauma, acute MI, pulmonary embolus, severe respiratory distress, progressive severe rheumatoid arthritis, psychiatric illness with potential threat to self or others, peritonitis, ARF • An abrupt change in neurologic status; e.g., seizure, TIA, weakness or sensory loss	• Cardiovascular imaging studies with contrast with identified risk factors • Cardiac electrophysiological tests • Diagnostic endoscopies w/identified risk factors • Discography	• Elective major surgery (open, percutaneous or endoscopic) w/ identified risk factors • Emergency major surgery (open, percutaneous, endoscopic) • Parenteral controlled substances • Drug therapy requiring intensive monitoring for toxicity • Decision not to resuscitate or to de-escalate care because of poor prognosis

D. DOCUMENTATION OF AN ENCOUNTER DOMINATED BY COUNSELING OR COORDINATION OF CARE

In the case where counseling and/or coordination of care dominates (more than 50%) of the physician/patient and/or family encounter (face-to-face time in the office or other outpatient setting or floor/unit time in the hospital or nursing facility), time is considered the key or controlling factor to qualify for a particular level of E/M services.

- *DG: If the physician elects to report the level of service based on counseling and/or coordination of care, the total length of time of the encounter (face-to-face or floor time, as appropriate) should be documented and the record should describe the counseling and/or activities to coordinate care.*

Index

subsequent nursing facility 241
 general guidelines 241
 issues 242
review of systems (ROS) 38

S

self-audit forms 421
shared E/M services 94
SNOCAMP format 32, 66
 assessment 67
 counseling and/or coordination of care 67
 medical decision making 67
 nature of presenting problem 67
 objective 67
 plan 68
 subjective 66
SOAP format 14, 31, 32, 65
 assessment 66
 objective 65
 plan 66
 subjective 65
social history 41, 66
split E/M services 94
student 90

subsequent care and discharge services 160
subsequent nursing facility
 annual assessment 241
subsequent nursing facility care 241
subsequent observation care 142, 436

T

Table of Risk 50, 52, 53, 98, 99, 175, 388
teaching physicians
 documentation 89, 90
 interns 84
 key portion 85
 physically present 85
 primary care 86
 psychiatry 88
 residents 84
 students 90
 time-based services 88
team conferences 295
third-party payers 16, 79
time 31
time-based services 88
transitional care management (TCM) 335